# Cambridge
# Handbook of Pain
# Medicine

T0198363

# Cambridge Handbook of Pain Medicine

Edited by

## Omar Viswanath
Clinical Professor of Anesthesiology, Creighton University School of Medicine, Phoenix, AZ, USA
Interventional Pain Medicine Physician, Innovative Pain and Wellness, Scottsdale, AZ, USA

## Ivan Urits
Interventional Pain Medicine Attending Physician, Southcoast Brain & Spine Center, Wareham, MA, USA

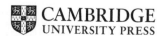

CAMBRIDGE
UNIVERSITY PRESS

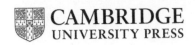

# CAMBRIDGE
## UNIVERSITY PRESS

Shaftesbury Road, Cambridge CB2 8EA, United Kingdom

One Liberty Plaza, 20th Floor, New York, NY 10006, USA

477 Williamstown Road, Port Melbourne, VIC 3207, Australia

314–321, 3rd Floor, Plot 3, Splendor Forum, Jasola District Centre, New Delhi – 110025, India

103 Penang Road, #05–06/07, Visioncrest Commercial, Singapore 238467

Cambridge University Press is part of Cambridge University Press & Assessment, a department of the University of Cambridge.

We share the University's mission to contribute to society through the pursuit of education, learning and research at the highest international levels of excellence.

www.cambridge.org
Information on this title: www.cambridge.org/9781108969826

DOI: 10.1017/9781108979849

© Cambridge University Press & Assessment 2024

First published 2024

Printed in the United Kingdom by CPI Group Ltd, Croydon CR0 4YY

*A catalogue record for this publication is available from the British Library.*

*Library of Congress Cataloging-in-Publication Data*
Names: Viswanath, Omar, editor. | Urits, Ivan, editor.
Title: Cambridge handbook of pain medicine / edited by Omar Viswanath, Ivan Urits.
Other titles: Handbook of pain medicine
Description: Cambridge, United Kingdom ; New York, NY : Cambridge University Press, 2023. | Includes bibliographical references and index.
Identifiers: LCCN 2023026414 (print) | LCCN 2023026415 (ebook) | ISBN 9781108969826 (paperback) | ISBN 9781108979849 (ebook)
Subjects: MESH: Chronic Pain – diagnosis | Chronic Pain – therapy | Pain Management – methods | Handbook
Classification: LCC RB127 (print) | LCC RB127 (ebook) | NLM WL 39 | DDC 616/.0472–dc23/eng/20230703
LC record available at https://lccn.loc.gov/2023026414
LC ebook record available at https://lccn.loc.gov/2023026415

ISBN 978-1-108-96982-6 Paperback

# Contents

# Contents

# Contributors

**Alaa Abd-Elsayed**
Department of Anesthesiology,
University of Wisconsin School of
Medicine and Public Health

**Shenwari R. Afredi**
University of Miami, Herbert
School of Business

**Kevin Bennett**
Herbert Wertheim College of
Medicine

**Pranav Bhargava**
LSUHSC-Shreveport School of
Medicine

**Karina Charipova**
Department of Plastic and
Reconstructive Surgery,
MedStar Georgetown University
Hospital

**Elyse M. Cornett**
Louisiana State University Health
Sciences Center Shreveport,
Department of Anesthesiology

**Zahaan Eswani**
LSUHSC-Shreveport School of
Medicine

**Clay Gibb**
Midwestern University Arizona
College of Osteopathic Medicine

**Jatinder Gill**
Beth Israel Deaconess Medical
Center, Department of Anesthesia,
Critical Care and Pain Medicine,
Harvard Medical School

**Kyle Gress**
Department of General Surgery,
MedStar Georgetown University
Hospital

**Andrew Han**
Georgetown University School of
Medicine

**Morgan Hasegawa**
University of Hawaii School of
Medicine, Department of
Orthopaedic Surgery

**Jamal Hasoon**
UT Houston McGovern Medical
School, Department of
Anesthesiology, Critical Care and
Pain Medicine

**Juyeon Kakazu**
Georgetown University School of
Medicine

**Hisham Kassem**
Advance Pain Management of
Florida

**Alan D. Kaye**
Louisiana State University Health
Sciences Center Shreveport,
Department of
Anesthesiology

**Ajay Kurup**
Mount Sinai Medical Center

**Vijay Kurup**
Chicago College of Osteopathic
Medicine of Midwestern
University

**Noushad Mamun**
Department of Physical
Medicine and Rehabilitation,
Memorial
Healthcare System

**Corey Moss**
LSUHSC-Shreveport School of
Medicine

**Nazir Noor**
Keck Medicine of USC,
Department of
Anesthesiology

**Vwaire Orhurhu**
University of Pittsburgh Medical
Center,
MVM Health

**Riki Patel**
UIC College of Medicine,
Department of
Anesthesiology

**Merlin Perez**
FIU Herbert Wertheim College of
Medicine

**Salomon Poliwoda**
Department of Anesthesiology,
Mount Sinai Medical Center

**Zohal Sarwary**
Creighton University School of
Medicine – Phoenix

**Ruben Schwartz**
Certified Spine and Pain Care

**Norris Talbot**
LSUHSC-Shreveport School of
Medicine

**Nolan Weinstein**
University of Arizona College of
Medicine – Phoenix

**Taylor Witten**
LSUHSC-Shreveport School of
Medicine

**Cyrus Yazdi**
Beth Israel Deaconess Medical
Center, Department of Anesthesia,
Critical Care and Pain Medicine,
Harvard Medical School

# Pain Handbook Introduction

To our readers,

Chronic pain is something that ALL medical professionals will encounter, no matter if they practice in primary care or a surgical/procedural specialty. Moreover, it is something that likely you will personally experience in your own life as well. To this point, we were not aware of a handbook that encapsulates the many pillars of Pain Medicine into a concise, easy-to-follow guide.

As double board-certified Anesthesiologists and Interventional Pain Medicine Physicians, we believe we have created just that: an easy-to-utilize handbook that covers all the major areas of pain medicine that will undoubtedly help you in your medical careers.

This handbook is appropriately set up in the following sections: Introduction to Pain and Pain Signaling Pathways, Common Categories of Pharmacologic Medications Utilized to Treat Chronic Pain, various Chronic Pain Conditions (in order from head and neck down to the lower extremities), Miscellaneous Pain Conditions, and finally Adjunctive/Complementary Modalities.

We believe that this handbook will provide you with all the pertinent information you will need to treat the vast majority of chronic pain issues, whether you are a physician, fellow, resident, medical student, nurse practitioner, nurse, nursing student, pharmacist, physician assistant, medical assistant, or any other medical professional in healthcare.

Thank you,

Omar Viswanath, MD
Ivan Urits, MD

# Central Neuropathic Pain Signaling Pathways

Karina Charipova and Kyle Gress

## Central Neuropathic Pain (CNP)

- A chronic neuropathic pain condition
- Results directly from injury to the central nervous system (CNS) or disease of the somatosensory nervous system (1)
- Pathophysiology of CNP is unclear, but the condition can likely be attributed to an increase in inflammatory mediators, voltage-gated ion channel dysfunction, and afferent nerve sensitization (1)
- Central pain syndromes included under the umbrella of CNP include central poststroke pain (CPSP), spinal cord injury (SCI) pain, and multiple sclerosis-related pain (1)
- Symptoms can be chronic or paroxysmal and may be provoked by various stimuli (e.g., mechanical touch, temperature) (2)
- Characterized by allodynia and spontaneous shooting, tingling, or burning pain that is moderate to severe in intensity and functionally limiting (2)
- Long-term pain relief and functional improvement are poor; symptoms are likely to worsen over time (3)

## Epidemiology and Risk Factors

- Symptom progression
  - Early development of symptoms is predictive of symptom persistence (4)
  - Of patients with symptoms 1 month after injury, 72% experienced persistence at 6 months and 69% at 12 months (4)
  - Neuropathic pain increases over time as musculoskeletal pain decreases (5)
- Common risk factors
  - Increased age (4)

- ○ Initial preservation of motor and sensory function following minor injury (6)
- ○ Early post-injury onset of allodynia (5)
- ○ Psychologic symptoms secondary to CNS injury (e.g., PTSD, anxiety, stress, depression, pain catastrophizing) (7)
- Characteristic EEG findings such as reduced alpha and absent theta and beta bands in response to eye openings may be predictive of CNP secondary to SCI (8)
- Biomarkers such as Differentially Expressed Genes and miRNAs have been proposed as predictors of CNP and have potential as therapeutic targets (9)

## Pathophysiology

### Altered Neuronal Cell Signaling

- Exact pathophysiology of CNP is still under investigation
- The condition is likely rooted in inflammation resulting from local glial and macrophage activation, migration, and proliferation resulting from a CNS insult (10, 11)
- Following injury, microglia cells produce proinflammatory markers such as brain-derived neurotrophic factor (BDNF), leading to increased neuronal excitability (10, 11)
- Colony-stimulating factor (CSF1R) signals microglial proliferation, which promotes an influx of $Ca^{2+}$ and increases tactile allodynia (12)
  - ○ CSF1R plays a similar role in macrophages by upregulating inflammatory cytokines (13)
- GABAergic neurotransmitters are also thought to be implemented in CNP (14)
  - ○ In the healthy spinal cord, $GABA_A$ and glycine exert an inhibitory effect on the firing of dorsal horn neurons (14)
  - ○ SCI has been shown to increase the concentration of alpha-2-delta-1 ($\alpha_2 \delta$-1) subunits of voltage-gated calcium channels in dorsal horn neurons, decreasing pain thresholds (14)
  - ○ Pregabalin has been shown to decrease tactile allodynia and $\alpha_2 \delta$-1 concentration, suggesting a direct effect on the neuropathic pain response (14)

- SCI downregulates expression of the potassium chloride cotransporter (KCC2), rendering $GABA_A$ and glycine ineffective and inducing spasticity and pain (15)
  - Downregulation of KCC2 also associated with decreased pain thresholds (15)
  - Treatment with TCB-2 [(4-bromo-3,6 dimethoxybenzocyclobuten-1-yl)methylamine hydrobromide] shown to upregulate KCC2 and decrease post-SCI allodynia (15)
  - TCB-2 also shown to decrease neuropathic pain targeting microRNA to prevent overexpression of inflammatory cytokines (16, 17)
- Essential oils have been implemented in preventing overactivation of inflammatory pathways and decreasing allodynia (18)

## Progression

- 23% of patients who initially screen negative for neuropathic pain shown to develop pain at 6 or 12 months after injury (19)
- The delayed development of CNP is not well understood (19)
- Delayed presentation of CNP may be linked to time required for neuroma development (19)
- Long-term follow-up is essential for patients who have suffered CNS injury (19)

## Sensitization

- Role of sensitization in the pathogenesis of CNP is unclear (20)
- Central sensitization involves structures in the anterior cingulate cortex (ACC), hippocampus, and amygdala (21)
- A study showed that following SCI patients experience central sensitization compared to controls but not compared to their own baselines (20)
- Varied dosages of opioid medication regimens do not appear to impact sensitization to pain or pressure post-SCI (20)

## Diagnosis

- Diagnosis is difficult, especially given delay in symptom onset (weeks to years)
- Detailed history and physical examination should help differentiate central and peripheral etiologies
- International Association for the Study of Pain diagnostic criteria require a history of CNS injury (22)

- ○ Imaging should be used to confirm history of stroke, SCI, MS, and other CNS lesions (22)
- ○ Pain and somatosensory changes must be distributed in body region affected by CNS injury (22)
- ○ Initial pain may be predominantly musculoskeletal, neuropathic pain becomes more prevalent over time (5)

# Pharmacologic Treatment Modalities

## First-Line Agents

- First-line interventions are similar to those used for peripheral neuropathy and include gabapentinoids, tricyclic antidepressants, SSRIs, and SNRIs (23)
  - ○ The efficacy of these first-line agents is highly individual-dependent
  - ○ These agents should be titrated to achieve clinically significant pain relief for each individual patient and account for comorbidities (i.e., depression)
  - ○ Patients with CNP may exhibit deficits in physical and cognitive function secondary to the original CNS injury with decreased tolerance for medications that cause sedation, dizziness, and ataxia (23)
  - ○ Since combination therapy is frequently required to achieve clinically meaningful pain relief, prescribers must be aware of drug interactions and polypharmacy

- **Gabapentin**
  - ○ Shown to be variably effective in post-SCI CNP at a dose of at least 1,800 mg/d (24)
  - ○ Typical starting dose of 300 mg daily
  - ○ Incremental increase by 300 mg every 4–7 days initially to a dosing of 3 times daily

- **Pregabalin**
  - ○ Two randomized controlled trials have shown pregabalin to be effective for post-SCI CNP at a mean dosage of 410–460 mg/d (25, 26)
  - ○ Shown to be variably efficacious in CPSP (27)
  - ○ Typical starting dose of 75 mg twice daily
  - ○ Incremental increase by 75 mg after 4–7 days to goal of 300 mg/d

- **Lamotrigine**
  - Shown to be effective in CPSP and in some forms of post-SCI CNP at mean dosages of 200–400 mg/d (28)
  - Typical starting dose of 25 mg/d for 2 weeks
  - Incremental weekly increase by 25 mg twice daily to goal of at least 100 mg twice daily

- **Amitriptyline**
  - Shown to be effective for CPSP at a dose of at least 75 mg/d (29)
  - Suggested to be variably effective in post-SCI pain with high dosages (up to 150 mg/d) proving effective in patients with comorbid depression (30)
  - Typical starting dose of 10–25 mg at bedtime
  - Incremental increase every 4–7 days to goal of 100 mg at bedtime

- **Duloxetine**
  - Shown to be effective in MS-related CNP at a dose of 60 mg/d (31)
  - Typical starting dose of 20–40 mg once daily
  - Incremental increase weekly by same dosage to goal of 60 mg/d

## Opioids

- Use of opioids for neuropathic pain control is not recommended given known risks associated with this drug class
  - Case reports indicate that some patients with refractory CNP secondary to CNS malignancy have achieved adequate pain control with combinations of high-dose oxycodone, methadone, and gabapentin (23)
  - Only one-third of patients with CNP experience up to a 50% decrease in pain with current pain regimens that implement opioids (32)
  - Opioids moderate pain through mu receptor pathways, but have been shown to increase neuropathic pain by increasing expression of toll-like receptor 4 (TLR4) (32)

## Cannabinoids

- Use of cannabinoids has proven efficacious in patients with CNP secondary to MS (33)

- ○ Dosing, relative proportion of cannabidiol and tetrahydro-cannabinol, and form of administration are highly variable, no formal recommendations are available

# Infusions

- **Methylprednisolone**
  - ○ A derivative of hydrocortisone and prednisolone, is a corticosteroid known to interfere with mediators of the inflammatory response (34)
  - ○ Can be given at higher doses than prednisone as an intravenous infusion for severe inflammation (34)
  - ○ A small study in China found that over 90% of patients with post-SCI CNP receiving a daily methylprednisolone infusion for 1 week experienced allodynia relief exceeding 50% (34)
    - These effects persisted during the 3-month follow-up; however, the data are underwhelming as the study was not placebo-controlled (34)

- **Baclofen**
  - ○ A gamma-aminobutyric acid (GABA) analog that acts by activating GABA receptors (35)
  - ○ A small placebo-controlled study found that intrathecal baclofen significantly decreases post-SCI CNP (35)
  - ○ Ability of baclofen to decrease spasticity gives it potential as an acute intervention (35)
  - ○ Endorsed by patients to improve function and decrease interference of chronic pain on daily life (35)

- **Ziconotide**
  - ○ An omega-conotoxin analog that blocks neuronal N-type voltage-sensitive calcium channels (36)
  - ○ A small study found that 70% of patients with post-SCI CNP experienced greater than 40% pain score reduction following intrathecal ziconotide injection (36)
  - ○ Analgesic effect is persistent, allowing patients to opt for placement of implanted ziconotide pumps (36)
  - ○ Further research is needed to evaluate both efficacy and toxicity of this drug

## Non-Pharmacologic Treatment Modalities

### Transcranial Magnetic Stimulation (TMS)

- TMS is a noninvasive form of brain stimulation that uses magnetic fields to stimulate specific areas of the brain (37)
- Thought to induce effects via manipulation of blood flow and neurotransmitter release (37)
- Has been successfully implemented in treatment of fibromyalgia, complex regional pain syndrome, and peripheral neuropathic pain (37)
- A randomized study found that TMS of the posterior superior insula induced analgesia and activation of the anterior cingulate cortex had an anxiolytic effect in patients with CPSP and post-SCI CNP (37)

### Transcranial Direct Current Stimulation (tDCS)

- An alternative to TMS that uses constant, direct low current to stimulate specific areas of the brain to modulate neuronal activity (21)
- There is evidence that tDCS directed at the primary motor cortex (M1) can achieve local and distant pain reduction (21)
- A randomized controlled study found that patients who underwent repeated stimulation with tDCS experienced significant pain reduction that persisted during follow-up (21)
- Effect of tDCS on pain is delayed, suggesting that pain reduction is a result of changes in cortical plasticity rather than immediate excitability (21)
- Treatment with tDCS requires an optimized protocol with repeated stimulation sessions (21)

### Breathing-Controlled Electrical Stimulation (BreEStim)

- BreEStim is a novel technique for treatment of neuropathic pain that modulates the autonomic system (38–40)
- BreEStim targets the pain-neuromatrix central autonomic network (PNM-CAN), which has been shown to be partially responsible for modulating pain (38–40)
- Activation of the PNM-CAN is quantified based on heartrate variability
- A small randomized controlled trial found that BreEStim was effective in decreasing post-SCI pain (31)

## Exercise

- Patients with CNP commonly experience a major decrease in quality of life due to not only pain but also a decrease in overall motor and sensory function
- A study conducted in mice found that exercise dampens microglial cell proliferation following spinal cord injury (11)
- A placebo-controlled study of post-SCI CNP patients found that exercise consisting of wheelchair propulsion resulted in subjective decreases of neuropathic pain on a numerical rating scale and an improvement of mood (42,43)
- EEG recordings of patients post-wheelchair exercise showed increased central peak alpha frequencies, correlating with a decrease in neuropathic pain (42,43)

## Conclusion

- CNP is a chronic pain condition resulting from injury to the central and specifically the somatosensory nervous system.
- Treatment of CNP is challenging, and patients should be educated that the goal is clinically meaningful pain relief rather than complete resolution of pain.
- Multimodal analgesia has been shown to be more effective than monotherapy and can be combined with advanced neuromodulation techniques such as TMS, tDCS, and BreEStim.
- Patients with refractory pain can benefit from referral to a multidisciplinary pain management team.

## References

1. Jensen TS, Baron R, Haanpää M et al. A new definition of neuropathic pain. *Pain.* 2011; 152(10): 2204–2205. doi: 10.1016/j.pain.2011.06.017.

2. Yekkirala AS, Roberson DP, Bean BP, Woolf CJ. Breaking barriers to novel analgesic drug development. *Nature Reviews Drug Discovery.* 2017; 16(8): 545–564. doi: 10.1038/nrd.2017.87.

3. Staudt MD, Clark AJ, Gordon AS et al. Long-term outcomes in the management of central neuropathic pain syndromes: A prospective observational cohort study. *Can J Neurol Sci.* 2018; 45(5): 545–552. doi: 10.1017/cjn.2018.55.

4. Warner FM, Cragg JJ, Jutzeler CR et al. Progression of neuropathic pain after acute spinal cord injury: A meta-analysis and framework for clinical trials. *J Neurotrauma.* 2019 15(1):40–48. doi: 10.1016/j.jpain.2013.09.008.

5. Finnerup NB, Norrbrink C, Trok K et al. Phenotypes and predictors of pain following traumatic spinal cord injury: A prospective study. *J Pain*. 2014;**15** (1):40–48. doi: 10.1016/j.jpain.2013.09.008.

6. Warner FM, Cragg JJ, Jutzeler CR et al. The progression of neuropathic pain after acute spinal cord injury: A meta-analysis and framework for clinical trials. *J Neurotrauma*. 2018;**36**(9):1461–1468.

7. Gruener H, Zeilig G, Laufer Y, Blumen N, Defrin R. Increased psychological distress among individuals with spinal cord injury is associated with central neuropathic pain rather than the injury characteristics. *Spinal Cord*. 2018;**56** (2):176–184. doi: 10.1038/s41393-017-0014-6.

8. Vuckovic A, Jajrees M, Purcell M, Berry H, Fraser M. Electroencephalographic predictors of neuropathic pain in subacute spinal cord injury. *J Pain*. 2018;**19**(11):1256.e1–1256.e17. doi: 10.1016/j .jpain.2018.04.011.

9. Wang Y, Ye F, Huang C et al. Bioinformatic analysis of potential biomarkers for spinal cord-injured patients with intractable neuropathic pain. *Clin J Pain*. 2018;**34**(9):825–830. doi: 10.1097/AJP.0000000000000608.

10. Tang Y, Liu L, Xu D et al. Interaction between astrocytic colony stimulating factor and its receptor on microglia mediates central sensitization and behavioral hypersensitivity in chronic post ischemic pain model. *Brain Behav Immun*. 2018;**68**:248–260.

11. Chhaya SJ, Quiros-Molina D, Tamashiro-Orrego AD, Houlé JD, Detloff MR. Exercise-induced changes to the macrophage response in the dorsal root ganglia prevent neuropathic pain after spinal cord injury. *J Neurotrauma*. 2019;**36**:877–890.

12. Du X-J, Chen Y-X, Zheng Z-C et al. Neural stem cell transplantation inhibits glial cell proliferation and P2X receptor-mediated neuropathic pain in spinal cord injury rats. *Neural Regen Res*. 2019;**14**(5):876–885.

13. Lee SH, Shi XQ, Fan A, West B, Zhang J. Targeting macrophage and microglia activation with colony stimulating factor 1 receptor inhibitor is an effective strategy to treat injury-triggered neuropathic pain. *Mol Pain*. 2018;**14**:1–12.

14. Kazuki K, Toshiya T, Yamanaka H et al. Upregulation of calcium channel alpha 2 delta 1 subunit in dorsal horn contributes to spinal cord injury-induced tactile allodynia- ClinicalKey. *Spinal J*. 2018;**18**(6):1062–1069.

15. Sánchez-Brualla I, Boulenguez P, Brocard C et al. Activation of 5-HT 2A receptors restores KCC2 function and reduces neuropathic pain after spinal cord injury. *Neuroscience*. 2018;**387**:48–57.

16. Li T, Wan Y, Sun L et al. Inhibition of microRNA-15a/16 expression alleviates neuropathic pain development through upregulation of G protein-coupled receptor kinase 2. *Biomol Ther*. 2019;**27**(4):414–422.

17. Yang Z, Xu J, Zhu R, Liu L. Down-regulation of miRNA-128 contributes to neuropathic pain following spinal cord injury via activation of P38. *Med Sci Monit.* 2017;**23**:405–411.

18. Sanna MD, Les F, Lopez V, Galeotti N. Lavender (Lavandula angustifolia Mill.) essential oil alleviates neuropathic pain in mice with spared nerve injury. *Front Pharmacol.* 2019;**10**:472. doi: 10.3389/fphar.2019.00472. eCollection 2019.

19. Warner FM, Cragg JJ, Jutzeler CR et al. The progression of neuropathic pain after acute spinal cord injury: A meta-analysis and framework for clinical trials. *J Neurotrauma.* 2018;**36**(9):1461–1468.

20. Rosendahl A, Krogh S, Kasch H. Pain assessment in hospitalized spinal cord injured patients–a controlled cross-sectional study. *Sc and J Pain.* 2018;**19**(2):299–307.

21. Thibaut A, Carvalho S, Morse L, Zafonte R, Fregni F. Delayed pain decrease following M1 tDCS in spinal cord injury: A randomized controlled clinical trial. *Neurosci Lett.* 2017;**658**:19–26.

22. Widerström-Noga E, Loeser JD, Jensen TS, Finnerup NB. AAPT diagnostic criteria for central neuropathic pain. *J Pain.* 2017;**18**(12):1417–1426. doi: 10.1016/j.jpain.2017.06.003.

23. Horan NA, Pugh TM. Intractable central pain in a patient with diffuse glioma. *Am J Phys Med Rehabil.* 2019;**98**:107–110.

24. Levendoglu F, Ogun CO, Ozerbil O, Ogun TC, Ugurlu H. Gabapentin is a first line drug for treatment of neuropathic pain in spinal cord injury. *Spine.* 2004;**29**:743–751.

25. Siddall PJ, Cousins MJ, Otte A et al. Pregabalin in central neuropathic pain associated with spinal cord injury: A placebo-controlled trial. *Neurol.* 2006;**67**:1792–1800.

26. Cardenas DD, Nieshoff EC, Suda K et al. A randomized trial of pregabalin in patients with neuropathic pain due to spinal cord injury. *Neurol.* 2013;**80**:533–539.

27. Vranken JH, Dijkgraaf MG, Kruis MR et al. Pregabalin in patients with central neuropathic pain: A randomized, double-blind, placebo-controlled trial of a flexible-dose regimen. *Pain.* 2008;**136**:150–157.

28. Finnerup NB, Sindrup SH, Bach FW, Johannesen IL, Jensen TS. Lamotrigine in spinal cord injury pain: A randomized controlled trial. *Pain.* 2002;**96**:375–383.

29. Leijon G, Boivie J. Central post-stroke pain – A controlled trial of amitriptyline and carbamazepine. *Pain.* 1989;**36**:27–36.

30. Rintala DH, Holmes SA, Courtade D et al. Comparison of the effectiveness of amitriptyline and gabapentin on chronic neuropathic pain in persons with spinal cord injury. *Arch Phys Med Rehabil.* 2007;**88**:1547–1560.

31. Vollmer TL, Robinson MJ, Risser RC, Malcolm SK. A randomized, double-blind, placebo-controlled trial of duloxetine for the treatment of pain in patients with multiple sclerosis. *Pain Pract*. 2014;**14**:732–744.

32. Ellis A, Grace PM, Wieseler J et al. Morphine amplifies mechanical allodynia via TLR4 in a rat model of spinal cord injury. *Brain Behav Immun*. 2016;**58**:348–356.

33. Svendsen KB, Jensen TS, Bach FW. Does the cannabinoid dronabinol reduce central pain in multiple sclerosis? Randomised double blind placebo controlled crossover trial. *BMJ*. 2004;**329**:253–260.

34. Li L, Han Y, Li T et al. The analgesic effect of intravenous methylprednisolone on acute neuropathic pain with allodynia due to central cord syndrome: A retrospective study. *J Pain Res*. 2018;**11**:1231–1238

35. Kumru H, Benito-Penalva J, Kofler M, Vidal J. Analgesic effect of intrathecal baclofen bolus on neuropathic pian in spinal cord injury patients. *Brain Res Bull*. 2018;**140**:205–211.

36. Brinzeu A, Berthiller J, Caillet J-B, Staquet H, Mertens P. Ziconotide for spinal cord injury-related pain. *Eur J Pain*. 2019;**23**(9):1688–1700.

37. Galhardoni R, da Silva VA, Garcia-Larrea L et al. Insular and anterior cingulate cortex deep stimulation for central neuropathic pain disassembling the percept of pain. *Neurol*. 2019;**92**(18):2165–2175.

38. Melzack R. Pain and neuromatrix in the brain. *J Dent Educ*. 2001;**65** (12):1378–1382.

39. Melzack R, Wall P. Pain mechanisms: a new theory. *Surv Anesth*. 1967;**11**:89–90.

40. Melzack R, Loeser J. Phantom body pain in paraplegics: Evidence for a central "pattern generating mechanism" for pain. *Pain*. 1977;**4**:195–210.

41. Karri J, Li S, Zhang L et al. Neuropathic pain modulation after spinal cord injury by breathing-controlled electrical stimulation (BreEStim) is associated with restoration of autonomic dysfunction. *J Pain Res*. 2018;**11**:2331–2341.

42. Boord P, Siddall P, Tran Y et al. Electroencephalographic slowing and reduced reactivity in neuropathic pain following spinal cord injury. *Spinal Cord*. 2008;**46**:118–123.

43. Wydenkeller S, Maurizio S, Dietz V, Halder P. Neuropathic pain in spinal cord injury: Significance of clinical and electrophysiological measures. *Eur J Neurosci*. 2009;**30**:91–99.

**Chapter 2**

# Cannabinoids Pain Signaling Pathways

Karina Charipova and Kyle Gress

## Endocannabinoid Pathways

- Endogenous cannabinoid system discovered in the early 1990s
- The endocannabinoid system includes cannabinoid receptors, ligands, and metabolic enzymes found within the central nervous system (CNS) (1)
- Inhibition or slowing of the degradation of endocannabinoids in select tissues may confer analgesic or anxiolytic effects (2,3)
- Cannabinoids are becoming increasingly prescribed and studied as potential analgesic agents (4)

## The Endocannabinoid System

### Endocannabinoids

- Endocannabinoids are bioactive lipids that bind to cannabinoid receptors (5)
- Endocannabinoids modulate neurotransmission and participate in pain perception, memory, mood, and appetite (6)
- Endocannabinoids are inactivated through both enzymatic degradation and transport after release into the synaptic cleft via influx of calcium (2,3)
- Noxious stimuli increase endocannabinoid release; decreasing endocannabinoid degradation may induce analgesia (6)
- Arachidonoylethanolamide (ADE), also known as anandamide, was the first isolated and characterized endocannabinoid (7)
  - Anandamide plays a role in higher cognitive process such as memory and movement control (5)
  - Anandamide also functions in pain, depression, fertility, and appetite (5)

- Other isolated endocannabinoids include 2-arachidonoylglycerol (2-AG), noladin ether, virodhamine, and N-arachidonoyldopamine (NADA) (6,8,9)

## Endogenous Cannabinoid Receptors

- Cannabinoid receptors are G protein-coupled receptors (GPCRs) composed of seven folded transmembrane helices (10)
- Two main cannabinoid receptor subtypes: type 1 (CB1) and type 2 (CB2); the WIN and abnormal-cannabinoid receptors are lesser-known subtypes (11–14)
- The CB1 receptor is primarily found in the nervous system, most heavily concentrated in the brain with lesser quantities located in the spine and peripheral nervous tissues (15)
  - CB1 receptors shown to modulate both peripheral and central pain perception
  - These receptors are highly expressed in the cortex, basal ganglia, hippocampus, and cerebellum (15–17)
  - They are also found in the thalamus, amygdala, midbrain periaqueductal gray matter (PAG), and substantial gelatinosa of the spinal cord, all of which play roles in nociceptive perception (12–16)
  - CB1 receptors are found mainly on neurons with myelinated A-fibers and much less commonly on C-fibers (17)
  - Immune cells and keratinocytes have also been shown to express CB1 receptors (18)
- The CB2 receptor is located primarily in the immune system (19)
  - They are also found in bone, liver, keratinocytes, hematopoietic cells, and brain microglia (20)
  - CB2 receptors have been shown to indirectly stimulate opioid receptors (5)
- Cannabinoids may also interact with other non-CB1/CB2 receptors such as GPR55/18 and opioid and serotonin receptors (21)

## Pharmacology

- The GPCR structure of CB1 and CB2 consists of 13 compounds thought to be orthosteric endocannabinoid ligands (22)
- GABA-ergic interneurons have been demonstrated to exhibit CB1 receptor activity (23)

- These interneurons have been found in the dorsal horn of the spinal cord (18)
- CB1 receptor agonists have been shown to reduce production of GABA (23)

- Several studies have demonstrated that presynaptic control of neurotransmitter release by CB1 is constitutively active (24)
- CB1 and CB2 signal transduction inhibits adenylyl cyclase, leading to a decrease in cyclic adenosine monophosphate (cAMP) production and stimulating mitogen-activated protein kinase (MAPK) (25)
- Inhibition of cytokine production and immune cell migration by CB2 receptors may enable attenuation of chronic pain and inflammation (26)

  - Inflammation in the dorsal root ganglia has been shown to have increased concentrations of CB2 receptor protein and mRNA (27)

- Off-target cannabinoid effects result from interaction with other receptor types such as the transient receptor potential vanilloid 1 (TRPV1) (28)

  - TRPV1 is involved in inflammation and nociception (28)
  - Endocannabinoids can agonize TRPV1, preventing the binding of higher efficacy agonists such as capsaicin (28)
  - TRPV1 is co-expressed with CB1 in certain cells, including in the CNS, and has been shown to demonstrate functional crosstalk (29)

## Analgesic Mechanism of Action

- Cannabinoid-induced analgesia was initially attributed to the action of CB1 in the CNS and CB2 in immune cells (30)
- Newer evidence suggests that additional target receptors exist in both the CNS and peripheral systems (21)

  - CB1 receptor activation is believed to reduce both acute and chronic pain by reducing inflammatory, visceral, and neuropathic pain (31)

- Studies of the use of cannabidiol (CBD) as early treatment in diabetic mice have demonstrated reductions in both microgliosis and tactile allodynia (32)
- Cannabinoid and opioid receptors share signaling pathways (4)

- ○ CB1 and CB2 agonists have been shown to improve release of endogenous opioids and to increase gene expression of opioid precursors (33)
- ○ There is evidence supporting the existence of cannabinoid receptor (CBR)-μ-opioid receptor (MOR) signaling complexes (34,35)
- ○ These complexes have been located in the dorsal horn of the spinal cord via CB1 and MORE colocalization (34,35)
- ○ Cannabinoids are thought to have a synergistic analgesic effect with opioids (33)
- ○ Activation of MORs induces analgesia, sedation, hypolocomotion, and respiratory depression (33)
- ○ Activation of cannabinoid receptors also induces analgesia and sedation, but does not produce respiratory depression (33)
- ○ Studies suggest that duration of analgesia can be increased by simultaneously administering a low-dose opioid and low-dose cannabinoid (33)

- Cannabinoid receptors, MORs, and adrenergic receptors in combination modulate opioid and norepinephrine release and function (33)

  - ○ Chronic pain has an interplay with underlying anxiety and depression (36)
  - ○ Modulation of the noradrenergic system can be important in the treatment of not only chronic anxiety and depression but also chronic pain and opioid withdrawal (36)
  - ○ The combination of a MOR agonist and an alpha-2 receptor agonist (e.g., clonidine, tizanidine, methylphenidate) synergistically produce analgesia (36)
  - ○ Synergism has also been seen in the combination of cannabinoid receptor agonists and alpha-adrenergic agonists (36)

- Prostaglandins are mediators of inflammation and nociception (37)

  - ○ Endocannabinoids are structurally similar to arachidonic acid (37)
  - ○ Cannabidiolic acid (CBDA) may be a selective inhibitor of COX-2, suggesting implications in the treatment of chronic pain such as arthritis (37)

# Therapeutic Applications

## Overview

- Cannabis has traditionally been ingested via smoke inhalation
  - This route is preferred due to rapidity of onset of action and increased control over ingested dose (38)
  - Effects secondary to inhalation are more predictable than those of oral ingestion (38)
  - Cannabis and cannabinoid agents have also been made available in the form of sublingual spray (38)
- Side effects of cannabis and cannabinoid agents manifest most significantly in the CNS (5)
  - These effects include drowsiness, dizziness, loss of focus, and xerostomia (5)
  - Cannabinoids have not been demonstrated to evoke long-term negative cognitive effects, but are believed to aggravate preexisting psychiatric conditions (5)
  - Addictive potential of medical cannabis is low (5)
  - A range of tolerance has been reported, with studies suggesting that 9–20% of regular users become dependent (5)
  - Cannabis use has not been associated with death (5)

## Cannabinoid Agents

- Studied cannabinoid receptor agonists include tetrahydrocannabinol (THC), CBD, and CB2 receptor activators (5)
- THC is a nonselective, lipophilic agent with significant potency as an analgesic and psychoactive substance (5)
  - Nabilone, dronabinol, levonantradol, and dexanabinol are synthetic THC analogs (5)
- CBD exhibits analgesic and anti-inflammatory properties similar to THC, but functions through a different mechanism (5)
  - CBD induces analgesia peripherally rather than centrally (5)
- CB2 agonists are suggested to have antinociceptive properties (5)
  - CB2 agonists are associated with fewer adverse cognitive and psychotic effects than CB1 agonists (5)
  - HU-308, a specific CB2 agonist, has been demonstrated to be an effective cannabimimetic not associated with behavioral changes (5)

## Antiemetic Properties

- The most widely accepted and documented therapeutic application of cannabis is as an antiemetic (5,39)
  - Cannabinoid therapy has specifically been used for the prevention of postoperative nausea and vomiting (PONV) (5)
  - Smoked cannabis or analogs of HTHC such as dronabinol and nabilone are used frequently in patients with cancer-suffering gastrointestinal distress (5)
  - Use of intravenous THC is limited by side effects and insufficient volume of evidence (40)

## Acute Pain Therapy

- Evidence of cannabinoid applications in the treatment of acute pain is lacking
  - Human studies have indicated effects ranging from analgesia to hyperalgesia (5)
  - Further studies are needed to evaluate efficacy of treatment in response to various modes of pain stimulation
- Efforts have been made to explore the applications of cannabinoids in the postoperative environment
  - 80% of patients endorse the belief that cannabis could be effective for the treatment of postsurgical pain and would use cannabinoid agents for this purpose if prescribed (41)
  - Given insufficient evidence of the efficacy of cannabinoids for the treatment of acute pain, the use of these agents postoperatively requires further investigation

## Chronic Pain Therapy

- The findings regarding the use of cannabinoids for chronic pain are mixed
  - Inhaled cannabis has consistently been found to reduce chronic noncancer pain (38)
  - Efficacy of oral cannabis in relieving chronic abdominal or arthritic pain is limited, but these agents may improve sleep and general quality of life (38)
- Despite heterogeneity across publications, there is moderate evidence that nabiximols are effective in reducing neuropathic pain (42)

- Some reports suggest that cannabinoids are more effective than opioids in reducing chronic neuropathic pain (43)
  - CT-3, an analog of THC-11-oic acid, has been shown to reduce chronic neuropathic pain when compared to placebo (44)
  - The implications of cannabinoids in the treatment of phantom pain are promising, but the current evidence is insufficient (45)
- Nabiximols are approved for treatment of opioid-resistant cancer pain in 30 countries (46,47)
  - THC and CBD have also been shown to have the potential to decrease cancer pain (47)
  - Synthetic cannabidiol has been tested in patients with breast cancer and glioma (48)
- There is an increasing body of evidence supporting the efficacy of cannabinoids in the treatment of migraines (49)
  - Assessment of THC in a rat model supported antimigraine effects (50)
  - Small studies have suggested that pain relief secondary to cannabinoids may be more significant than that of ergotamine and aspirin (51)
- Cannabinoids have been assessed in the treatment of multiple sclerosis (MS)
  - These agents are safe but minimally effective in management of some symptoms (i.e., bladder dysfunction) (52)
  - The effects of cannabinoids on spasticity are still under investigation, with studies currently producing mixed findings (53)
  - Cannabinoids are variably effective in relieving MS-associated chronic neuropathic pain (54)
- Cannabinoids are frequently used in patients with fibromyalgia, but evidence supporting their use is currently inadequate (55)

## Conclusion

- Cannabinoid therapy may offer a viable alternative to opioids for management of chronic pain
- Studies have demonstrated the presence of endocannabinoids and cannabinoid receptors throughout the nervous system

- Cannabinoids have been shown to induce analgesic effects through mechanisms different from traditional antinociceptive pathways
- Investigations of the clinical applications of cannabinoids have been limited
- Clinical trials suggest that extracts containing THC or its derivatives may be efficacious in the treatment of inflammatory, neuropathic, and oncologic pain
- Pharmacologic agents aimed at increasing levels of endogenous endocannabinoids may represent an alternative way of producing analgesia
- There is a need for further double-blinded placebo-controlled clinicals to support the use of cannabinoids for pain control

# References

1. Starowicz K, Finn DP. Cannabinoids and pain: Sites and mechanisms of action. *Adv Pharmacol Sci.* 2017;**80**:437–475.

2. Di Marzo V, Fontana A, Cadas H, Schinelli S, Cimino G, Schwartz J-C, Piomelli D. Formation and inactivation of endogenous cannabinoid anandamide in central neurons. *Nature.* 1994;**372**(6507):686–691.

3. Giuffrida A, Beltramo M, Piomelli D. Mechanisms of endocannabinoid inactivation: Biochemistry and pharmacology. *J Pharmacol Exp Ther.* 2001;**298**(1):7–14.

4. Parolaro D, Realini N, Vigano D, Guidali C, Rubino T. The endocannabinoid system and psychiatric disorders. *Exp Neurol.* 2010;**224**(1):3–14.

5. Manzanares J, Julian M, Carrascosa A. Role of the cannabinoid system in pain control and therapeutic implications for the management of acute and chronic pain episodes. *Curr Neuropharmacol.* 2006;**4**(3):239–257.

6. Walker JM, Krey JF, Chu CJ, Huang SM. Endocannabinoids and related fatty acid derivatives in pain modulation. *Chem Phys Lipids.* 2002;**121**(1–2):159–172.

7. Devane WA, Hanus L, Breuer A, Pertwee RG, Stevenson LA, Griffin G, Gibson D, Mandelbaum A, Etinger A, Mechoulam R. Isolation and structure of a brain constituent that binds to the cannabinoid receptor. *Science.* 1992;**258**(5090):1946–1949.

8. Mechoulam R, Ben-Shabat S, Hanus L, Ligumsky M, Kaminski NE, Schatz AR, Gopher A, Almog S, Martin BR, Compton DR. Identification of an endogenous 2-monoglyceride, present in canine gut, that binds to cannabinoid receptors. *Biochem Pharmacol.* 1995;**50**(1):83–90.

9. Porter AC, Sauer J-M, Knierman MD, Becker GW, Berna MJ, Bao J, Nomikos GG, Carter P, Bymaster FP, Leese AB, Felder CC. Characterization

of a novel endocannabinoid, virodhamine, with antagonist activity at the CB1 receptor. *J Pharmacol Exp Ther.* 2002;**301**(3):1020–1024.

10. Mackie K. Cannabinoid receptors: Where they are and what they do. *J Neuroendocrinol.* 2008;**20**(s1):10–14.

11. Sañudo-Peña MC, Strangman NM, Mackie K, Walker JM, Tsou K. CB1 receptor localization in rat spinal cord and roots, dorsal root ganglion, and peripheral nerve. *Zhongguo Yao Li Xue Bao.* 1999;**20**(12):1115–1120.

12. Manning BH, Martin WJ, Meng ID. The rodent amygdala contributes to the production of cannabinoid-induced antinociception. *Neuroscience.* 2003;**120**(4):1157–1170.

13. Martin WJ, Hohmann AG, Walker JM. Suppression of noxious stimulus-evoked activity in the ventral posterolateral nucleus of the thalamus by a cannabinoid agonist: Correlation between electrophysiological and antinociceptive effects. *J Neurosci.* 1996;**16**(20):6601–6611.

14. Lichtman AH, Cook SA, Martin BR. Investigation of brain sites mediating cannabinoid-induced antinociception in rats: Evidence supporting periaqueductal gray involvement. *J Pharmacol Exp Ther.* 1996;**276**(2):585–593.

15. Luo C, Kumamoto E, Furue H, Chen J, Yoshimura M. Anandamide inhibits excitatory transmission to rat substantia gelatinosa neurones in a manner different from that of capsaicin. *Neurosci Lett.* 2002;**321**(1–2):17–20.

16. Morisset V, Urban L. Cannabinoid-induced presynaptic inhibition of glutamatergic EPSCs in substantia gelatinosa neurons of the rat spinal cord. *J Neurophysiol.* 2001;**86**(1):40–48.

17. Bridges D, Rice ASC, Egertová M, Elphick MR, Winter J, Michael GJ. Localisation of cannabinoid receptor 1 in rat dorsal root ganglion using in situ hybridisation and immunohistochemistry. *Neuroscience.* 2003;**119**(3):803–812.

18. Hill KP, Palastro MD, Johnson B, Ditre JW. Cannabis and pain: A clinical review. *Cannabis cannabinoid Res.* 2017;**2**(1):96–104.

19. Ibrahim MM, Porreca F, Lai J, Albrecht PJ, Rice FL, Khodorova A, Davar G, Makriyannis A, Vanderah TW, Mata HP, Malan TP. CB2 cannabinoid receptor activation produces antinociception by stimulating peripheral release of endogenous opioids. *Proc Natl Acad Sci.* 2005;**102**(8):3093–3098.

20. Abrams D, Guzman M. Cannabis in cancer care. *Clin Pharmacol Ther.* 2015;**97**(6):575–586.

21. Scavone JL, Sterling RC, Van Bockstaele EJ. Cannabinoid and opioid interactions: Implications for opiate dependence and withdrawal. *Neuroscience.* 2013;**248**:637–654.

22. Pertwee RG. Endocannabinoids and their pharmacological actions. *Handb. Exp. Pharmacol.* 2015;**231**:1–37. doi: 10.1007/978-3-319-20825-1_1.

23. Katona I, Sperlágh B, Maglóczky Z, Sántha E, Köfalvi A, Czirják S, Mackie K, Vizi ES, Freund TF. GABAergic interneurons are the targets of cannabinoid actions in the human hippocampus. *Neuroscience.* 2000;**100**(4):797–804.

24. Schlicker E, Kathmann M. Modulation of transmitter release via presynaptic cannabinoid receptors. *Trends Pharmacol Sci.* 2001;**22**(11):565–572.

25. Ibsen MS, Connor M, Glass M. Cannabinoid CB $_1$ and CB $_2$ receptor signaling and bias. *Cannabis Cannabinoid Res.* 2017;**2**(1):48–60.

26. Niu J, Huang D, Zhou R, Yue M, Xu T, Yang J, He L, Tian H, Liu X, Zeng J. Activation of dorsal horn cannabinoid CB2 receptor suppresses the expression of P2Y12 and P2Y13 receptors in neuropathic pain rats. *J Neuroinflammation.* 2017;**14**(1):185.

27. Fine PG, Rosenfeld MJ. The endocannabinoid system, cannabinoids, and pain. *Rambam Maimonides Med J.* 2013;**4**(4):e0022.

28. Lowin T, Straub RH. Cannabinoid-based drugs targeting CB1 and TRPV1, the sympathetic nervous system, and arthritis. *Arthritis Res Ther.* 2015;**17**(1):226.

29. Cristino L, de Petrocellis L, Pryce G, Baker D, Guglielmotti V, Di Marzo V. Immunohistochemical localization of cannabinoid type 1 and vanilloid transient receptor potential vanilloid type 1 receptors in the mouse brain. *Neuroscience.* 2006;**139**(4):1405–1415.

30. Rahn EJ, Hohmann AG. Cannabinoids as pharmacotherapies for neuropathic pain: from the bench to the bedside. *Neurotherapeutics.* 2009;**6**(4):713–737.

31. Gui H, Liu X, Liu L-R, Su D-F, Dai S-M. Activation of cannabinoid receptor 2 attenuates synovitis and joint destruction in collagen-induced arthritis. *Immunobiology.* 2015;**220**(6):817–822.

32. Toth CC, Jedrzejewski NM, Ellis CL, Frey WH. Cannabinoid-mediated modulation of neuropathic pain and microglial accumulation in a model of murine type I diabetic peripheral neuropathic pain. *Mol Pain.* 2010;**6**:1744–8069.

33. Nielsen S, Sabioni P, Trigo JM, Ware MA, Betz-Stablein BD, Murnion B, Lintzeris N, Khor KE, Farrell M, Smith A, Le Foll B. Opioid-sparing effect of cannabinoids: A systematic review and meta-analysis. *Neuropsychopharmacology.* 2017;**42**(9):1752–1765.

34. Hojo M, Sudo Y, Ando Y, Minami K, Takada M, Matsubara T, Kanaide M, Taniyama K, Sumikawa K, Uezono Y. μ-Opioid receptor forms a functional heterodimer with cannabinoid CB1 receptor: Electrophysiological and FRET assay analysis. *J Pharmacol Sci.* 2008;**108**(3):308–319.

35. Salio C, Fischer J, Franzoni MF et al. CB1-cannabinoid and μ -Opioid receptor co-localization on postsynaptic target in the rat dorsal horn. *Neuroreport*. 2001;**12**(17):3689–3692.

36. Cathel AM, Reyes BAS, Wang Q et al. Cannabinoid modulation of alpha2 adrenergic receptor function in rodent medial prefrontal cortex. *Eur J Neurosci*. 2014;**40**(8):3202–3214.

37. Takeda S, Misawa K, Yamamoto I, Watanabe K. Cannabidiolic acid as a selective cyclooxygenase-2 inhibitory component in cannabis. *Drug Metab Dispos*. 2008;**36**(9):1917–1921.

38. Romero-Sandoval EA, Kolano AL, Alvarado-Vázquez PA. Cannabis and cannabinoids for chronic pain. *Curr Rheumatol Rep*. 2017;**19**(11):67.

39. Rai A, Meng H, Weinrib A, Englesakis M. A review of adjunctive CNS medications used for the treatment of post-surgical pain. *CNS Drugs*. 2017;**31**(7):605–615.

40. Kleine-brueggeney M, Greif R, Brenneisen R et al. Intravenous delta-9-tetrahydrocannabinol to prevent postoperative nausea and vomiting: A randomized controlled trial. *Anesth Analg*. 2015;**121**(5).

41. Khelemsky Y, Goldberg AT, Hurd YL et al. Perioperative patient beliefs regarding potential effectiveness of marijuana (cannabinoids) for treatment of pain: A prospective population survey. *Reg Anesth Pain Med*. 2017;**42**(5):652–659.

42. Meng H, Johnston B, Englesakis M et al. Selective cannabinoids for chronic neuropathic pain: A systemic review and meta-analysis. *Anesth Analg*. 2017;**125**(5):1638–1652.

43. Fitzcharles M-A, Baerwald C, Ablin J, Häuser W. Efficacy, tolerability and safety of cannabinoids in chronic pain associated with rheumatic diseases (fibromyalgia syndrome, rheumatoid arthritis): A systematic review of randomized controlled trials. *Schmerz (Berlin, Germany)*. 2016;**30**(1):47–61.

44. Karst M, Salim K, Burstein S et al. Analgesic effect of the synthetic cannabinoid CT-3 on chronic neuropathic pain. *JAMA*. 2003;**290**(13):1757.

45. Hall N, Eldabe S. Phantom limb pain: A review of pharmacological management. *Br J Pain*. 2018;**12**(4):202–207.

46. Russo EB. Cannabis Therapeutics and the Future of Neurology. *Front Integr Neurosci*. 2018;**12**:51.

47. Davis MP. Cannabinoids for symptom management and cancer therapy: The evidence. *J Natl Compr Canc Netw*. 2016;**14**(7):915–922.

48. Kenyon J, Liu W, Dalgleish A. Report of objective clinical responses of cancer patients to pharmaceutical-grade synthetic cannabidiol. *Anticancer Res*. 2018;**38**(10):5831–5835.

49. Baron EP. Medicinal properties of cannabinoids, terpenes, and flavonoids in cannabis, and benefits in migraine, headache, and pain: An update on current

evidence and cannabis science. *Headache J Head Face Pain*. 2018;**58** (7):1139–1186.

50. Kandasamy R, Dawson CT, Craft RM, Morgan MM. Anti-migraine effect of Δ 9-tetrahydrocannabinol in the female rat. *Eur J Pharmacol*. 2018;**818**:271–277.

51. Pamplona FA, Phytolab E, Giniatullin Rashidginiatullin R et al. Emerging role of (endo)cannabinoids in migraine. *Front Pharmacol*. 2018;**9**:420.

52. Torres-moreno MC, Papaseit E, Torrens M, Farré M. Assessment of efficacy and tolerability of medicinal cannabinoids in patients with multiple sclerosis: A systematic review and meta-analysis. *JAMA*. 2018;**1**(6):1–16.

53. Smith PF. Therapeutics and clinical risk management new approaches in the management of spasticity in multiple sclerosis patients: Role of cannabinoids. *Ther Clin Risk Manag*. 2010;**6**:6–59.

54. Langford RM, Mares J, Novotna A et al. A double-blind, randomized, placebo-controlled, parallel-group study of THC/CBD oromucosal spray in combination with the existing treatment regimen, in the relief of central neuropathic pain in patients with multiple sclerosis. *J Neurol*. 2013;**260** (4):984–997.

55. Russo EB. Clinical endocannabinoid deficiency reconsidered: Current research supports the theory in migraine, fibromyalgia, irritable bowel, and other treatment-resistant syndromes. *Cannabis Cannabinoid Res*. 2016;**1** (1):154–165.

# Chapter 3

# The Microbiome and Chronic Pain Syndromes

Karina Charipova, Alaa Abd-Elsayed, and Kyle Gress

## The Microbiome

- The gut microbiome is the community of organisms that occupies the human gastrointestinal tract
- The human microbiome consists of approximately $10^{14}$ microbes, including bacteria, bacteriophages, archaea, eukaryotic viruses, fungi, and protozoa (1)
- The microbiome is influenced by genetic and environmental factors, most clearly diet
- The gut microbiome has been implemented in several physiologic processes (e.g., homeostasis, metabolism, immune activity)
  - Dysbiosis refers to negative changes to the gut microbiome
  - Dysbiosis is thought to be associated with the pathogenesis of disease states (e.g., autoimmune disorders, inflammatory bowel disease (IBD), metabolic syndrome, malignancy) (2–7)
  - The exact mechanisms by which dysbiosis leads to disease are being investigated
- A bidirectional relationship between the gut microbiota and the brain, known as the gut–brain axis, has been proposed to be implemented in neurobehavioral development (8–10)
- Role of diet in the microbiome leaves room for socioeconomic implications
  - Soluble dietary fiber is believed to play key role in dictating makeup of microbiota (11)
  - Short chain fatty acids produced from soluble fiber may contribute to improved immunologic functioning (11)
  - Higher-income families shown to consume diets richer in soluble fiber (11)
  - Diet adjustments and the incorporation of supplementation can be both challenging and costly
  - Income inequality may predispose to dysbiosis (12)

# Experimental Evidence

## Vitamin D and Chronic Pain

- There is evidence that vitamin D plays a role in the development of pain
- Vitamin D has been demonstrated to modulate pain through action on the gut microbiome via the endocannabinoid system
  - In a mouse model, an association was demonstrated between vitamin D deficiency and allodynia, spinal neuronal sensitization, and modifications in endocannabinoid pathways in the spinal cord and the gut (13)
  - Pain and inflammation associated with vitamin D deficiency may result from decreased endocannabinoid signaling at CB1 and CB2 receptors (13)
- There may be a relationship between pain perception and the composition of the gut biome; dietary interventions may change intestinal flora (13)

## Diversity of Gut Microbiota

- Research suggests that increased species diversity of the bacteria in the gut may be protective against disease
- Adult rat models show that animals treated with a 6-week antibiotic course experience changes in microbial diversity and a concurrent change in neurotransmitter release (14)
  - Diversity of the gut microbiome decreased following antibiotic treatment (14)
  - Antibiotic treatment was associated with reduced 5-HT, increased 5-HIAA/5-HT turnover in the hippocampus, increased tryptophan, increased noradrenaline, and increased L-DOPA (14)
  - These changes reflect dysregulation of monoamine synthesis and degradation (14)
  - Antibiotic-induced microbiota depletion is correlated with a phenotype of depressive-like behaviors and impaired cognition (14)
  - Microbiota depletion was not associated with an anxiety-like phenotype (15,16)
  - The association between microbiota and the development of a depression-like state may help elucidate the link between depression and chronic pain syndromes

- Antibiotic-treated rats have been shown to have reduced visceral hypersensitivity (14)
  - Antibiotics have traditionally been associated with decreased pain thresholds (15,16)
  - These findings may be linked to the timing of microbiota depletion (i.e., during adolescence vs. adulthood)

## Role of Infection

- Foodborne diarrheal and parasitic infections can contribute to dysbiosis
- Suckling rats infected with *Giardia* exhibited increased visceral hypersensitivity compared to controls (17)
  - This change correlated with changes in colonic structure (i.e., villus height, crypt depth, mucus layer thinning) (17)
  - Changes also observed remote from active colonization in the rectum (17)
- Human microbiome research proposes "the leaky gut" hypothesis
  - Intestinal permeability is regulated by tight junctions
  - Increased permeability can enable bacterial translocation, resulting in chronic pain and inflammation
  - Gastrointestinal infection is thought to disrupt colonic structure, increasing inflammation and hypersensitivity
  - More evidence is needed to support this causal relationship

## Interplay with Opioids

- Dysregulation of gut flora by opioids may help to explain link between microbiome and chronic pain
- Studies have endorsed a link between opioid use and increased bacterial translocation
  - Toll-like receptors (TLRs) may be implicated in this mechanism (18–20)
  - TLRs are believed to mediate the relationship between morphine, dysbiosis, altered metabolism, increased gut intestinal permeability, and inflammation (19)
  - Fecal transplantation from placebo and TLR knockout mice has been shown to allow microbial reconstitution
  - Mouse models suggest that changes in the microbiome may occur after as little as one day of opioid use (20)

- Decreased microbiome diversity and increased colonization by potentially pathogenic species have been noted with morphine administration in mice (20)
  - *Enterococcus faecalis* has been observed to accelerate opioid tolerance (20)
  - Microbes may decrease morphine deconjugation and entero-hepatic recirculation (20)
  - Intestinal barrier dysfunction may be linked to changes in microbiome metabolism and increased TLR-4 signaling (20)

## Osteoarthritis

- Gut dysbiosis is thought to accelerate joint degeneration
- Obesity is a known key risk factor in the development of osteoarthritis
- Obesity is associated with increased local and systemic inflammation (21)
  - Mouse model has been used to evaluate contribution of obesity-related dysbiosis to osteoarthritis (OA) (21)
  - Obesity shown to be associated with decrease in beneficial *Bifidobacteia* and a concurrent increase in proinflammatory species (21)
  - Oligofructose supplementation reverses effects of obesity on gut microbiome and reduces systemic inflammation (21)
- Gut dysbiosis may directly facilitate inflammatory changes in knee joints
  - Obese mice found to have a fivefold increase in macrophage infiltration into the joint space (21)
  - Obese mice also have increase of gene expression related to macrophage lineages (21)
  - Obesity is linked to increase in infiltrating macrophages, but not resident tissue macrophages (21)
  - Systemic inflammation seen in obesity may promote chemokine-mediated migration of monocytes to the knee (21)
  - Oligofructose reduces proliferation of infiltrating macrophages (21)
- Oligofructose supplementation may protect against OA-related degeneration and improve histomorphometric outcomes

## Clinical Evidence

- Majority of studies of the microbiome are currently limited to animal models
- Most areas of microbiome research in humans has focused on its role in gastrointestinal and autoimmune disorders (e.g., rheumatoid arthritis, juvenile idiopathic arthritis)

## Chronic Pelvic Pain Syndrome

- Chronic pelvic pain syndrome (CPPS) refers to persistent pelvic pain and discomfort; it is often associated with urologic symptoms like urgency (22)
  - CPPS is noninflammatory
  - CPPS has been seen in association with other chronic conditions such as IBD and fibromyalgia
  - Most beneficial treatment has been found to be multimodal
- Gut microbiome in patients with CPPS has been proposed to be different from healthy controls
  - Study evaluated this hypothesis by comparing bacterial sRNA of CPPS patients and healthy controls (22)
  - CPPS found to be associated with significantly decreased diversity of intestinal microbiota (22)
  - Increased duration of CPPS associated with more significantly decreased bacterial diversity (22)
  - *Prevotella* counts found to be particularly decreased in CPPS (22)
  - *Prevotella* known to be associated with higher diets and thought to be protective from inflammation; may be a marker for cases of CPPS

## Fibromyalgia

- Fibromyalgia is a disorder characterized by widespread musculoskeletal pain that can be accompanied by mood disturbances, fatigue, insomnia, and other symptoms (23)
  - Musculoskeletal pain frequently manifests as localized tender points
  - Psychiatric comorbidities are frequently observed
  - The condition lacks biomarkers and has historically been challenging to diagnose and treat

- When compared to healthy age-matched controls, metabolic profiles of fibromyalgia patients differed (23)
  - Fibromyalgia patients had elevated hippuric, succinic, and lactic acid metabolites (23)
  - Elevations of these metabolites are suggested to be linked to the gut microbiome
  - By the Fibromyalgia Impact Questionnaire, the biosignatures of creatine, taurine, and succinic acid served as predictors of pain and fatigue symptoms (23)
  - Urinary metabolite analysis may help to diagnose fibromyalgia and guide treatment
- A group at McGill University developed an algorithm that could diagnose the presence of fibromyalgia and severity of disease with 87% accuracy based on microbiome abnormalities (24)

## Myalgic Encephalomyelitis

- Myalgic encephalomyelitis, or chronic fatigue syndrome (ME/CFS), is associated with a constellation of symptoms, the most notable of which is overwhelming, often debilitating, fatigue
  - Other symptoms include sleep disturbances, orthostatic intolerance, muscle pain, and lymphadenia
  - Symptoms frequently worsen after exertion
- Significant differences in microbiomes have been shown to exist between ME/CFS patients and healthy controls (25)
  - The counts of bacteria have been shown to increase in both the gut and the blood in ME/CFS after exertion (25)
  - Changes occurred in controls as well, but were less extreme (25)
  - ME/CFS is also associated with delayed clearance of these bacteria from blood (25)
- A hypothesis for ME/CFS pathogenesis involves translocation of gram-negative bacteria across tight junctions to trigger inflammation (26)
  - Exertion is thought to worsen symptoms by increasing translocation across tight junctions (25)
  - Inflammation may result specifically from lipopolysaccharides in the outer membrane of gram-negative bacteria (26)
  - The immune responses of ME/CFS patients are thought to be more robust than those of healthy controls

- Blood assays of ME/CFS patients in response to gram-negative commensal bacteria were compared to those of controls (26)
  - The study group had significantly elevated levels of IL-1, TNFα, neopterin, and elastase (26)
  - Peak immune (IgM and IgA) responses were higher in ME/CFS patients (26)
  - ME/CFS patients were found to have exaggerated responses compared to not only healthy controls but also patients with chronic fatigue not meeting ME/CFS thresholds (26)
  - Specific immune responses also correlated more directly with discrete symptoms (e.g., increased IgA associated with increased fatigue, autonomic dysregulation, gastrointestinal symptoms, malaise)
- Treatments aimed at decreasing bacterial translocation may help to both improve gut barrier functioning and manage ME/CFS and other disorders

## Treatments

### Probiotics

- Supplementation with probiotics has been suggested to facilitate shift of the microbiome to a less-inflammatory state
- Six months of supplementation with probiotic *Lactobacillus casei* Shirota (LeS) was shown to significantly decrease Visual Analog Scale (VAS) and Western Ontario and McMaster Universities Osteoarthritis Index (WOMAC) scores in patients with OA (27)
  - Pain and physical function also significantly decreased with probiotic use (27)
  - Decreases in both VAS and WOMAC scores were strongly correlated with a decrease in serum CRP levels (27)
- A pilot 8-week randomized controlled trial found that use of a daily multispecies probiotic by patients with fibromyalgia improves impulsivity and decision-making (28)
  - Pain was not significantly improved (28)
  - Changes in most other cognitive measures were not significant (28)
- Gastrointestinal disorders (e.g., celiac disease, *Helicobacter pylori* infections, gastroparesis) have been shown to be associated with migraine frequency (29)

- ○ A survey study demonstrated that 80% of patients with migraine experienced improved quality of life following a 90-day trial of a daily probiotic cocktail (29)
- ○ A randomized controlled study of 63 migraine patients did not support a significant difference between probiotics and placebo in migraine frequency reduction (30)
- ○ The potential association between dysbiosis, probiotic use, and headache/migraine reduction requires further study

- Supplementation with DSF (probiotic, 450 billion bacteria per sachet) was tested as a treatment for chemotherapy-induced peripheral neuropathy (CIPN) (31)

- ○ Paclitaxel-induced CIPN is thought to be caused in part by increased expression of TRPV1 and TRPV4 pain receptors (31)
- ○ DSF was found to restore baseline levels of expression of both TRPV1 and TRPV2, counteracting CIPN (31)

- It has been demonstrated that, in a spared nerve injury model, antibiotic-treated rats displayed a pain-prone phenotype (32)

- ○ Fecal transplantation could be used to induce the pain-prone phenotype (32)
- ○ The microbiome may have a role in modulating pain secondary to nerve trauma

- A probiotic mixture of *Lactobacillus reuteri* and *Bifidobacterium* did not yield any measurable pain relief in thermal and mechanically nerve injuries (33)
- Probiotic mixtures may play a role in modulating pain processes, but these effects are likely highly disease-specific

## Dietary Interventions

- Neck and shoulder pain is a complaint endorsed by patients with several chronic conditions including fibromyalgia and ME/CFS
- Fermented foods have been recommended as a method of introducing beneficial bacteria into the gut biome
- A double-blind, placebo-controlled randomized crossover study evaluated changes in the microbiome resulting from the introduction of NKCP into the diet (34)

- ○ Natto is a Japanese fermented soybean dish known to contain *Bacillus subtilis*, which produces NKCP (34)

- ○ NKCP has been shown to have anticoagulant and thrombolytic properties (34)
- ○ The small 30-subject study found that ingestion of 200 mg of NKCP was associated with significantly lower VAS scores for neck and shoulder stiffness and improved headache scores (34)
- ○ Bacterial metabolites may affect disease outcomes
- Natural anti-inflammatory and anti-oxidative substances (NAIOs) include zinc, glutamine, taurine, L-carnitine, N-acetyl-cysteine, and lipoic acid (35)
- A 10- to 14-month study of 41 ME/CFS patients evaluated outcomes of a lactose-free, gluten-free, and low-carb diet with incorporation of NAIOs (35)
  - ○ IgA and IgM responses were found to normalize and correlated with clinical improvement (35)
  - ○ Good response to treatment was associated with younger age and shorter illness duration (35)

## Conclusion

- Microbiome research is becoming increasingly robust as the microbiome becomes increasingly linked with various disease states and potential therapies
- The majority of research to date has focused on exploring the role of microbiota and dysbiosis in various autoimmune disorders, but interest has grown in their interplay with chronic pain disorders
- The microbiome has primarily been linked to human disorders through modulation of inflammatory pathways
- Most studies have taken place in animal models, introducing the challenge of translating this research to human interventional models
- Pre/probiotics, fermented foods, dietary fiber, NAIOSs, fecal transplants, and novel therapies have been proposed to treat dysbiosis
- Further investigation of the link between the microbiome and nociception may help with diagnosis and management of conditions like OA, fibromyalgia, and neuropathic pain

## References

1. Zhang Y-J, Li S, Gan R-Y et al. Impacts of gut bacteria on human health and diseases. *Int J Mol Sci.* 2015;**16**(12):7493–7519.

2. Sheflin AM, Whitney AK, Weir TL. Cancer-promoting effects of microbial dysbiosis. *Curr Oncol Rep.* 2014;**16**(10):406.

3.  Vuong HE, Hsiao EY. Emerging roles for the gut microbiome in autism spectrum disorder. *Biol Psychiatry*. 2017;**81**(5):411–423.

4.  Geurts L, Neyrinck AM, Delzenne NM et al. Gut microbiota controls adipose tissue expansion, gut barrier and glucose metabolism: Novel insights into molecular targets and interventions using prebiotics. *Benef Microbes*. 2014;**5**(1):3–17.

5.  Rigoni R, Fontana E, Guglielmetti S et al. Intestinal microbiota sustains inflammation and autoimmunity induced by hypomorphic RAG defects. *J Exp Med*. 2016;**213**(3):355–375.

6.  Gagnière J, Raisch J, Veziant J et al. Gut microbiota imbalance and colorectal cancer. *World J Gastroenterol*. 2016;**22**(2):501–518.

7.  Schulberg J, De Cruz P. Characterisation and therapeutic manipulation of the gut microbiome in inflammatory bowel disease. *Intern Med J*. 2016;**46**(3):266–273.

8.  Nicholson JK, Holmes E, Kinross J et al. Host-gut microbiota metabolic interactions. *Science*. 2012;**336**(6086):1262–1267.

9.  Cryan JF, Dinan TG. Mind-altering microorganisms: The impact of the gut microbiota on brain and behaviour. *Nat Rev Neurosci*. 2012;**13**(10):701–712.

10. Hsiao EY, McBride SW, Hsien S et al. Microbiota modulate behavioral and physiological abnormalities associated with neurodevelopmental disorders. *Cell*. 2013;**155**(7):1451–1463.

11. So D, Whelan K, Rossi M et al. Dietary fiber intervention on gut microbiota composition in healthy adults: A systematic review and meta-analysis. *Am J Clin Nutr*. 2018;**107**(6):965–983.

12. Harrison CA, Taren D. How poverty affects diet to shape the microbiota and chronic disease. *Nat. Rev. Immunol*. 2018;**18**:279–287.

13. Shipton EA, Shipton EE. Vitamin D and pain: Vitamin D and its role in the aetiology and maintenance of chronic pain states and associated comorbidities. *Pain Res Treat*. 2015;**2015**: 904967.

14. Hoban AE, Moloney RD, Golubeva AV et al. Behavioural and neurochemical consequences of chronic gut microbiota depletion during adulthood in the rat. *Neurosci*. 2016;**339**:463–477.

15. O'Mahony SM, Felice VD, Nally K et al. Disturbance of the gut microbiota in early-life selectively affects visceral pain in adulthood without impacting cognitive or anxiety-related behaviors in male rats. *Neurosci*. 2014;**277**:885–901.

16. Verdú EF, Bercik P, Verma-Gandhu M et al. Specific probiotic therapy attenuates antibiotic induced visceral hypersensitivity in mice. *Gut*. 2006;**55**(2):182–190.

17. Halliez MCM, Motta J-P, Feener TD et al. Giardia duodenalis induces paracellular bacterial translocation and causes postinfectious visceral hypersensitivity. *Am J Physiol Gastrointest Liver Physiol.* 2016;**310**(8):G574–G585.

18. Meng J, Yu H, Ma J et al. Morphine induces bacterial translocation in mice by compromising intestinal barrier function in a TLR-dependent manner. *PLoS One.* 2013;**8**(1):e54040.

19. Banerjee S, Sindberg G, Wang F et al. Opioid-induced gut microbial disruption and bile dysregulation leads to gut barrier compromise and sustained systemic inflammation. *Mucosal Immunol.* 2016;**9**(6):1418–1428.

20. Wang F, Meng J, Zhang L et al. Morphine induces changes in the gut microbiome and metabolome in a morphine dependence model. *Sci Rep.* 2018;**8**(1):1–15.

21. Schott EM, Farnsworth CW, Grier A et al. Targeting the gut microbiome to treat the osteoarthritis of obesity. *JCI Insight.* 2018;**3**(8):e95997.

22. Shoskes DA, Wang H, Polackwich AS et al. Analysis of gut microbiome reveals significant differences between men with chronic prostatitis / chronic pelvic pain syndrome and controls. *J Urol.* 2016;**196**(2):435–441.

23. Malatji BG, Meyer H, Mason S et al. A diagnostic biomarker profile for fibromyalgia syndrome based on an NMR metabolomics study of selected patients and controls. *BMC Neurol.* 2017;**17**(1):1–15.

24. Minerbi A, Gonzalez E, Brereton NJB et al. Altered microbiome composition in individuals with fibromyalgia. *Pain.* 2019;**160**(11):2589–2602.

25. Shukla SK, Cook D, Meyer J et al. Changes in gut and plasma microbiome following exercise challenge in myalgic encephalomyelitis / chronic fatigue syndrome (ME / CFS). *PLoS One.* 2015;**10**:1–15.

26. Maes M, Twisk FNM, Kubera M et al. Increased IgA responses to the LPS of commensal bacteria is associated with inflammation and activation of cell-mediated immunity in chronic fatigue syndrome. *J Affect Disord.* 2012;**136**(3):909–917.

27. Lei M, Guo C, Wang D, Zhang C, Hua L. The effect of probiotic Lactobacillus casei Shirota on knee osteoarthritis: A randomised double-blind, placebo-controlled clinical trial. *Benef Microbes.* 2017;**8**(5):697–703.

28. Roman P, Estévez AF, Miras A et al. A pilot randomized controlled trial to explore cognitive and emotional effects of probiotics in fibromyalgia. *Sci Rep.* 2018;**8**(1):1–9.

29. Cámara-Lemarroy CR, Rodriguez-Gutierrez R, Monreal-Robles R, Marfil-Rivera A. Gastrointestinal disorders associated with migraine: A comprehensive review. *World J Gastroenterol.* 2016;**22**:8149–8160.

30. Naghibi MM, Day R. The microbiome, the gut-brain axis and migraine. *Gastrointest Nurs*. 2019;**17**(8):38–45.

31. Zhong S, Zhou Z, Liang Y et al. Targeting strategies for chemotherapy-induced peripheral neuropathy: Does gut microbiota play a role? *Crit. Rev. Microbiol*. 2019;**45**:369–393.

32. Yang C, Fang X, Zhan G et al. Key role of gut microbiota in anhedonia-like phenotype in rodents with neuropathic pain. *Transl Psychiatry*. 2019;**9**(1):57.

33. Huang J, Zhang C, Wang J, Guo Q, Zou W. Oral *Lactobacillus reuteri* LR06 or *Bifidobacterium* BL5b supplement do not produce analgesic effects on neuropathic and inflammatory pain in rats. *Brain Behav*. 2019;**9**(4):e01260.

34. Sunagawa Y, Okamura N, Miyazaki Y et al. Effects of products containing *Bacillus subtilis* var. *natto* on healthy subjects with neck and shoulder stiffness, a double-blind, placebo-controlled, randomized crossover study. *Biol Pharm Bull*. 2018;**41**(4):504–509.

35. Maes M, Leunis J-C. Normalization of leaky gut in chronic fatigue syndrome (CFS) is accompanied by a clinical improvement: Effects of age, duration of illness and the translocation of LPS from gram-negative bacteria. *Neuro Endocrinol Lett*. 2008;**29**(6):902–910.

**Chapter 4**

# Nonsteroidal Anti-inflammatory Drugs (NSAIDs)

Andrew Han and Alan D. Kaye

## Medication Class: NSAIDs

### Introduction

- Nonsteroidal anti-inflammatory drugs (NSAIDs) are a class of medications used to treat pain, inflammation, and fevers
- There are many over-the-counter (OTC) drugs that are easily accessible

### List of Medications (1)

- Nonselective
  - Diclofenac
  - Diflunisal
  - Etodolac
  - Fenoprofen
  - Flurbiprofen
  - Ibuprofen
  - Indomethacin
  - Ketoprofen
  - Ketorlac
    Mefenamic acid
  - Meloxicam
  - Nabumetone
  - Naproxen
  - Piroxicam
  - Sulindac
  - Tolmetin
- Nonselective (irreversible)
  - Aspirin
- COX-2 selective
  - Celecoxib

### Indications

- NSAIDs are the mainstay as both first-line and multimodal treatment of a wide range of conditions as an analgesic, anti-inflammatory, and antipyretic

- ○ Migraines (2–5)
- ○ Musculoskeletal pain (6,7)
- ○ Dysmenorrhea (8)
- ○ Gout (9)
- ○ Pyrexia (10)
- ○ Arthritis (11)
- ○ Postoperative pain (12)

## Mechanism(s) of Action (13–16)

- COX-1 is constitutively expressed and involved in synthesis of prostaglandins and thromboxane A2 (platelets)
- COX-2 is expressed in response to inflammation or injury and is primarily responsible for analgesia
- Most NSAIDs are nonselective inhibitors of cyclooxygenase-1 (COX-1) and cyclooxygenase-2 (COX-2) resulting in inhibition of prostaglandin synthesis
- Aspirin is an NSAID that has an *irreversible* nonselective inhibition effect of COX-1 and COX-2
  - ○ COX inhibition prevents thromboxane synthesis so aspirin is used as an antiplatelet therapy at low doses (16,17)

## Routes of Administration

- Oral (18)
- Topical (19,20)
  - ○ Cream, gel, foam, spray formulations

## Dosing

- Ibuprofen (18)
  - ○ 200mg oral tablets
  - ○ Maximum recommended daily dose of 2,400 mg
- Naproxen (3)
  - ○ Oral free acid form
  - ○ Oral sodium salt form
    - ▪ More quickly absorbed by gastrointestinal tract, preferred for analgesia
    - ▪ Immediate-release (IR) and delayed-release (DR) formulations
    - ▪ 250 mg, 220 mg, or 500 mg

- Aspirin (4)
  - 500–1000mg for pain relief

## Side Effects/Adverse Reactions (3,21)

- Gastric discomfort
- Gastric ulcers
- Rash
- Heartburn
- Nausea
- Vomiting
- Dizziness
- Headaches
- Bruising
- Gastrointestinal bleeding

## Contraindications (18,22)

- Hypersensitivity to NSAIDs or aspirin
- NSAID-/aspirin-induced asthma
- Active gastrointestinal bleeding or peptic ulceration
- Third trimester of pregnancy

## Metabolism (23)

- Most NSAIDs are metabolized by the liver, specifically the CYP2C9 enzyme

## References

1. Ghlichloo I, Gerriets V. Nonsteroidal anti-inflammatory drugs (NSAIDs). *Treatment of Chronic Pain Conditions: A Comprehensive Handbook*. 2021;1:77–79.

2. Worthington I, Pringsheim T, Gawel MJ et al. Canadian headache society guideline: Acute drug therapy for migraine headache. *Can J Neurol Sci*. 2016;**40**(S3):S1–S3.

3. Moyer S. Pharmacokinetics of naproxen sodium. *Cephalalgia*. 1986;**6**(Suppl. 4):77–80.

4. Altabakhi IW, Zito PM. *Acetaminophen/Aspirin/Caffeine*. Treasure Island, FL; 2019.

5. Schramm SH, Moebus S, Ozyurt Kugumcu M et al. Use of aspirin combinations with caffeine and increasing headache frequency: A prospective population-based study. *Pain*. 2015;**156**(9):1747–1754.

6. Järvinen TA, Järvinen TL, Kääriäinen M et al. Muscle injuries: Optimising recovery. *Best Pract Res Clin Rheumatol.* 2007;**21**(2):317–331.

7. Casazza BA. Diagnosis and treatment of acute low back pain. *Am Fam Physician.* 2012;**85**(4):343–350.

8. Dawood MY. Primary dysmenorrhea: Advances in pathogenesis and management. *Obstet. Gynecol.* 2006;**108**(2):428–441.

9. Shekelle Paul G, Newberry Sydne J, FitzGerald John D et al. Management of gout: A systematic review in support of an American College of Physicians Clinical Practice Guideline. *Ann. Intern. Med.* 2017;**166**(1):37–51.

10. Bartfai T, Conti, B. Fever. *Sci. World J.* 2010;**10**:490–503.

11. Krasselt M, Baerwald C. Celecoxib for the treatment of musculoskeletal arthritis. *Expert Opin Pharmacother.* 2019;**20**(14):1689–1702.

12. Gupta A, Bah M. NSAIDs in the treatment of postoperative pain. *Curr Pain Headache Rep.* 2016;**20**(11):62. doi: 10.1007/s11916-016-0591-7.

13. Bushra R, Aslam N. An overview of clinical pharmacology of ibuprofen. *Oman Med. J.* 2010;**25**(3):155–1661.

14. Vane JR, Botting RM. Mechanism of action of nonsteroidal anti-inflammatory drugs. *Am. J. Med.* 1998;**104**(3):2S–8S.

15. Romsing J, Moiniche S. A systematic review of COX-2 inhibitors compared with traditional NSAIDs, or different COX-2 inhibitors for post-operative pain. *Acta Anaesthesiologica Scandinavica.* 2004;**48**(5):525–546.

16. Altabakhi IW, Zito PM. *Acetaminophen/Aspirin/Caffeine.* Treasure Island, FL: StatPearls Publishing; 2019.

17. Perneby C, Wallen NH, Rooney C, Fitzgerald D, Hjemdahl P. Dose- and time-dependent antiplatelet effects of aspirin. *Thrombosis and Haemostasis.* 2006;**95**(4):652–658.

18. Bushra R, Aslam N. An overview of clinical pharmacology of ibuprofen. *Oman Med J.* 2010;**25**(3):155–1661.

19. McPherson ML, Cimino NM. Topical NSAID formulations. *Pain Medicine.* 2013; **14**(1);S35–S39. doi: 10.1111/pme.12288. PMID: 24373109.

20. Irvine J, Afrose A, Islam N. Drug development and industrial pharmacy formulation and delivery strategies of ibuprofen: Challenges and opportunities. *Drug development and industrial pharmacy.* 2017; **44**(2):173–183.

21. Mills RFN, Adams SS, Cliffe EE, Dickinson W, Nicholson JS. The metabolism of ibuprofen. *Xenobiotica: The Fate of Foreign Compounds in Biological Systems.* 2008; **3**(9):589–598. doi: 10.3109/00498257309151547. PMID: 4202799.

22. Sutton LB. Naproxen sodium: Pharmacists should counsel patients to determine whether self-medication with OTC NSAIDs is contraindicated. *J. Am. Pharm. Assoc.* 1996;**36**(11):663–667.

23. Wyatt JE, Pettit WL, Harirforoosh S. Pharmacogenetics of nonsteroidal anti-inflammatory drugs. *Pharmacogenomics J.* 2012;**12**(6):462–467.

**Chapter**

**5**

# Acetaminophen

Andrew Han and Alan D. Kaye

## Acetaminophen (APAP)

- Antipyretic agent
- Non-opioid analgesic

## Indications (1–3)

- Mild to moderate pain
  - Muscle, joint, peripheral nerve
- Fever
- Headaches
  - Migraines

## Mechanism(s) of Action(s) (1–3)

- COX inhibition
  - Although the mechanism of action is not fully elucidated, acetaminophen is known to inhibit cyclooxygenase (COX-1 and COX-2), resulting in inhibition of prostaglandin synthesis
  - Also theorized to inhibit splice variant of COX-1, COX-3
- Central nervous system-acting
  - Para-acetyl-aminophenol (acetaminophen) acts as a reducing agent and inactivates the oxidized cyclooxygenase enzyme
  - Peroxides counteract the reducing mechanism of acetaminophen
    - Peroxides are elevated in peripheral inflammation sites
    - Brain has low peroxide concentration
      - This means that acetaminophen has more central-acting effects

- Endogenous opioid pathway
  - Potentially involved in the endogenous opioid pathway by activating the descending pathway and synergistically interacting at the level of the spinal cord
- Nitric oxide pathway
  - Acetaminophen inhibits nitric oxide synthase activity by inhibiting substance P-mediate hyperanalgesia, ultimately producing analgesia
- Cannabinoid CB1 receptors
  - Acetaminophen can indirectly activate cannabinoid CB1 receptors in the central nervous system

## Routes of Administration (5,6)

- Oral
- Rectal
- Intravenous

## Dosing (6)

- Oral, adults (7)
  - 0.5–1.0 g every 4–6 hours
  - Maximum of 4 g over 24 hours
  - Exceeding 5 g can lead to hepatotoxicity
- IV, adults (8,9)
  - 1,000 mg every 6 hours or 650 mg every 4 hours
  - Maximum single dose of 1,000 mg
  - Minimum dosing interval of 4 hours
  - Do not exceed maximum daily dose of IV acetaminophen of 4,000 mg/d
- Rectal, children only
  - Do not exceed 4 g over 24 hours

## Side Effects/Adverse Reactions (7–9)

- Hepatotoxicity and acute liver failure
  - Most common in overdose
  - Toxicity due to metabolism of acetaminophen by liver and oxidative stress

- Dangerous symptoms of hepatotoxicity: hyperammonemia, somnolence, stupor, coma, lactic acidosis, cerebral edema, brain stem herniation, vascular collapse
  - Acute kidney injury can also occur with acute liver failure
- Common, mild
  - Headaches
  - Insomnia
  - Nausea, vomiting
  - Constipation
  - Itching
  - Atelectasis
- Rare, severe
  - Toxic epidermal necrolysis
  - Acute generalized exanthematous pustulosis
  - Stevens–Johnson syndrome
  - Pneumonitis

## Contraindications (11–16)
- Hypersensitivity to acetaminophen
- Hepatic impairment
- Active hepatic disease
- Renal impairment
- Acute and/or chronic alcohol use
- CYP2E1 metabolized drugs
  - Anticonvulsant drugs
  - Tuberculosis drugs

## Metabolism (7,17)
- Acetaminophen is primarily metabolized via glucuronidation and sulfation by liver
- Also metabolized by CYP450 (CYP2E1) enzymes
  - NAPQ1 is the metabolite produced by CYP450 enzymes
  - NAPQ1 is toxic
- Metabolites are excreted in the urine
- Half-life varies from 1 to 4 hours

# References

1. Marmura MJ, Silberstein SD, Schwedt TJ. The acute treatment of migraine in adults: The American Headache Society evidence assessment of migraine pharmacotherapies. *Headache: The Journal of Head and Face Pain.* 2015;**55** (1):3–20.

2. Shankar K, Mehendale HM. Acetaminophen. *Encyclopedia of Toxicology.* 2005:18–23. www.sciencedirect.com/referencework/9780123864550/encyclopedia-of-toxicology

3. Graham GG, Scott KF. Mechanism of action of paracetamol and related analgesics. *InflammoPharmacology.* 2003;11(4–6):401–413.

4. Ovid: Mechanism of Action of Paracetamol. [Internet]. [cited November 4, 2021]. https://ovidsp.dc1.ovid.com/ovid-a/ovidweb.cgi?Linkshib%3Adc1%3A0xe085521d29c94f38a5378afabd394240&PASSWORD=0xe08571d29c94f38a5378afabd394240&CSC=Y&T=JS&D=ovft&SEARCH=1075-2765.an+d+%2212%22.vo+and+%221%22.ip+and+%2246%22.pg+or+%2210.1097%2F00045391-200501000–00008%22.di&NEWS=N&PAGE=fulltext&entityID=https%3A%2F%2Fidp.georgetown.edu%2Fopenathens.

5. Bannwarth B, Péhourcq FB. [Pharmacologic basis for using paracetamol: pharmacokinetic and pharmacodynamic issues] – PubMed [Internet]. [cited November 3, 2021]. https://pubmed.ncbi.nlm.nih.gov/14758786/.

6. Gerriets V, Anderson J, Nappe TM. Acetaminophen (Oral Route, Rectal Route) Proper Use – Mayo Clinic [Internet]. [cited November 5, 2021]. www.mayoclinic.org/drugs-supplements/acetaminophen-oral-route-rectal-route/proper-use/drg-20068480.

7. What dose of paracetamol for older people? *Drug and Therapeutics Bulletin.* 2018;56(6):69–72. https://dtb.bmj.com/content/56/6/69.citation-tools

8. Malaise O, Bruyere O, Reginster JY. Intravenous paracetamol: A review of efficacy and safety in therapeutic use. *Future Neurol.* 2007;2(6):673–688.

9. Shastri N. Intravenous acetaminophen use in pediatrics. *Pediatr. Emerg.* 2015;**31**(6):444–448.

10. Acetaminophen. *Dynamed plus.* EBSCO Information Services; 2018.

11. Gerriets V, Anderson J, Nappe TM. Acetaminophen. *Liver Pathophysiology: Therapies and Antioxidants.* 2021;101–112.

12. Barrett BJ. Acetaminophen and adverse chronic renal outcomes: An appraisal of the epidemiologic evidence. *Am J Kidney Dis.: Off. J Natl. Kidney Fou.* 1996;**28**(1 Suppl 1):S14–S19.

13. Dart RC, Erdman AR, Olson KR et al. Acetaminophen poisoning: An evidence-based consensus guideline for out-of-hospital management. *Clinical Toxicology (Philadelphia, Pa).* 2006;**44**(1):1–18.

14. Zimmerman HJ, Maddrey WC. Acetaminophen (paracetamol) hepatotoxicity with regular intake of alcohol: Analysis of instances of therapeutic misadventure. *Hepatology*. 1995;**22**(3):767–773.

15. Bray GP, Harrison PM, O'Grady JG, Tredger JM, Williams R. Long-term anticonvulsant therapy worsens outcome in paracetamol-induced fulminant hepatic failure. *Hum Exp Toxicol*. 1992;**11**(4):265–270.

16. Nolan CM, Sandblom RE, Thummel KE, Slattery JT, Nelson SD. Hepatotoxicity associated with acetaminophen usage in patients receiving multiple drug therapy for tuberculosis. *Chest*. 1994;**105**(2):408–411.

17. Wang X, Wu Q, Liu A, et al. Paracetamol: Overdose-induced oxidative stress toxicity, metabolism, and protective effects of various compounds in vivo and in vitro. *Drug Metab. Rev*. 2017;**49**(4):395–437.

**Chapter 6**

# Topicals
## Topical: Lidocaine, Capsaicin, Diclofenac

Juyeon Kakazu and Elyse M. Cornett

## Introduction

- Oral medication has been the mainstay of therapy; however, the use of topical formulation for chronic pain can reduce serious systemic side effects caused by oral medications (1)
- Topical administration of medication via patches, gels, creams, ointments, and solutions can provide local anesthesia and bypass major organ system (2)

## Medication and Mechanism of Action

- Lidocaine (3)
  - Amide-type local anesthetic agent stabilizing the neuronal membranes by inhibiting the ionic fluxes required for initiation and conduction of impulses
- Capsaicin (3,4)
  - Selective agonist for TRPV1 receptor expressed in afferent neuronal C fibers and Aδ fibers resulting in loss of receptor functionality causing impaired local nociception
- Diclofenac (5)
  - Inhibition of prostaglandin synthesis by blocking COX-1 and COX-2

## Indications (1,6–7)

- Chronic neuropathic pain
- Strains/sprains/contusions
- Osteoarthritis
- Postherpetic neuralgia

## Dosing/Routes of Administration

- Lidocaine
  - 5% patch
  - 1–3 patches applied once daily and to be removed after 12 hours
- Capsaicin (4)
  - Patch
    - 8% patch up to four patches at a time
  - Cream
    - 0.025%, 0.075%, and 0.1% creams
    - Applied four times a day
- Diclofenac
  - Gel
    - 1% solution; 2 g dose four times daily
    - No more than 16 g should be applied
  - Patch (7)
    - 1.3% patch containing 180 mg of diclofenac epolamine
    - Apply to painful areas twice a day
  - Topical Solution (8)
    - 1.5% solution: apply 40 drops of solution to painful areas four times daily
    - 2% solution: use twice daily to affected areas

## Side Effects/Adverse Reactions

- Lidocaine
  - Dry skin
  - Hives/itching/skin rash
  - Irritation
  - Swelling
- Capsaicin (4)
  - Erythema
  - Burning/stinging
  - Itching
- Diclofenac (8)
  - Pruritus

- ○ Dry skin
- ○ Contact dermatitis
- ○ Cardiovascular risk
- ○ GI risk

## Contraindications

- Lidocaine
  - ○ Heart condition
  - ○ Infected/open skin
  - ○ Allergic reaction to food/dyes or preservatives
  - ○ Pregnant
  - ○ Breastfeeding
- Capsaicin (4)
  - ○ Sensitivity to fruits or spices
- Diclofenac (8)
  - ○ Known hypersensitivity to diclofenac, aspirin, or other NSAIDs
  - ○ Asthma
  - ○ Urticaria
  - ○ Hepatic disease
  - ○ Perioperative period

## References

1. Stanos SP, Galluzzi KE. Topical therapies in the management of chronic pain. *Postgrad Med*. 2013;**125**(4 Suppl 1):25–33. https://doi.org/10.1080/00325481.2013.1110567111.

2. Barkin RL. The pharmacology of topical analgesics. *Postgrad Med*. 2013;**125**(4 Suppl 1):7–18. https://doi.org/10.1080/00325481.2013.1110566911.

3. Derry S, Lloyd R, Moore RA, McQuay HJ. Topical capsaicin for chronic neuropathic pain in adults. *Cochrane Database Syst. Rev*. 2009;(**4**):CD007393. https://doi.org/10.1002/14651858.CD007393.PUB2.

4. Groninger H, Schisler RE. Topical capsaicin for neuropathic pain #255. *J. Palliat. Med*. 2012;**15**(8):946. https://doi.org/10.1089/JPM.2012.9571.

5. Gan TJ. Diclofenac: an update on its mechanism of action and safety profile. *Curr Med Res Opin*. 2010;**26**(7):1715–1731. https://doi.org/10.1185/03007995.2010.486301.

6. Sarbacker GB. Topical Therapies for Chronic Pain Management: A Review of Diclofenac and Lidocaine. *Postgrad Med*. 2013;125(4 Suppl 1):25–33. Accessed

November 5, 2021. www.uspharmacist.com/article/topical-therapies-for-chronic-pain-management-a-review-of-diclofenac-and-lidocaine

7. Fda, Cder. Flector Patch (diclofenac epolamine) label. 2011. Accessed November 5, 2021. www.fda.gov/medwatch.

8. Fda, Cder. Pennsaid (diclofenac sodium) solution label. 2009. Accessed November 5, 2021. www.fda.gov/medwatch.

# Muscle Relaxants

Merlin Perez and Nazir Noor

## Cerebral Palsy

### Introduction

- CNS disease that begins in children and leads to neuromuscular and neurocognitive disabilities
- Most common cause of childhood disability (5)
- Common etiologies include CNS infections, CNS vascular insufficiency, and CNS trauma (5)
- Signs and symptoms include micro- or macrocephaly, muscle weakness, the persistence of primitive reflexes, and abnormal motor development (5)
- Hypotonia, spasticity, and dystonia are diagnostic of cerebral palsy (6)
- CP is classified by topographical categories as well as by type of neuromuscular dysfunction (6)
- Therapy for CP focuses on the management of pain, physical therapy, and surgery for musculoskeletal abnormalities (6)

### Oral Muscle Relaxants for Chronic Pain Management (8)

- Anticholinergics
- Baclofen
- Benzodiazepines
- Dopamine-related treatments

### Baclofen

- MOA (6)
  - GABA-B agonist
  - At presynaptic neurons: decreases excitatory neurotransmitter release

- At postsynaptic neurons: leads to hyperpolarization and inhibits neurotransmission
- Decreases substance P release
- Reduces spasticity and abnormal muscle tone by working at the cerebral and spinal cord levels
- Indications (3)
  - FDA-approved for managing reversible spasticity in several conditions such as multiple sclerosis and spinal cord lesions
- Adverse Reactions
  - Common: drowsiness, dizziness, and weakness, nausea, headache, hypotension, paresthesia (6)
  - Abrupt discontinuation may lead to seizures and hallucinations (3)
- Overall recommendation (6)
  - Current evidence has shown baclofen to be effective in improving muscle tone and strength; however, this effect can be short term, and prolonged use may lead to increased weakness

## Diazepam

- MOA
  - Binds to BNZ1 and BNZ2 receptors and increases the affinity of GABA for GABA receptors (6)
  - Binding to BNZ2 receptors inhibits monosynaptic and polysynaptic pathways (6)
- Indications (2)
  - FDA approved for management of anxiety disorders, spasticity associated with upper motor neuron disorders, management of certain refractory epilepsy patient
- Adverse reactions (2)
  - Common: confusion, sedation, fatigue, tremor, headache, ataxia, anterograde amnesia, depression, dystonia
- Overall recommendations (6)
  - Diazepam is an effective short-term treatment for spasticity in children with cerebral palsy
  - It improves symptoms with a dose response, meaning it should be given as recommended at 0.2–0.8 mg/kg and dosed 3 to 4 times a day (9)

# Tizanidine

- MOA (6)
  - Alpha 2 noradrenergic agonist
  - Causes hyperpolarization and prevents release of norepinephrine and substance P, inhibiting excess stimulation when spasticity occurs and attenuating painful stimuli
- Indications (4)
  - FDA approved for spasticity management associated with multiple sclerosis, spinal cord injury, ALS, brain injury
- Adverse reactions
  - Common: drowsiness, blurred vision, asthenia, constipation, dyskinesia, nervousness
- Overall recommendation (4)
  - Studies have shown the efficacy of tizanidine in the reduction of spasticity in childhood cerebral palsy
  - Treatment before the age of 4–5 shows the most significant reduction in limb deformities

# Flexeril

- MOA
  - Centrally acting muscle relaxant that antagonizes reserpine, enhances anticholinergic effects, and induces sedation (6)
- Indications
  - FDA approved in adjunct to rest and physical therapy to relieve muscle spasms associated with acute, painful musculoskeletal conditions, and for short-term use
- Adverse reactions (7)
  - Common: dry mouth, somnolence, dizziness, and confusion
- Overall recommendation (6)
  - Effective in the treatment of peripheral muscle spasm and pain in acute muscle injury
  - Patients should be monitored as it has an increased risk for serotonin syndrome and prolonged QT interval

## Dantrolene

- MOA (6)
  - Antagonizes the ryanodine receptor within the sarcoplasmic reticulum, inhibiting the release of calcium from the sarcoplasmic reticulum and reducing actin-myosin cross bridge formation
- Indications (6)
  - Main indication is for the treatment of malignant hyperthermia
  - Also treats muscle spasticity associated with upper motor neuron disorders, traumatic brain injury, cerebral palsy, and multiple sclerosis
- Adverse reactions (1)
  - Black box warning for hepatotoxicity
  - Common: drowsiness, diarrhea, dizziness, weakness, and fatigue
- Overall recommendation (6)
  - Dantrolene causes less sedation than other muscle relaxants
  - Studies have shown the efficacy of dantrolene in the reduction of muscle spasticity, although most studies are outdated. Further research is needed to understand its efficacy in treating CP

## References

1. *Dantrium Capsules.* (2011, October). www.accessdata.fda.gov/drugsatfda_docs/label/2012/017443s043s046s048s049lbl.pdf.

2. Dhaliwal JS, Rosani A, Saadabadi A. Diazepam. *XPharm: The Comprehensive Pharmacology Reference*, 2022;1–7. https://doi.org/10.1016/B978-008055232-3.61585-5.

3. Lomanto, M. (2010). Baclofen. In R. Sinatra, J. Jahr, and J. Watkins-Pitchford (eds.), *The Essence of Analgesia and Analgesics*, pp. 379–382. Cambridge: Cambridge University Press. doi:10.1017/CBO9780511841378.095

4. Malik, T. (2010). Tizanidine. In R. Sinatra, J. Jahr, and J. Watkins-Pitchford (eds.), *The Essence of Analgesia and Analgesics*, pp. 375–378. Cambridge: Cambridge University Press. doi:10.1017/CBO9780511841378.094

5. Hallman-Cooper JL, Cabrero FR. Cerebral palsy. *StatPearls*. 2021. www.ncbi.nlm.nih.gov/books/NBK538147/.

6. Jacki Peck B, Urits I, Crane J et al. Oral muscle relaxants for the treatment of chronic pain associated with cerebral palsy. *PsychoPharmacology Bulletin.* 2020;**50**(4):142–162.

7. Zegarra, M. (2010). Cyclobenzaprine. In R. Sinatra, J. Jahr, & J. Watkins-Pitchford (Eds.), *The Essence of Analgesia and Analgesics*, pp. 370–371. Cambridge: Cambridge University Press. doi:10.1017/CBO9780511841378.092

8. Termsarasab P, Thammongkolchai T, Frucht SJ. Correction to: Medical treatment of dystonia. *J Clin Mov Disord.* 2018;**5**(1):8.

9. Tilton A. Management of spasticity in children with cerebral palsy. *Semin Pediatr Neurol.* 2009;**16**(2):82–89.

**Chapter 8**

# Opioids

Merlin Perez and Nazir Noor

## Introduction

- A class of analgesics structurally similar to the natural alkaloids derived from the resin of the opium poppy (3)
- Natural alkaloids are known as opiates, and they include morphine and other similarly structured drugs, such as codeine, hydrocodone, and oxycodone (3)
- Synthetic derivatives include hydromorphone, fentanyl, and heroin, among others (3)

## Full and Partial Agonists (3)

- Alfentanil
- Buprenorphine
- Butorphanol
- Oxycodone
- Codeine
- Diphenoxylate
- Loperamide
- Tramadol
- Fentanyl
- Morphine
- Heroin
- Hydrocodone
- Sufentanil
- Hydromorphone
- Levorphanol
- Meperidine
- Methadone
- Opium
- Oxymorphone

- Pentazocine
- Remifentanil

# Opiate Antagonists (3)

- Naldemedine
- Nalmefene
- Naloxegol
- Naloxone
- Naltrexone

# MOA

- Three opiate receptors, μ, κ, and δ, are found predominantly in the CNS. Most analgesic effect of opioids is mediated by the μ receptors
- Decrease presynaptic calcium influx and increase postsynaptic potassium efflux, leading to inhibition of neuronal firing and neurotransmitter release

# Metabolism (4)

- Metabolized by the liver, mainly by the CYP3A4 and CYP2D6 enzymes

# Indications (1)

- Chronic pain
- Relief from diarrhea (diphenoxylate, loperamide)
- Cough suppression (dextromethorphan)
- Anesthesia

# Adverse Reactions (1)

- Dysphoria
- Urinary retention
- Nausea
- Respiratory depression
- Constipation
- Sedation
- Hypotension
- Potential for addiction

## Contraindications (2)

- Pregnancy
- Respiratory instability
- Psychiatric instability
- Active diversion of controlled substances
- Potential drug–drug interaction
- Use caution if given to patients with liver or kidney dysfunction
- Overdose can be fatal due to respiratory depression, especially when used concomitantly with alcohol and benzodiazepines
- Withdrawal syndrome can occur if suddenly stopped

## References

1. Cohen B, Ruth LJ, Preuss CV. *Opioid Analgesics– StatPearls – NCBI Bookshelf.* (n.d.). Retrieved August 6, 2022, from www.ncbi.nlm.nih.gov/books/NB K459161/.

2. Grewal N, Huecker MR. *Opioid Prescribing– StatPearls – NCBI Bookshelf.* (n.d.). Retrieved August 6, 2022, from www.ncbi.nlm.nih.gov/books/NB K551720/.

3. LiverTox: Clinical and Research Information on Drug-Induced Liver Injury. Bethesda (MD): National Institute of Diabetes and Digestive and Kidney Diseases; 2012. Opioids. www.ncbi.nlm.nih.gov/books/NBK547864/.

4. Smith, HS. Opioid metabolism. *Mayo Clinic Proceedings.* 2009;*84*(7):613. htt ps://doi.org/10.1016/S0025-6196(11)60750-7.

# Chapter 9

# Antineuropathic Medications

Juyeon Kakazu and Alan D. Kaye

## Introduction

- Neuropathic pain (NP)
  - Subtype of chronic pain syndrome defined by the International Association of the Study of Pain (IASP) as a "pain caused by a lesion or disease of the somatosensory system" (1)
  - Consequence of CNS or PNS lesions
  - Activities are generated in the somatosensory system without peripheral afferent stimulation
- Etiologies/Classification
  - Central
    - Vascular, inflammatory, traumatic, epileptic, degenerative changes, and syringomyelia (2,3)
- Peripheral
    - Entrapment syndromes, phantom limb pain, trigeminal neuralgia, diabetic mononeuropathy, ischemic neuropathy, acute zoster-postherpetic neuralgia, and drug-induced peripheral neuropathy (2,3)
  - Episodic vs. continuous pain
- Risk factors
  - Cancer (40%) (4)
  - Diabetes (25%) (5)
  - Elderly (6)
  - Children (7)
  - Dental procedures (8)

- Pathophysiology
  - ○ Somatosensory system injury causing complex ectopic signaling between neuronal pathways (9)

## Medications and MOA for NP

- SNRIs (e.g., duloxetine, venlafaxine)
  - ○ Inhibits reuptake of serotonin and norepinephrine in the synaptic clefts (10)
- TCAs
  - ○ Block the reuptake of serotonin and norepinephrine in pre-synaptic terminals via blocking the serotonin transporter (SERT) and norepinephrine transporter (NET) (10)
- Anticonvulsants (Gabapentin/Pregabalin)
  - ○ Gabapentin
    - Gamma-aminobutyric acid (GABA) analog targeting voltage-gated $Ca^{2+}$ channels to inhibit neurotransmitter release (11)
  - ○ Pregabalin
    - MOA is similar to that of gabapentin with a higher affinity to the calcium channels and has a linear pharmacokinetics (11)

## Indications (12)

- Trigeminal neuralgia
- Postherpetic neuralgia (PHN)
- Painful diabetic neuropathy
- Phantom limb pain (PLN)
- Spinal cord injury
- Chemotherapy-induced peripheral neuropathy (CIPN)

## Dosing/Routes of Administration (11)

- SNRIs (e.g., duloxetine, venlafaxine)
  - ○ Duloxetine
    - 30 mg PO once a day and titrate up to 60 mg twice daily with or without meals for 4 weeks
  - ○ Venlafaxine
    - Immediate release: 75 mg/day in 2 or 3 divided doses; titrate up to 225 mg/day

- Extended release: 37.5 mg or 75 mg once daily; titrate up to 225 mg once daily
- TCAs (e.g., amitriptyline/nortriptyline)
  - 10–25 mg at bedtime and titrate up to a maximum of 150 mg/day) for 6–8 weeks
- Anticonvulsants (gabapentin/pregabalin)
  - Pregabalin
    - 50 mg 3 times a day or 75 mg 2 times a day for 4 weeks; titrate up to 300–600 mg/day
  - Gabapentin
    - 100–300 mg/day; titrate up to 300–600 mg/day for 5–10 weeks

## Side Effects/Adverse Reactions (11)

- SNRIs (e.g., duloxetine, venlafaxine)
  - Hyponatremia
  - Tachycardia
  - Increased suicidal behavior
  - Hypertension
  - Serotonin syndrome
  - Sexual dysfunction
- TCAs
  - Blurred vision
  - Dry mouth
  - Constipation
  - Weight gain or loss
  - Serotonin syndrome
  - Fatal cardiac dysrhythmias (QTc prolongation)
  - Increased suicidal behavior
- Gabapentin/pregabalin (13)
  - Dizziness
  - Sedation
  - Dose-dependent edema
  - Stevens–Johnson syndrome
  - Toxic epidermal necrolysis
  - Respiratory depression

## Contraindications/Metabolization

- SNRIs (11,14)
  - Dose tapering due to serotonin syndrome
  - Suicidal thoughts
  - Manic depression
  - SIADH
- TCAs (11,14)
  - ECG abnormalities
  - Depression
  - Glaucoma
  - Acute porphyria
- Anticonvulsants (13)
  - Depression
  - Chronic kidney disease (CKD)
  - Chronic heart failure

## References

1. Jensen TS, Baron R, Haanpää M et al. A new definition of neuropathic pain. *Pain.* 2011;**152**(10):2204–2205. https://doi.org/10.1016/J.PAIN.2011.06.017.

2. Jones MR, Urits I, Wolf J et al. Drug-induced peripheral neuropathy: A narrative review. *Current Clinical Pharmacology.* 2020;**15**(1):38–48. https://doi.org/10.2174/1574884714666190121154813.

3. Gierthmühlen J, Baron R. Neuropathic pain. *Seminars in Neurology.* 2016;**36**(5):462–468. https://doi.org/10.1055/S-0036-1584950.

4. Bennett MI, Rayment C, Hjermstad M et al. Prevalence and aetiology of neuropathic pain in cancer patients: A systematic review. *Pain.* 2012;**153**(2):359–365. https://doi.org/10.1016/J.PAIN.2011.10.028.

5. Hébert HL, Veluchamy A, Torrance N, Smith BH. Risk factors for neuropathic pain in diabetes mellitus. *Pain.* 2017;**158**(4):560. https://doi.org/10.1097/J.PAIN.0000000000000785.

6. Davis MP. Cancer-related neuropathic pain: Review and selective topics. *Hematology/Oncology Clinics of North America.* 2018;**32**(3):417–431. https://doi.org/10.1016/J.HOC.2018.01.005.

7. Howard RF, Wiener S, Walker SM. Neuropathic pain in children. *Archives of Disease in Childhood.* 2014;**99**(1):84–89. https://doi.org/10.1136/ARCHDISCHILD-2013-304208.

8. Tınastepe N, Oral K. Neuropathic pain after dental treatment. *Agri: Agri (Algoloji) Dernegi'nin Yayin organidir = The Journal of the Turkish Society of Algology.* 2013;**25**(1):1–6. https://doi.org/10.5505/AGRI.2013.55477.

9. Scholz J, Woolf CJ. The neuropathic pain triad: Neurons, immune cells and glia. *Nature Neuroscience.* 2007;**10**(11):1361–1368. https://doi.org/10.1038/NN1992.

10. Fornasari D. Pharmacotherapy for neuropathic pain: A review. *Pain and Therapy.* 2017;**6**(Suppl 1):25. https://doi.org/10.1007/S40122-017-0091-4.

11. Zilliox LA. Neuropathic pain. *Continuum (Minneapolis, Minn).* 2017;**23**(2):512–532. https://doi.org/10.1212/CON.0000000000000462.

12. Cruccu G, Truini A. A review of neuropathic pain: From guidelines to clinical practice. *Pain Ther.* 2017;**6**(Suppl 1):35. https://doi.org/10.1007/S40122-017-0087-0.

13. Pregabalin (Oral Route) Side Effects – Mayo Clinic. 2023. Accessed October 13, 2021. www.mayoclinic.org/drugs-supplements/pregabalin-oral-route/side-effects/drg-20067411?p=1.

14. Side Effects – Antidepressants – NHS. 2021. Accessed October 13, 2021. www.nhs.uk/mental-health/talking-therapies-medicine-treatments/medicines-and-psychiatry/antidepressants/side-effects/.

# Chapter 10

# Cannabinoids

Juyeon Kakazu and Jamal Hasoon

## Introduction (1)

- The use of cannabinoids and its derivatives for chronic pain is increasing
- Two most well-known and clinically relevant forms of cannabinoids are delta-9-tetrahydrocannabinol (THC) and cannabidiol (CBD)
- Main receptors targeted are cannabinoid receptor 1 (CB1) and CB2

## Medications and Mechanism(s) of Action

- Nabiximols: Sativex (2)
  - 1:1 combination ratio of THC and CBD
  - Partial agonist of CB1 and CB2 via THC and simultaneous antagonism of CB1 and CB2 receptors via CBD

- Epidiolex (3)
  - The only plant-derived CBD
  - Acts on CB receptors, a type of G-protein-coupled receptor, of the endocannabinoid system throughout the body
  - Negative allosteric modulator of CB receptors

- Marinol (Dronabinol) (4)
  - Synthetic form of THC
  - Psychoactive component acting as a weak partial agonist of CB1 and CB2 receptors

- Cesamet (Nabilone) (5)
  - Synthetic cannabinoid similar to THC
  - Similar to Marinol; agonist at CB1 and CB2 receptors
  - Twice as active as THC

## Indications (6)

- Multiple sclerosis
- Cancer-related pain/cancer-related nausea and vomiting (anti-emetic)

- Peripheral neuropathic pain
- HIV-associated weight loss

# Dosing/Routes of Administration (3,6)

- Nabiximols: Sativex
    - Oromucosal cannabinoid spray; administered to the buccal mucosa
    - Eacy spray delivers 2.7 mg of THC and 2.5 mg of CBD
    - Daily dose not to exceed 12 sprays
- Epidiolex
    - PO liquid solution of 100 mg/ml concentrate
- Marinol (Dronabinol)
    - PO 2.5 mg BID
    - Maximum dose to 10 mg BID
- Cesamet (Nabilone)
    - PO 1–2 mg BID
    - May be administered two to three times a day during the course of chemotherapy
    - Maximum recommended daily dose is 6 mg TID

# Side Effects/Adverse Reactions

- Nabiximols: Sativex (7,8)
    - Dizziness
    - Diarrhea
    - Headaches
- Epidiolex (3)
    - Somnolence
    - Diarrhea
    - Fatigue
    - Decreased appetite
    - Hepatotoxicity
- Marinol (Dronabinol) (4)
    - Dizziness/lightheadedness
    - Nausea/vomiting
    - Abdominal pain
    - Mental/mood changes
- Cesamet (Nabilone) (5)
    - Vertigo

- ○ Drowsiness
- ○ Euphoria
- ○ Dry mouth
- ○ Ataxia
- ○ Anorexia

## Contraindications (9)

- Addiction
- Heart disease
- HTN
- Seizures
- Eating disorders
- Psychiatric disorders

## References

1. Kumar RN, Chambers WA, Pertwee RG. Pharmacological actions and therapeutic uses of cannabis and cannabinoids. *Anaesthesia*. 2001;**56**(11):1059–1068. https://doi.org/10.1046/J.1365-2044.2001.02269.X.

2. Malfitano AM, Proto MC, Bifulco M. Cannabinoids in the management of spasticity associated with multiple sclerosis. *Neuropsychiatr. Dis. Treat.* 2008;**4**(5):847. https://doi.org/10.2147/NDT.S3208.

3. EPIDIOLEX® (cannabidiol) | Greenwich Biosciences. 2021. Accessed November 5, 2021. www.greenwichbiosciences.com/epidiolex.

4. O'Donnell B, Meissner H, Gupta V. Dronabinol. *Pharma-Kritik*. 2021;**24**(8):29–31. Accessed November 5, 2021. www.ncbi.nlm.nih.gov/books/NBK557531/.

5. Ware MA, Daeninck P, Maida V. A review of nabilone in the treatment of chemotherapy-induced nausea and vomiting. *Ther. Clin. Risk Manag.* 2008;**4**(1):99. https://doi.org/10.2147/TCRM.S1132.

6. Grotenhermen F, Müller-Vahl K. The Therapeutic Potential of Cannabis and Cannabinoids. *Deutsches Ärzteblatt International*. 2012;**109**(29–30):495. https://doi.org/10.3238/ARZTEBL.2012.0495.

7. Russo M, Naro A, Leo A et al. Evaluating Sativex® in neuropathic pain management: A clinical and neurophysiological assessment in multiple sclerosis. *Pain Med. (Malden, Mass)*. 2016;**17**(6):1145–1154. https://doi.org/10.1093/PM/PNV080.

8. Serpell MG, Notcutt W, Collin C. Sativex long-term use: An open-label trial in patients with spasticity due to multiple sclerosis. *J. Neurol.* 2013;**260**(1):285–295. https://doi.org/10.1007/S00415-012-6634-Z.

9. Sheikh NK, Dua A. Cannabinoids. Published online July 25, 2021. Accessed November 5, 2021. www.ncbi.nlm.nih.gov/books/NBK556062/.

Chapter

# 11

## Post-dural Puncture Headache

Nolan Weinstein and Jatinder Gill

- Common adverse complication following dural puncture (DP) during epidural or spinal anesthesia
- Dull throbbing headache
- Fronto-occipital distribution
- Worse in seated position
- Alleviated when supine
  - Other symptoms include: nausea, vomiting, neck stiffness, tinnitus, hypoacusia
- Symptoms develop spontaneously within five days of DP
  - Symptoms resolve within one week
  - Treatment with an epidural patch may shorten symptom duration to 48 hours (1)

## Epidemiology and Risk Factors

- Post-dural puncture headache (PDPH) incidence varies from 0.38% to 6.3% (1)
- DP occurs in approximately 1.5% of epidural procedures
- 76–85% of patients with dural puncture experience symptoms of PDPH (2)
- In 29% of patients the only symptom is headache (2)
- Common risk factors for PDPH:
  - Female gender
  - Younger age
  - Low CSF opening pressure
  - Pregnancy and vaginal delivery (4)
  - Prior headache
  - Low BMI

- ○ Obesity is a protective factor due to elevated CSF pressures (5,6)

## Pathophysiology

- Precise mechanism is unclear
- Hypotheses:
  - ○ Loss of CSF relative to spinal fluid production
  - ○ Low CSF pressures lead to intracranial hypotension
    - Unable to support the brain
    - Traction shifts the brain caudally pressuring pain-sensitive structures (7)
  - ○ Central venous dilation compensates for the loss of CSF, resulting in pressure sensation (8)
    - Positional relief supports this hypothesis

## Diagnosis

- Presence of post-dural headache in the setting of DP is sufficient
- Differential diagnosis (9,10):
  - ○ Intracranial hypotension
  - ○ Infection
  - ○ Eclampsia
  - ○ Central venous thrombosis
  - ○ Intracranial tumors
  - ○ Pituitary apoplexy
  - ○ Non-specific headache
  - ○ Migraine
- ICHD-3 criteria for specific diagnosis of PDPH:
  - ○ Visualization of CSF leak on MRI
  - ○ CSF opening pressure <60 mm Hg
- Neuroimaging is usually not necessary unless there are complications or uncertainties

## Treatment Modalities

- First step is conservative management (8)
  - ○ Supine positioning is often sufficient to alleviate pain (11)
  - ○ Increased fluids used in practice, uncertain efficacy (12)
  - ○ More than 85% of cases resolve without medical management (13)

- Medical management:
  - Caffeine is safe and effective
    - Offers headache relief by blocking adenosine
    - Results in arterial vasoconstriction and decreased blood flow
    - Also increases CSF production via sodium pump activation (14)
    - 500 mg of caffeine in 1 L saline has proven effective in the prevention of PDPH (15)
  - Acetaminophen and NSAIDs are commonly used (13)
    - Often good first step in medical management
    - Augment with increased fluid rehydration
  - Combination analgesics often used, such as butalbital-acetaminophen-caffeine
    - Evidence in support is lacking
  - Oral theophylline has proven effective (16)
  - Hydrocortisone shown to significantly decrease pain (17)
  - Little evidence supporting the use of sumatriptan
  - If medical management with the above medication does not work within 72 hours, further treatment may be necessary (18)
- **Epidural blood patch** (EBP) — gold standard in treating PDPH
  - Procedure to inject small amounts of autologous blood into the epidural space
  - Very well tolerated overall
  - Provides relief in 61–98% of patients (1)
  - Complete relief was observed in 35–75% of obstetrical cases (19)
    - Lower success rate than general population likely due to larger-gauge needles used (20)
  - Proposed MOA of EBP: increases CSF pressure and volume (21)
    - Assists in plugging dural leak
    - Increased CSF volume and pressure reduce traction on pain-sensitive regions (8)
  - Patients often experience immediate relief

- ○ Indicated in patients who fail conservative and medical management
- ○ Contraindications for procedure: infection, anticoagulation, coagulopathy
- ○ Complications:
  - ▪ Back pain by injection site is most common (22)
  - ▪ Other far rarer complications (23–26):
    - • Meningitis
    - • Intrathecal hematoma
    - • Arachnoiditis
    - • Subdural abscess
    - • Cauda equine syndrome
    - • Facial nerve palsy
- ○ Recent study found 20 ml to be the optimal volume of blood injected (27)
- ○ EBP should be reserved for patients in high need, as PDPH is a self-limiting condition

## Conclusion

- Adverse event is seen commonly in patients receiving epidural or spinal neuraxial anesthesia
- Occurs following inadvertent puncture of the dura
- Conservative treatment is often adequate in the majority of patients, but medical management can be used liberally with a variety of safe, well-studied pharmacologic options
- Epidural blood patch is the gold standard in treating unremitting PDPH but should be used cautiously due to the potential for rare but serious complications

## References

1. Kwak K-H. Postdural puncture headache. *Korean J Anesthesiol.* 2017;**70**(2):136–143.

2. Morewood GH. A rational approach to the cause, prevention and treatment of postdural puncture headache. *CMAJ.* 1993;**149**(8):1087–1093.

3. Amorim JA, Gomes De Barros MV, Valença MM. Post-dural (post-lumbar) puncture headache: Risk factors and clinical features. *Cephalalgia.* 2012;**32**(12):916–923.

4. Haller G, Cornet J, Boldi M-O, Myers C, Savoldelli G, Kern C. Risk factors for post-dural puncture headache following injury of the dural membrane: A

root-cause analysis and nested case-control study. *Int J Obstet Anesth.* 2018;**36**:17–27.

5.  Liu H, Kalarickal PL, Rosinia F. A case of paradoxical presentation of postural postdural puncture headache. *J Clin Anesth.* 2012;**24**(3):255–256.

6.  Faure E, Moreno R, Thisted R. Incidence of postdural puncture headache in morbidly obese parturients. *Reg Anesth.* 1994;**19**(5):361–363.

7.  Candido KD, Stevens RA. Post-dural puncture headache: Pathophysiology, prevention and treatment. *Best Pract Res Clin Anaesthesiol.* 2003;**17** (3):451–469.

8.  Gaiser RR. Postdural puncture headache. *Anesthesiol Clin.* 2017;**35** (1):157–167.

9.  Lim G, Zorn JM, Dong YJ, DeRenzo JS, Waters JH. Subdural hematoma associated with labor epidural analgesia. *Reg Anesth Pain Med.* 2016;**41** (5):628–631.

10. Darvish B, Dahlgren G, Irestedt L et al. Auditory function following post-dural puncture headache treated with epidural blood patch. A long-term follow-up. *Acta Anaesthesiol Scand.* 2015;**59**(10):1340–1354.

11. Salzer J, Rajda C, Sundström P et al. How to minimize the risk for headache? A lumbar puncture practice questionnaire study = Hogyan csökkenthető a posztpunkciós fejfájás? Kérdőíves vizsgálat a lumbálpunkciós gyakorlatról. *Ideggyogy Sz.* 2016;**69**(11–12):397–402.

12. Arevalo-Rodriguez I, Ciapponi A, Roqué i Figuls M, Muñoz L, Bonfill Cosp X. Posture and fluids for preventing post-dural puncture headache. *Cochrane Database Syst Rev.* 2016;**3**:CD009199.

13. Choi A, Laurito CE, Cunningham FE. Pharmacologic management of postdural puncture headache. *Ann Pharmacother.* 1996;**30**(7–8):831–839.

14. Baratloo A, Rouhipour A, Forouzanfar MM et al. The role of caffeine in pain management: A brief literature review. *Anesthesiol Pain Med.* 2016;**6**(3): e33193.

15. Yücel A, Ozyalçin S, Talu GK, Yücel EC, Erdine S. Intravenous administration of caffeine sodium benzoate for postdural puncture headache. *Reg Anesth Pain Med.* 1999;**24**(1):51–54.

16. Feuerstein TJ, Zeides A. Theophylline relieves headache following lumbar puncture: Placebo-controlled, double-blind pilot study. *Klin Wochenschr.* 1986;**64**(5):216–218.

17. Noyan Ashraf MA, Sadeghi A, Azarbakht Z, Salehi S, Hamediseresht E. Evaluation of intravenous hydrocortisone in reducing headache after spinal anesthesia: A double blind controlled clinical study [corrected]. *Middle East J Anaesthesiol.* 2007;**19**(2):415–422.

18. Ahmed S V, Jayawarna C, Jude E. Post lumbar puncture headache: Diagnosis and management. *Postgrad Med J.* 2006;**82**(973):713–716.

19. Scavone BM, Wong CA, Sullivan JT et al. Efficacy of a prophylactic epidural blood patch in preventing post dural puncture headache in parturients after inadvertent dural puncture. *Anesthesiology.* 2004;**101**(6):1422–1427.

20. Safa-Tisseront V, Thormann F, Malassiné P et al. Effectiveness of epidural blood patch in the management of post-dural puncture headache. *Anesthesiology.* 2001;**95**(2):334–339.

21. Kroin JS, Nagalla SKS, Buvanendran A et al. The mechanisms of intracranial pressure modulation by epidural blood and other injectates in a postdural puncture rat model. *Anesth Analg.* 2002;**95**(2):423–429.

22. Booth JL, Pan PH, Thomas JA, Harris LC, D'Angelo R. A retrospective review of an epidural blood patch database: The incidence of epidural blood patch associated with obstetric neuraxial anesthetic techniques and the effect of blood volume on efficacy. *Int J Obstet Anesth.* 2017;**29**:10–17.

23. Roy-Gash F, Engrand N, Lecarpentier E, Bonnet MP. Intrathecal hematoma and arachnoiditis mimicking bacterial meningitis after an epidural blood patch. *Int J Obstet Anesth.* 2017;**32**:77–81.

24. Rucklidge M. All patients with a postdural puncture headache should receive an epidural blood patch. *Int J Obstet Anesth.* 2014;**23**(2):171–174.

25. Devroe S, Van de Velde M, Demaerel P, Van Calsteren K. Spinal subdural haematoma after an epidural blood patch. *Int J Obstet Anesth.* 2015;**24**(3):288–289.

26. Urits I, Viswanath O, Petro J, Aner M. Management of dural puncture headache caused by caudal epidural steroid injection. *J Clin Anesth.* 2019;**52**:67–68.

27. Paech MJ, Doherty DA, Christmas T, Wong CA, Epidural blood patch trial group: The volume of blood for epidural blood patch in obstetrics. *Anesth Analg.* 2011;**113**(1):126–133.

# 12

# Migraines

Noushad Mamun and Ruben Schwartz

## Migraine Headaches

- Migraine headache is a highly prevalent and disabling neurological primary headache disorder
- It is characterized by disabling, throbbing, episodic, unilateral headaches associated with neurologic features such as photophobia, phonophobia, or autonomic symptoms like nausea and vomiting lasting 4 to 72 hours at a time (headache committee)
- Patients will often avoid bright lights or loud noises
- 30% of migraine patients experience auras which are unilateral focal neurological disturbances prior to the headache onset, often manifested as visual, sensory, or motor symptoms (10)

## Epidemiology and Risk Factors

- Migraine headache is common and affects about 12% of the US population.
- At the level of specific diseases, migraine was the second most disabling condition after low back pain (4)
- An analysis of 2016 GBD data estimated that migraine caused 45.1 million years lived with disability (YLDs) in that year (4)
- Migraine headaches predominantly affect women (3)
- Of all women, 18% have migraine headaches, and 5% of that of men (2)
- Chronic headaches affect 1.4% to 2.2% globally (2)
- There are several neurological medical conditions that have been found to be more common in individuals with migraine headaches when compared to the general population (2)
- Conditions associated with migraine headaches include multiple sclerosis, epilepsy, restless leg syndrome, strokes, systemic lupus erythematosus, posttraumatic stress disorder, and depression (5)

- There are implications of 38 migraine-associated gene poly-morphisms that harbor 44 independent susceptibility markers for the prevalent forms of migraine which have been validated based on population studies (6)
- Migraine headaches involve interactions among multiple genes and epigenetic factors (1)

## Pathophysiology

- Pathophysiology of migraine headache is still unclear and being studied; however, calcitonin gene-related peptide (CGRP) is believed to play a major and important role; therefore, it has become a primary therapeutic target (8,19)
- This was supported by the finding of CGRP release during acute migraine attacks and then subsequent normalization of CGRP levels after efficacious sumatriptan treatment (9)
- These findings have been a focal point in recent pharmacological developments in managing migraine headaches
- Trigeminovascular pathways also play a role in neuropeptide release and symptomology
  - CGRP is secreted in trigeminal ganglion neurons. It is a strong vasodilator of cerebral and dura mater vessels, therefore a component of neurogenic inflammation and trigeminal pain signaling (11)
- Cortical spreading depression is hypothesized to be the reason for aura experiences

## Diagnosis

- Typically, migraine headaches are diagnosed clinically in accord-ance with international classification of headache disorders (13,14)
- Diagnosis of migraine headaches is based on patient history, physical exam, and fulfilling diagnostic criteria according to the international classification of headache disorders
- The international classification of headache disorders describes migraine headaches in two main categories: migraine with aura and migraine without aura. There are also criteria for acute versus chronic migraine headaches
- Typically, migraine headaches are pulsatile, unilateral, have mod-erate to severe pain intensity, and they are aggravated by physical activity, often resulting in avoidance behavior

- During these headaches, neurological phenomenon is usually associated such as nausea/vomiting, photophobia, and phonophobia
- Migraine headache that has associated auras which are reversible unilateral neurological deficits affecting vision, brainstem, speech and language, and sensory
- Migraine headaches are considered chronic migraines if the patient has been suffering migraine episodes for more than 15 days per month for 6 consecutive months (7,12)

# Treatment

- Migraine management can be divided by acute/abortive treatment versus chronic prophylactic treatment
- Acute or abortive treatment aims to stop progression of the active headache (12,15,16)
  - Oral agents usually non-steroidal anti-inflammatory drugs (e.g. ibuprofen, naproxen), triptans, and anti-emetics have been used with variable relief in pain
  - Anti-emetics
    - used as conjunctive therapy with NSAIDs
  - Selective serotonin 1F receptor agonists
    - Lasmiditan FDA approved in October 2019
    - Effective in patients who cannot use triptans due to underlying cardiovascular risks
  - Ergots
    - Ergotamine and dihydroergotamine can be given IV, IM, subcutaneous, and intranasal
  - CGRP-related therapies (17,19)
    - Development of this medication in recent years has shown efficacy in management of migraine headaches
    - Small-molecule CGRP receptor antagonists, GEPANTS are effective for acute relief of migraine headaches (18)
    - Monoclonal antibodies against CGRP (Eptinezumab, Fremanezumab, and Galcanezumab) or the CGRP receptor (Erenumab) effectively prevent migraine attacks

- Selective monoclonal antibodies that bind either CGRP or the CGRP receptor
  - Anti-receptor antibody, Erenumab, is human IgG2 monoclonal antibody that targets CGRP binding site on CGRP receptor
    - FDA approved May 2018 and EMA approved for Europe
    - Administered once a month by subcutaneous injection
  - Anti-CGRP antibodies show similar efficacy and safety profiles
    - Fremanezumab
      - FDA approved September 2018
      - Fully humanized IgG2a monoclonal antibody administered once per month by subcutaneous injection
    - Galcanezumab
      - FDA approved September 2018
      - Fully humanized IgG4 monoclonal antibody administered once per month by subcutaneous injection
    - Eptinezumab is a genetically engineered humanized IgG1 monoclonal antibody that is formulated for intravenous administration and intended for once every three months dosing
      - Successful in therapeutic goal for migraine prophylaxis in decreasing frequency of migraine attacks
      - Antibodies have demonstrated efficacy in reducing migraine days in patients with episodic or chronic migraine
- Transcutaneous supraorbital nerve stimulation
  - Known to reduce the intensity of headaches
- Transcranial magnetic stimulation
  - Contraindicated in patients with epilepsy
- Peripheral nerve blocking versus stimulation
  - Occipital plexus nerve block
  - Sphenopalatine ganglion block

- Prophylactic/Preventive treatment
  - Beta-blockers, metoprolol, and propranolol are commonly used
    - Hypertensive and non-smoker patients
  - Antidepressants – amitriptyline and venlafaxine
  - anticonvulsants
  - Calcium-channel blockers

# References

1. Charles A. The pathophysiology of migraine: Implications for clinical management. *Lancet Neurol.* 2018;**17**(2):174–182. https://doi.org/10.1016/S1474-4422(17)30435-0.

2. Burch RC, Buse, DC, Lipton RB. Migraine: Epidemiology, burden, and comorbidity. *Neurol. Clin.* 2019;**37**(4): 631–649. https://doi.org/10.1016/j.ncl.2019.06.001.

3. Buse DC, Loder EW, Gorman JA et al. Sex differences in the prevalence, symptoms, and associated features of migraine, probable migraine and other severe headache: Results of the American Migraine Prevalence and Prevention (AMPP) Study. *Headache.* 2013;**53**(8):1278–1299. https://doi.org/10.1111/head.12150.

4. GBD 2016 Headache Collaborators. Global, regional, and national burden of migraine and tension-type headache, 1990–2016: A systematic analysis for the global burden of disease study 2016. *Lancet Neurol.* 2018;**17**(11):954–976. https://doi.org/10.1016/S1474-4422(18)30322-3.

5. Scher AI, Bigal ME, Lipton RB. Comorbidity of migraine. *Curr. Opin. Neurol.* 2005;**18**(3), 305–310. https://doi.org/10.1097/01.wco.0000169750.52406.a2.

6. Gormley P, Anttila V, Winsvold BS et al. Meta-analysis of 375,000 individuals identifies 38 susceptibility loci for migraine. *Nat. Genet.* 2016;**48**(8):856–866. https://doi.org/10.1038/ng.3598.

7. Cribbin CL, Dani KA, Tyagi A. Chronic Migraine: An Update on Diagnosis and Management. *Neurol India.* n.d.;**69**(Supplement):S67–S75. https://doi.org/10.4103/0028-3886.315972.

8. Deen M, Correnti E, Kamm K et al. Blocking CGRP in migraine patients – a review of pros and cons. *J. Headache Pain.* 2017;**18**(1):96. https://doi.org/10.1186/s10194-017-0807-1.

9. Goadsby PJ, Edvinsson L. The trigeminovascular system and migraine: Studies characterizing cerebrovascular and neuropeptide changes seen in humans and cats. *Ann. Neurol.* 1993;**33**(1):48–56. https://doi.org/10.1002/ana.410330109.

10. Goadsby PJ, Holland PR. An update: Pathophysiology of migraine. *Neurol. Clin.* 2019;37(4):651–671. https://doi.org/10.1016/j.ncl.2019.07.008.

11. Iyengar S, Johnson KW, Ossipov MH, Aurora SK. CGRP and the trigeminal system in migraine. *Headache.* 2019;59(5):659–681. https://doi.org/10.1111/head.13529

12. Mungoven TJ, Henderson LA, Meylakh N. Chronic migraine pathophysiology and treatment: A review of current perspectives. *Front. Pain Res. (Lausanne, Switzerland).* 2021;2:705276. https://doi.org/10.3389/fpain.2021.705276.

13. Khan J, Asoom LIal, Sunni Aal et al. Genetics, pathophysiology, diagnosis, treatment, management, and prevention of migraine. *Biomed. Pharmacother.* 2021;139:111557. https://doi.org/10.1016/j.biopha.2021.111557.

14. Headache Classification Committee of the International Headache Society (IHS) The International Classification of Headache Disorders, 3rd ed. *Cephalalgia: J Headache Pain.* 2018;38(1):1–211. https://doi.org/10.1177/0333102417738202

15. Hsu Y-C, Lin K-C, Taiwan HST. Medical treatment guidelines for acute migraine attacks. *Acta Neurologica Taiwanica.* 2017;26(2):78–96.

16. Cameron C, Kelly S, Hsieh S-C et al. Triptans in the acute treatment of migraine: A systematic review and network meta-analysis. *Headache.* n.d.;55 (Suppl 4):221–235. https://doi.org/10.1111/head.12601.

17. Lee S, Staatz CE, Han N, Baek IH. Safety evaluation of oral calcitonin-gene-related peptide receptor antagonists in patients with acute migraine: A systematic review and meta-analysis. *Eur. J. Clin. Pharmacol.* 2022;78(9):1365–1376. https://doi.org/10.1007/s00228-022-03347-6.

18. Dodick DW, Lipton RB, Ailani J et al. Ubrogepant for the treatment of migraine. *New England J. Med.* 2019;381(23): 2230–2241. https://doi.org/10.1056/NEJMoa1813049

19. Edvinsson L. Role of CGRP in migraine. *Handb. Exp. Pharmacol.* 2019;255:121–130. https://doi.org/10.1007/164_2018_201

# Chapter 13

# Trigeminal Neuralgia

Karina Charipova and Kyle Gress

- Trigeminal neuralgia (TN), or *tic douloureux*, is characterized by recurrent attacks of lancinating, neuropathic facial pain in the dermatomal distribution of the trigeminal nerve (1)
- First described as early as in the first century, but accurate descriptions were not documented until the 1700s (6)
  - First fully described by John Fothergill in 1773, is sometimes referred to as "Fothergill's Disease"
  - *Tic douloureux* refers to the distinctive facial muscle spasms associated with the condition (7)
- In patients with TN, minimal stimulation (e.g., light touch, tooth brushing, chewing, talking, wind) causes debilitating pain

## Epidemiology and Risk Factors

- TN is the most common facial pain syndrome
- Incidence of TN is 4–13 people per 100,000 (1)
- Prevalence estimated to be 0.015% in the general population (8)
- TN can resolve spontaneously with as many as 63% of patients reporting total resolution of symptoms for several years (5)
- There is no significant mortality associated with TN, but the condition has high morbidity and is detrimental to the quality of life
- Risk factors include:
  - Advanced age (1)
    - Most affected individuals are over the age of 50
    - Incidence up to 25.9 per 100,000 in individuals over 80
    - Cases in children are very rare (9)
  - Female sex, with female preponderance of 1.7 to 1.5 to 1 (8)
  - Rare familial inheritance, most cases are sporadic
  - No racial predilection

- Some cases of TN are associated with multiple sclerosis, chronic sinusitis, and diabetes (1)

## Pathophysiology

- The trigeminal (CN V) controls facial sensation and motor function (2)
  - It has three terminal branches: ophthalmic (V1, sensory), maxillary (V2, sensory), and mandibular (V3, sensory and motor)
  - TN may be idiopathic or associated with compression of the trigeminal nerve by a vessel, tumor, or arteriovenous malformation
- There is controversy surrounding the pathogenesis of TN, but neurovascular compromise is presently the most widely accepted theory
  - Neurovascular compromise may be primary or secondary (1)
    - Primary compression involves direct compression independent of another pathology
    - Secondary compression refers to the involvement of a tumor (e.g., meningioma, vestibular schwannoma), aneurysm, or cyst
  - It is thought that TN involves compression of the nerve root at the prepontine cistern (1)
- Pain occurs in varying distributions, in at least one unilateral dermatome and usually in the maxillary (V2) and mandibular (V3) distributions (11)
  - Less than 5% of patients experience symptoms in the ophthalmic (V1) distribution (11)
  - Rare cases involve bilateral pain (10)
- Autonomic symptoms (e.g., ptosis, miosis, tearing, sweating) occur in up to 30% of TN patients unilaterally, ipsilateral to side of facial pain (11)
- Imaging tests such as MRI, functional MRI (fMRI), diffusion tensor imaging, and three-dimensional time-of-flight MRA can be used to determine functional pathology (1)
  - Functional MRI can evaluate brain activity in response to activation of TN trigger zones (1)

- ○ Studies using fMRI have demonstrated that patients with TN display increased sensitization of trigeminal nociceptive systems to various types of stimuli (1)
- ○ Trigeminal evoked potentials and neurophysiologic recordings of trigeminal reflexes are options for patients who cannot undergo MRI (5)

# Diagnosis

- International Headache Society (IHS) divides TN into two forms: "classical" and "symptomatic" (3)
  - ○ Classic form (Type 1, TN1) induces sporadic pain characterized by severe episodic burning typically lasting up to two minutes but at times occurring in clusters that can span up to several hours (3)
  - ○ Atypical or symptomatic (Type 2, TN2) is associated with less severe but constant dull aching and burning pain (4)
  - ○ A third form, idiopathic trigeminal neuralgia, is diagnosed when there is no evidence of neurovascular compression or secondary causes
- Both types of TN can occur in the same individual, even at the same time
- The diagnosis of TN is largely clinical (3)
  - ○ Relies on identification of a paroxysmal occurrence of each episode
  - ○ Each episode must have clear onset and termination
  - ○ Some patients cannot identify an inciting event
- TN is traditionally diagnosed after three episodes of unilateral pain that satisfy the following characteristics (4):
  - ○ Pain occurs along at least one trigeminal nerve division; pain is not associated with a neurologic deficit and does not radiate beyond the trigeminal distribution
  - ○ Pain can be provoked by an innocuous stimulus to dermatomes on the unilateral side of the face involving the pain (4)
  - ○ Pain must be two of the following:
    - Severely intense
    - Sharp, electric, stabbing, or shock-like in quality
    - Paroxysmal, lasting one second up to two minutes; pain should not be continuous

- New proposed classification aims to streamline diagnosis and triage for clinical trials; patients must satisfy all three criteria (5):
  - Unilateral pain
  - Paroxysmal pain
  - Trigeminal distribution of pain
- Imaging and other testing can be conducted to rule out alternative diagnoses (e.g., herpes zoster, trigeminal nerve trauma, migraine, cluster headache) (12)
  - Once TN diagnosis is made, neuroimaging is recommended to distinguish between TN1 and TN2 (13)
  - MRI with or without contrast is preferred to improve visualization of trigeminal nerve and adjacent structures that may be involved in secondary TN (13)
    - Classic TN is diagnosed if changes in trigeminal root are seen secondary to neurovascular compression on MRI
    - Secondary TN is diagnosed when MRI shows a cause of nerve compression such as a brain tumor or arteriovenous malformation
    - Idiopathic TN is diagnosed in the setting of a negative MRI

## Treatment

- Mainstays
  - Medication (i.e., antiepileptics, tricyclic antidepressants, etc.)
  - Surgery
  - Complementary approaches
- Surgical management is indicated for those who have:
  - Failed medical treatment with ≥3 medications
  - Suffer from intolerable side effects
  - Have intractable symptoms
- Surgical intervention is categorized as destructive or non-destructive
- Deep brain and motor cortex neuromodulation are off-label, emerging techniques that may offer relief for patients with refractory TN

## References

1.  Montano N, Conforti G, Di Bonaventura R et al. Advances in diagnosis and treatment of trigeminal neuralgia. *Ther Clin Risk Manag.* 2015;**11**:289–299.

2.  Walker HK. Cranial nerve V: The trigeminal nerve. *Clin. Methods Hist. Phys. Lab. Exam.*1990.

3.  Krafft RM. Trigeminal neuralgia. *Am Fam Physician*. 2008;**77**:1291–1296.

4.  McMillan R. Trigeminal neuralgia – A debilitating facial pain. *Rev Pain*. 2011;**5**:26–34.

5.  Cruccu G, Finnerup NB, Jensen TS et al. Trigeminal neuralgia: New classification and diagnostic grading for practice and research. *Neurology*. 2016;**87**:220–228.

6.  Pearce JMS. Trigeminal neuralgia (Fothergill's disease) in the 17th and 18th centuries. *J Neurol Neurosurg Psychiatry*. 2003;**74**:1688.

7.  Rose FC. Trigeminal neuralgia. *Arch Neurol*. 1999;**56**:1163.

8.  Katusic S, Beard CM, Bergstralh E, Kurland LT. Incidence and clinical features of trigeminal neuralgia, Rochester, Minnesota, 1945–1984. *Ann Neurol*. 1990;**27**:89–95.

9.  Childs AM, Meaney JF, Ferrie CD, Holland PC. Neurovascular compression of the trigeminal and glossopharyngeal nerve: three case reports. *Arch Dis Child*. 2000;**82**:311–315.

10. Zakrzewska JM, Linskey ME. Trigeminal neuralgia. *BMJ*. 2015;**350**:h1238.

11. Maarbjerg S, Gozalov A, Olesen J, Bendtsen L. Trigeminal neuralgia – a prospective systematic study of clinical characteristics in 158 patients. *Headache*. 2014;**54**:1574–1582.

12. Bope ET, Kellerman RD, Conn's current therapy. *Faculty Bookshelf*. 2016; 70.

13. Gronseth G, Cruccu G, Alksne J et al. Practice parameter: The diagnostic evaluation and treatment of trigeminal neuralgia (an evidence-based review): Report of the Quality Standards Subcommittee of the American Academy of Neurology and the European Federation of Neurological Societies. *Neurology*. 2008;**71**:1183–1190.

**Chapter 14**

# Occipital Neuralgia

Noushad Mamun

- Occipital neuralgia (ON) is a rare headache disorder mainly affecting the posterior upper neck and posterior head region (1)
- By definition, ON is characterized by paroxysmal shooting or stabbing, sudden-onset pain that has frequent recurrence, lasting for a few minutes at a time (3)
- This pain syndrome is related to the nerve distribution that involves spinal nerves emerging from the upper cervical region that traverse to the base of the neck and run up the posterior scalp
- Involves compression, injury, or trauma to greater occipital nerve (GON), lesser occipital nerve (LON), and then rarely, due to third occipital nerve (TON) (1,2)
- Conceptually, nerve entrapment between anatomical structures has been hypothesized to be a large contributing factor to the pathophysiology of ON (1)

## Epidemiology and Risk Factors

- There are no recent dedicated epidemiological studies that document the incidence or prevalence of ON (4–7)
  - However, a 2009 Dutch study on the incidence of facial pain in general population found that ON had an incidence rate of 3.2 per 100,000 (7)
  - Same study showed an increased incidence rate in women in comparison to men, but was not statistically significant (7)
- **Risk factors**
  - Head trauma
  - Cervical osteoarthritis
  - Cervical disc degeneration
  - Gout
  - Diabetes

# Etiology

- Most cases of ON are idiopathic with no clear etiology that is structurally identifiable (8,9)
- Proposed etiologies causing ON can be divided into sub-categories, osteogenic, neurogenic, vascular, muscular, and tendinous (2)
    - Osteogenic causes include C1–C2 arthrosis, atlantodental sclerosis, callus formation at C1–C2 fracture, hypermobile C1 posterior arch
    - Neurogenic causes include schwannoma located in the craniocervical junction or of the occipital nerves (12,13). Also, C2 myelitis and multiple sclerosis have been reported
    - Vascular causes include giant cell arteritis, compression of GON due to occipital artery, C2 posterior column spinal infarction (4,10)
    - Musculoskeletal causes reported include neck strain and whiplash injuries

# Pathophysiology

- It is hypothesized that the pain from ON is due to compression, injury, or irritation (e.g. chronic instability, entrapment, trauma, inflammation) of the greater occipital nerve, lesser occipital nerve, and/or the third occipital nerve (5,11)
    - Greater occipital nerve
        - Greater occipital nerve (GON) is the most commonly affected nerve causing ON (reference). It arises from the medial division of dorsal ramus of C2, purely an afferent nerve that runs posteriorly between the C1 and C2 vertebrae (need reference)
        - GON is the affected nerve in 90% of patients with ON (1)
            - Pathophysiology includes
                - Compression of GON between atlas and axis / causing severe pain upon head rotation (4)
                - Compression of GON due to close proximity to occipital artery (4)
                - Chronically contracted muscles and spondylosis of the upper cervical spine leading to GON irritation are often implicated (8,9)
                - GON schwannoma (12,13)

- Lesser occipital nerve
  - ○ Lesser occipital nerve (LON) arises from C2 and C3 ventral rami, and travels along the posterior portion of the sterno-cleidomastoid muscle up to the occipital region, lateral to the GON (14)
    - ▪ LON is affected in 10% of patients with ON (1)
    - ▪ Pathophysiology
      - • Stretching of the C2 ventral ramus by the obliquus capitis inferior muscle during forceful movements (15)
      - • compression of the C2 ventral ramus as it crosses atlanto-axial junction
      - • LON compression secondary to vertebral artery (16)
- Third occipital nerve
  - ○ Third occipital nerve (TON) arises from the dorsal ramus of the C3 spinal nerve and travels up to the occipital region at midline (14)
    - ▪ TON is rarely affected in the diagnosis of ON (1)
    - ▪ Pathophysiology
      - • Presumed secondary to C2 to C3 facet joint TON entrapment (17)

## Diagnosis

- ON is predominantly a clinical diagnosis based on history and physical exam
- According to the international classification of headache disorder (ICHD-III), diagnosis of ON must meet the following criteria (3):
  - ○ Unilateral or bilateral pain in the distribution of greater, lesser, and/or third occipital nerves with fulfillment of
    - ▪ Two of the following three pain characteristics:
      - • Recurring paroxysmal painful attacks lasting seconds to minutes
      - • Severe intensity
      - • Stabbing, sharp, or shooting in quality
  - ○ Pain associated with both
    - ▪ Allodynia and/or dysaesthesia during light stimulation of scalp and/or hair

- Tenderness or trigger points over the affected nerve distributions
  - Pain is temporarily relieved by local anesthetic block of suspected nerve (5)
- Once there is a high clinical suspicion for ON, diagnostic anesthetic block of suspected nerve confirms the diagnosis, per ICHD-III guidelines (1,4)
  - One diagnostic nerve block has a false-positive rate of 40%; therefore, a second diagnostic block is needed for a more definitive diagnosis (1,4)
  - Use of ultrasonography can be useful in that swelling associated with the nerve can help identify the specific level of nerve entrapment or damage (4,18)
- Imaging can be helpful in determining etiology of ON
  - For example, plain radiograph/X-rays can unveil underlying degenerative vertebral changes near C1 to C2 (19)
  - CT scan can help reveal degenerative osseous pathology or identify possible masses compressing the occipital nerves (20)
- MRI can be done to visualize surrounding cervical and occipital issues to aid in determining etiology of occipital nerve compression or cervical spine pathology (5)

## Treatment

- Conservative management
  - Nonpharmacological management
    - Many conservative measures such as immobilization, cervical collar, physical therapy, or cryotherapy have not been found to be effective in managing patients with ON (1,21)
    - Acupuncture has shown promising results for the treatment of ON as a conservative option for management (5)
  - Pharmacologic management
    - Nonsteroidal anti-inflammatory agents provide alleviation in pain for patients; however, overall, have shown transient long-term effects (21)
    - Tricyclic antidepressants and anticonvulsants can be trialed initially to treat ON as well

- Interventional management
  - In cases of refractory ON, more invasive and interventional treatments are
    - Greater occipital nerve block
    - Local anesthetic in conjunction with corticosteroid used for peripheral nerve block
      - Generally, 1–2% lidocaine or 0.25–0.5% bupivacaine is utilized along with corticosteroids, such as dexamethasone, methylprednisolone, or betamethasone (4)
    - Choice of procedure for diagnostic and therapeutic purposes (4)
  - Botulinum Toxin A injection (BTX)
    - Reported to relieve sharp pain for months; however, dull pain usually remains (5)
  - Radiofrequency ablation (RFA)
    - Temperature-dependent neurolysis (22)
    - Used after adequate pain relief from local anesthetic block
    - Beyond six months, RFA has shown to have superior results in comparison to botulinum toxin injections or nerve stimulation (21)
  - Cryoneurolysis (24)
    - Form of thermal neurolysis involving application of cold temperatures onto the suspected occipital nerve causing ON (23)
    - Nitrous oxide is used, cryoneurolysis is achieved at a temperature of −20°C to −100°C (24)
    - Reduced risk of neuroma when compared to RFA (25)
  - Neuromodulation
    - Occipital nerve stimulation
      - Nerve stimulator leads are placed in the subcutaneous layer where the occipital nerve emerges at the base of the skull (4)
      - Treatment is considered successful if the patient achieves greater than 50% pain relief for more than 24 hours

- No statistical difference when compared to Botulinum toxin injections; however, patients have reportedly preferred the occipital nerve stimulation route as it is a reversible approach (18)
  - Pulsed radiofrequency (PRF)
    - Unlike radiofrequency ablation, PRF is hypothesized to act through a temperature-independent neuromodulatory process (22)
    - To date, various clinical studies have demonstrated improvement in pain and quality of life; however, there has not yet been conclusive evidence in support of long-term therapeutic efficacy (26)
- Refractory occipital neuralgia
  - Surgical decompression of occipital nerve
    - Often chosen for refractory chronic occipital neuralgia with associated headaches (5)
    - ON patients who have previously responded well to greater occipital nerve blocks, Botulinum toxin injections (27)
  - Surgical decompression procedure through resection of obliquus capitis inferior muscle is the definitive treatment; however, it is associated with significant risks (4)
    - This option is often efficacious for those patients whose pain increases with flexion of the cervical spine (5,21)

# References

1. Djavaherian DM, Guthmiller KB. *Occipital Neuralgia – StatPearls – NCBI Bookshelf.* (n.d.). Retrieved August 22, 2022, from www.ncbi.nlm.nih.gov/books/NBK538281/.

2. Vanelderen P, Lataster A, Levy R et al. 8. Occipital neuralgia. *Pain Pract.: Off. J World Inst. Pain.* n.d.;**10**(2):137–144. https://doi.org/10.1111/j.1533-2500.2009.00355.x.

3. Headache Classification Committee of the International Headache Society (IHS). The international classification of headache disorders, 3rd ed. *Cephalalgia.* 2018;**38**(1):1–211. https://doi.org/10.1177/0333102417738202.

4. Swanson D, Guedry R, Boudreaux M et al. An update on the diagnosis, treatment, and management of occipital neuralgia. *Journal of Craniofacial Surgery,* 2022;**33**(3):779–783. https://doi.org/10.1097/SCS.0000000000008360.

5. Choi I, Jeon, SR. Neuralgias of the head: Occipital neuralgia. *J. Korean Med. Sci.* 2016;31(4):479–488. https://doi.org/10.3346/jkms.2016.31.4.479.

6. Dougherty C. Occipital neuralgia. *Curr Pain Headache Rep.* 2014;18(5):411. https://doi.org/10.1007/s11916-014-0411-x.

7. Koopman JSHA, Dieleman JP, Huygen FJ et al. Incidence of facial pain in the general population. *Pain.* 147(1–3):122–127. https://doi.org/10.1016/j .pain.2009.08.023.

8. Magnússon T, Ragnarsson T, Björnsson A. Occipital nerve release in patients with whiplash trauma and occipital neuralgia. *Headache.* 1996; **36**: 32–36.

9. Cohen SP, Plunkett AR, Wilkinson I et al. Headaches during war: Analysis of presentation, treatment, and factors associated with outcome. *Cephalalgia.* 2012; **32**:94–108.

10. Cornely C, Fischer M, Ingianni G, Isenmann S. Greater occipital nerve neuralgia caused by pathological arterial contact: Treatment by surgical decompression. *Headache.* 2011;51(4):609–612. https://doi.org/10.1111/j .1526-4610.2010.01802.x.

11. Elias WJ, Burchiel KJ. Trigeminal neuralgia and other neuropathic pain syndromes of the head and face. *Curr Pain Headache Rep.* 2002;6(2):115–124. https://doi.org/10.1007/s11916-002-230007-238.

12. Ural A, Ceylan A, Inal E, Celenk F. A case of greater occipital nerve schwannoma causing neuralgia. *Kulak Burun Bogaz Ihtisas Dergisi: KBB = Ear Nose Throat J.* n.d.;18(4):253–256.

13. Ballesteros-Del Rio B, Ares-Luque A, Tejada-Garcia J, Muela-Molinero A. Occipital (Arnold) neuralgia secondary to greater occipital nerve schwannoma. *Headache.* n.d.;43(7):804–807. https://doi.org/10.1046/j.1526-4610.2003.03142.x.

14. Yu M, Wang S-M. Anatomy, head and neck, occipital nerves. *StatPearls.* 2021, www.ncbi.nlm.nih.gov/books/NBK542213/.

15. de Araújo Lucas G, Laudanna A, Chopard RP, Raffaelli, E. Anatomy of the lesser occipital nerve in relation to cervicogenic headache. *Clin Anat.* 1994;7 (2):90–96. https://doi.org/10.1002/ca.980070207.

16. Hunter CR, Mayfield FH. Role of the upper cervical roots in the production of pain in the head. *Am. J. Surg.* 1949;78(5):743–751. https://doi.org/ 10.1016/0002–9610(49)90316–5.

17. Bogduk N, Marsland A. On the concept of third occipital headache. *J. Neurol. Neurosurg. Psychiatry.* 1986;49(7):775–780. https://doi.org/10.1136/jnnp .49.7.775.

18. Narouze S. Occipital neuralgia diagnosis and treatment: The role of ultrasound. *Headache.* 2016;56(4):801–807. https://doi.org/10.1111/head .12790.

19. Ehni G, Benner B. Occipital neuralgia and the C1-2 arthrosis syndrome. *J. Neurosurg.* 1984;**61**(5):961–965. https://doi.org/10.3171/jns .1984.61.5.0961.

20. Kapoor V, Rothfus WE, Grahovac SZ, Amin Kassam SZ, Horowitz, MB. Refractory occipital neuralgia: preoperative assessment with CT-guided nerve block prior to dorsal cervical rhizotomy. *AJNR. Am. J. Neuroradiol.* n.d.;**24**(10):2105–2110.

21. Finiels P-J, Batifol D. The treatment of occipital neuralgia: Review of 111 cases. *Neuro-Chirurgie.* 2016;**62**(5):233–240.

22. Manolitsis N, Elahi F. Pulsed radiofrequency for occipital neuralgia. *Pain Physician.* n.d.;**17**(6):E709-E717.

23. Kastler A, Attyé A, Maindet C et al. Greater occipital nerve cryoneurolysis in the management of intractable occipital neuralgia. *J. Neuroradiol.* 2018;**45** (6):386–390. https://doi.org/10.1016/j.neurad.2017.11.002.

24. Ilfeld BM, Preciado J, Trescot AM. Novel cryoneurolysis device for the treatment of sensory and motor peripheral nerves. *Expert Rev. Med. Devices.* 2016;**13**(8):713–725. https://doi.org/10.1080/17434440.2016.1204229.

25. Hsu M, Stevenson FF. Wallerian degeneration and recovery of motor nerves after multiple focused cold therapies. *Muscle & Nerve.* 2015;**51**(2):268–275. https://doi.org/10.1002/mus.24306

26. Vanelderen P, Rouwette T, de Vooght P et al. Pulsed radiofrequency for the treatment of occipital neuralgia: a prospective study with 6 months of follow-up. *Reg. Anesth. & and Pain Med.* n.d.;**35**(2):148–151. https://doi.org /10.1097/aap.0b013e3181d24713.

27. Jose, A, Nagori, SA, Chattopadhyay, PK, Roychoudhury, A. Greater occipital nerve decompression for occipital neuralgia. *J. Craniofac. Surg.* 2018;**29**(5): e518–e521. https://doi.org/10.1097/SCS.0000000000004549.

# Chapter 15

# Chronic Neuraxial Spine Pain

Nazir Noor and Shenwari R. Afredi

- Three sources of pain (1):
  1. Axial pain (e.g., axial lumbosacral)
  2. Radiculopathic pain (e.g., lumbosacral radiculopathy)
  3. Referred pain
- Axial low back pain is pain that is localized to the low back and does not radiate in a known dermatomal pattern; however, it can radiate down the thighs in a non-dermatomal pattern
- Lumbosacral radiculopathy or radicular pain is low back pain that travels into one or both lower extremities along a dermatomal distribution
- Referred pain is pain that spreads to a region remote from sources but in a non-dermatomal fashion
- Low back pain is the fifth most common chief complaint
- US annual and lifetime prevalence of low back pain is 10–30% and 65–80%, respectively
- Acute = <6 weeks, subacute = 6–12 weeks, chronic = >12 weeks (2,3)
- Oftentimes, a multidisciplinary approach to treatment is most effective (i.e., medical, psychological, physical, interventional management) (4)

## Clinical Presentation

- History
  - 85% of low back pain is nonspecific (5,6)
  - Duration of symptoms, location, radiation, severity (e.g., visual analog scale), description of pain (e.g., burning, lancinating, numbness), alleviating/aggravating factors, history of similar symptoms, other associated symptoms (5,7)
  - 15% of low back pain results from serious etiology (6)

- History of cancer is the strongest risk factor for back pain due to bone metastasis (7–9)
- Bone metastasizing cancers include breast, lung, renal cell, and prostate cancers (6)
  - Important to inquire about the type of cancer, location, treatments, recent weight loss, worsening pain at night, and inability to attain relief at rest or supine position (5,7)
- History of injection
  - Important to inquire about fever, malaise, spinal injection, epidural catheter placement, IV drug use, immunosuppression, and other concurrent infections (5,6)
- History of recent or substantial trauma (7,10)
  - Important to inquire about the mechanism of traumatic injury and possible structural damage (e.g., ligamentous tear, vertebral compression fracture) (11)
- History of neurologic compromise
  - Important to inquire about bowel/bladder control changes (e.g., spinal cord or cauda equina compression can lead to urinary retention followed by urinary and/or fecal incontinence), recent numbness (i.e., bilateral leg numbness with saddle anesthesia is an indication of cauda equina syndrome), gait instability, weakness in lower extremities (5,7,10)
- History of social and/or psychological distress
  - Important to inquire about history of substance abuse, disability compensation, work status, and symptoms of depression (10)
  - Psychiatric comorbid conditions, somatization, and/or maladaptive coping strategies are associated with poorer outcomes in neuraxial pain (7)
  - Utilize questionnaires to assess these aspects of pain management (e.g., Opioid Risk Tool, Patient Health Questionnaire-9, Current Opioid Misuse Measure) (11)
- Physical Examination
  - Essential part of management of neuraxial and low back pain (10)

- General physical examination with thorough neurological examination (i.e., motor strength of back and lower extremity muscles, deep tendon reflex testing, upper motor neuron reflexes, etc.), inspection of thoracolumbar spine, palpation of over spinous processes, range of motion movements, and test for specific disorders (6,8,12)
- Focus on abnormal kyphosis, lordosis, and scoliosis (11)
- Skin evaluation for rashes, scars, swelling, signs of trauma or inflammation (6)
- Palpation over spinous processes may reveal localized tenderness that is consistent with abscess, epidural tumor, and vertebral compression fractures (12)
- Tenderness of paraspinal region consistent with facet arthropathy and myofascial pain (13)
- Pain provoked by a range of motion is a nonspecific finding but may be helpful in the differential diagnosis

  - Pain provoked by lateral rotation and/or extension of the back is suggestive of facet arthropathy (14)
  - Pain provoked by forward flexion of back is suggestive of discogenic or vertebrogenic pathology because flexion of lumbar spine causes axial loading (15)
  - Examples of special range of motion tests:
    - Sacroiliac joint provocative tests (Gaenslen's, thigh thrust, distraction, FABER/Patrick's), straight leg raise, facet loading test, FADDIR (5,7,12,16,17)

# Diagnostic Testing

- Seldom required for treatment of lower back pain (7,10)
  - Laboratory studies, such as ESR and/or CRP, for suspected malignancy, infection
  - Plain radiographs help determine the need for advanced imaging, such as CT and/or MRI (7,8)
- Electrodiagnostic testing
  - Electromyography and nerve conduction velocity studies
    - Help differentiate chronic from acute radiculopathy, localize pathologic lesion, and determine if observed radiologic abnormalities are likely sources of symptoms (7)

- Imaging
  - X-rays, CT, MRI
    - After failed medical-directed conservative care of lower back pain → imaging (preferably start with weight-bearing radiographs of lumbar spine (AP and lateral) (8)
    - CT and/or MRI are useful. If radiographs do not explain unremitting lower back pain or there are red flags (6,8,18)
    - MRI without contrast is considered best initial test for most (19)
    - MRI with gadolinium allows distinction of scar from disc in patient with prior back surgery (19)
    - CT is useful for patients who cannot have MRI (e.g., patient has an MRI-incompatible permanent pacemaker or spinal cord stimulator implant)
  - Most lower back pain of <4 weeks does not require imaging (8)
  - Imaging is useful when severe or progressive neurologic deficits present or when serious neurologic disease is suspected (red flags) (8)
  - Spinal stenosis and radiculopathy patients receive imaging if they are good candidates for surgery or minimally invasive interventions, such as minimally invasive lumbar decompression

## Etiology

- History, physical, and imaging help differentiate neuraxial pain
- Myofascial pain
  - Myofascial trigger points in fascia, tendons, and muscles (20–22)
  - Localized tender spots in a taut band, pain on palpation, decreased range of motion (6,22)
- Facet-mediated pain
  - Degeneration of intervertebral discs → lumbar facet joint degeneration (14)
  - Osteoarthritis of facet joints or stress in facet joint capsules (23)
- Discogenic pain
  - 39% of lower back pain is attributed to intervertebral disc (24)

- ○ Disc disruption is mainly due to the degradation of disc and its nuclear components
  - ▪ Complicated by radial fissures extending from nucleus to annulus (25)
- Lumbar post-laminectomy syndrome (26)
  - ○ Incidence 10–40% (27)
  - ○ Etiology based on preoperative, intraoperative, and postoperative factors
    - ▪ Preoperative risk
      - • History of anxiety, depression, poor coping strategies, pursuing litigation, and worker's compensation (28)
    - ▪ Intraoperative risk
      - • Poor surgical technique, surgery at incorrect level/site of spine, inability to achieve an anticipated surgical goal (29)
    - ▪ Postoperative risk
      - • Surgical complications, rate of disease progression, epidural fibrosis, new instability, development of myofascial pain syndrome (30)
- Spinal stenosis
  - ○ Degenerative changes leading to decreased space for neurovascular elements
    - ▪ Symptoms of gluteal and lower extremity pain, fatigue with or without lower back pain occur with upright exercise, walking, lumbar extension → causing neurogenic claudication (31)
  - ○ Spinal canal narrowing or nerve root impingement (12,32)
- Sacroiliac join pain
  - ○ Sacroiliac joint is diathrodial synovial joint with profuse innervation, thus it is capable of being source of lower back pain (33)
  - ○ No existing historical, physical, or radiographical features provide definitive diagnosis (17)
  - ○ Moderate evidence for the use of fluoroscopic CT-guided intraarticular joint injection; lateral branch blocks may provide therapeutic pain relief in some patients (34,35)

# Treatment Modalities

- Management individually tailored to each patient
- Pharmacologic
  - Nonsteroidal anti-inflammatory drugs (NSAIDs) and acetaminophen
    - For acute and chronic low back pain
    - NSAIDs – nonselective (e.g., ibuprofen, meloxicam, naproxen) and selective COX-2 inhibitors (e.g., celecoxib) (10,36)
      - Adverse effects involve renal, cardiovascular, and gastrointestinal systems (8,10)
      - Recommend the lowest effective dose and shortest duration possible (8,10)
      - NSAIDs are shown to be slightly better for chronic lower back pain when compared to acetaminophen (7)
  - Skeletal muscle relaxants
    - Useful in acute low back pain (7,10)
    - Adverse effects – CNS sedation, increased risk of falls (7)
  - Opioids
    - Mechanism – mu receptor agonists
    - Adverse effects – respiratory depression, constipation, long-term use causes hyperalgesia, tolerance, addiction
    - Judiciously used, only for severe, debilitating pain uncontrolled with nonopioid medications (8)
    - Patient evaluation for risk of addiction or aberrant behavior (e.g., personal or family history of addiction, poorly controlled psychological comorbidity, sexual abuse history, age <45) (7)
  - Tricyclic antidepressants (TCA)
    - Mechanism – serotonin and norepinephrine reuptake inhibition, sodium channel blockade, NMDA antagonism (7)
    - Adverse effects – dry mouth/constipation (anticholinergic), dizziness/drowsiness (antihistaminergic)
  - Serotonin norepinephrine reuptake inhibitors (SNRIs)
    - Duloxetine, venlafaxine (duloxetine often better tolerated) (7)

- Mechanism – serotonin and norepinephrine reuptake inhibition, which is important for descending pain inhibition (11)
- Adverse effects – dry mouth, self-limited nausea, dizziness, headache, insomnia (11)

○ Antiepileptics (e.g., gabapentin, pregabalin, topiramate)

- Gabapentin and pregabalin mechanism – alpha-2-delta voltage-gated calcium channel blockers (37)
- Topiramate mechanism – voltage-gated sodium channel blocker, enhance GABA receptor activity (38)
  - Topiramate is only antiepileptic evidenced to provide analgesia and improved quality of life for low back pain (39)
  - Adverse effects – weight loss (may be considered advantageous side effect), dizziness, somnolence, rare nephrolithiasis (39)

- Psychological treatments
  ○ Multidisciplinary approach for analgesic efficacy and reduction of disability
  ○ Types of psychological treatment include:
    - Cognitive behavioral therapy (CBT), progressive relaxation, biofeedback (11)
    - CBT – goal-oriented approach targeting maladaptive thinking and coping strategies to change behavior and improve mood (7)
    - Progressive relaxation – muscle tension-reducing technique involving systemic flexing and relaxing of specific muscles with the aim of achieving profound relaxation; provides short-term improvement in pain and function (40)
    - Biofeedback – relaxation approach utilizing auditory and visual feedback from muscle activity to reduce muscle tension (40)

- Physical and rehabilitation
  ○ Specific movements and exercise to train the body to promote good physical health (5,8)
  ○ Stretching exercises are most associated with pain reduction; strengthening exercises are most associated with functional improvement (5,8)

- Other forms of physical therapies include: (11)
  - Lumbar support
  - Transcutaneous electrical nerve stimulation (TENS) unit
  - Superficial heat and/or cold application
  - Massage therapy
- Interventions
  - Lumbar facet (zygapophyseal) joint interventions
    - Lumbar facet joints are innervated by medial branches of the dorsal rami, with nerve endings within the facet joints (14)
    - Medial branch nerve blocks and radiofrequency ablations, the latter of which can provide 6–12 months of improved pain and function (14)
  - Sacroiliac joint interventions
    - Innervated by ventral and dorsal sacral rami
      - Posterior sacroiliac joint (site of sacroiliac joint steroid injection) – innervated by lateral branches of sacral dorsal rami (34,41)
    - Intra-articular sacroiliac joint steroid injections
    - Sacral lateral branch radiofrequency ablation targeting posterior sacroiliac joint and ligaments
      - Diagnostic blocks of sacroiliac joint intra-articular injections or L5 dorsal ramus plus S1-S3 lateral branch blocks, followed by radiofrequency ablation, which can provide three to six months of improved function (35)
  - Epidural steroid injections
    - Indications – cervical/thoracic/lumbar radicular pain, spinal stenosis (31)
    - Provide significant, though temporary (<3 months) analgesia (31)
    - Pain reduction and improved function in spinal stenosis (31)
    - Local anesthetic alone improves analgesia by increasing blood flow to ischemic nerve roots, suppressing nociceptive transmission, and washing out inflammatory mediators (31)
  - Spinal cord stimulation
    - Mechanism – delivers electrical impulses via epidural electrodes at vertebral levels associated with pain, either

overlapping pain with masking paresthesia (traditional low-frequency SCS devices) or through high-frequency (10 kHz) non-paresthesia neuromodulation (42)

○ Other interventions for low back pain

- Dorsal root ganglion stimulation (43)
- Peripheral nerve stimulation implants (44)
- Minimally invasive lumbar decompression (45)

# References

1. Bogduk N. On the definitions and physiology of back pain, referred pain, and radicular pain. *Pain.* 2009;**147**(1–3):17–19. https://pubmed.ncbi.nlm.nih.gov/19762151/.

2. Atlas SJ, Deyo RA. Evaluating and managing acute low back pain in the primary care setting. *J Gen Intern Med.* 2001;**16**(2):120–131. https://pubmed.ncbi.nlm.nih.gov/11251764/.

3. Heuch I, Foss IS. Acute low back usually resolves quickly but persistent low back pain often persists. *J Physiother.* 2013;**59**(2):127. https://pubmed.ncbi.nlm.nih.gov/23663799/.

4. Elkayam O, Ben Itzhak S, Avrahami E et al. Multidisciplinary approach to chronic back pain: Prognostic elements of the outcome. *Clin Exp Rheumatol.* 1996;**14**(3):281–288. https://pubmed.ncbi.nlm.nih.gov/8809442/.

5. Deyo R, Weinstein J. Low back pain. *N Engl J Med.* 2001;**344**(5):363–70. https://www-nejm-org.libproxy1.usc.edu/doi/pdf/10.1056%252FNEJM200102013440508.

6. Deyo RA, Rainville J, Kent DL. What can the history and physical examination tell us about low back pain? *JAMA J Am Med Assoc.* 1992;**268**(6):760–765.

7. Chou R. Low back pain. *Ann Intern Med.* 2021;**174**(8):ITC113–ITC128. https://pubmed.ncbi.nlm.nih.gov/34370518/.

8. Chou R, Qaseem A, Snow V et al. Diagnosis and treatment of low back pain: A joint clinical practice guideline from the American College of Physicians and the American Pain Society. *Ann Intern Med.* 2007;**147**(7):478–491 https://pubmed.ncbi.nlm.nih.gov/17909209/.

9. Deyo RA, Diehl AK. Cancer as a cause of back pain: Frequency, clinical presentation, and diagnostic strategies. *J Gen Intern Med.* 1988;**3**(3):230–238. https://pubmed.ncbi.nlm.nih.gov/2967893/.

10. Van Tulder M, Becker A, Bekkering T et al. Chapter 3. European guidelines for the management of acute nonspecific low back pain in primary care.

*Eur Spine J.* 2006;**15**(Suppl 2):S169–S191. https://pubmed.ncbi.nlm.nih.gov/16550447/.

11. Urits I, Burshtein A, Sharma M et al. Low back pain, a comprehensive review: Pathophysiology, diagnosis, and treatment. *Curr Pain Headache Rep [Internet].* 2019;**23**(3):23. https://pubmed.ncbi.nlm.nih.gov/30854609/.

12. Rubinstein SM, van Tulder M. A best-evidence review of diagnostic procedures for neck and low-back pain. *Best Pract Res Clin Rheumatol.* 2008;**22**(3):471–482. https://pubmed.ncbi.nlm.nih.gov/18519100/.

13. Partanen J V, Ojala TA, Arokoski JPA. Myofascial syndrome and pain: A neurophysiological approach. *Pathophysiol Off J Int Soc Pathophysiol.* 2010;**17**(1):19–28. https://pubmed.ncbi.nlm.nih.gov/19500953/.

14. Kalichman L, Hunter DJ. Lumbar facet joint osteoarthritis: A review. *Semin Arthritis Rheum.* 2007;**37**(2):69–80. https://pubmed.ncbi.nlm.nih.gov/17379279/.

15. Park WM, Kim K, Kim YH. Effects of degenerated intervertebral discs on intersegmental rotations, intradiscal pressures, and facet joint forces of the whole lumbar spine. *Comput Biol Med.* 2013;**43**(9):1234–1240. https://pubmed.ncbi.nlm.nih.gov/23930818/.

16. Bagwell JJ, Bauer L, Gradoz M, Grindstaff TL. The reliability of Faber test hip range of motion measurements. *Int J Sports Phys Ther.* 2016;**11**(7):1101–1105. www.ncbi.nlm.nih.gov/pubmed/27999724.

17. Zelle BA, Gruen GS, Brown S, George S. Sacroiliac joint dysfunction: Evaluation and management. *Clin J Pain.* 2005;**21**(5):446–455. https://pubmed.ncbi.nlm.nih.gov/16093751/.

18. Chou R, Qasseem A, Owens D, Shekelle P. Diagnostic imaging for low back pain: advice for high-value health care from the American College of Physicians. *Ann. Intern. Med.* 2011;**154**(3):181–189. https://web-s-ebscohost-com.libproxy1.usc.edu/ehost/pdfviewer/pdfviewer?vid=0&sid=a46376cb-0b2a-4f25-adcf-ed190625a0f0%40redis.

19. Wilkinson LS, Elson E, Saifuddin A, Ransford AO. Defining the use of gadolinium enhanced MRI in the assessment of the postoperative lumbar spine. *Clin Radiol.* 1997;**52**(7):530–534. https://pubmed.ncbi.nlm.nih.gov/9240706/.

20. Simons DG. New views of myofascial trigger points: etiology and diagnosis. *Arch Phys Med Rehabil.* 2008;**89**(1):157–159. https://pubmed.ncbi.nlm.nih.gov/18164347/.

21. Lucas N, MacAskill P, Irwig L, Moran R, Bogduk N. Reliability of physical examination for diagnosis of myofascial trigger points: A systematic review of the literature. *Clin J Pain.* 2009;**25**(1):80–89. https://pubmed.ncbi.nlm.nih.gov/19158550/.

22. Giamberardino MA, Affaitati G, Fabrizio A, Costantini R. Myofascial pain syndromes and their evaluation. *Best Pract Res Clin Rheumatol.* 2011;**25** (2):185–198. https://pubmed.ncbi.nlm.nih.gov/22094195/.

23. Bogduk N. Evidence-informed management of chronic low back pain with facet injections and radiofrequency neurotomy. *Spine J.* 2008;**8**(1):56–64. https://pubmed.ncbi.nlm.nih.gov/18164454/.

24. Comer C, Conaghan PG. Tackling persistent low back pain in primary care. *Practitioner.* 2009;**253**:32–34.

25. Aprill C, Bogduk N. High-intensity zone: A diagnostic sign of painful lumbar disc on magnetic resonance imaging. *Br J Radiol.* 1992;**65**(773):361–369. https://pubmed.ncbi.nlm.nih.gov/1535257/.

26. Taylor RS, Taylor RJ. The economic impact of failed back surgery syndrome. *Br J Pain.* 2012;**6**(4):174–181. https://pubmed.ncbi.nlm.nih.gov/26516490/.

27. Waguespack A, Schofferman J, Slosar P, Reynolds J. Etiology of long-term failures of lumbar spine surgery. *Pain Med.* 2002;**3**(1):18–22. https://pubmed.ncbi.nlm.nih.gov/15102214/.

28. Orhurhu V, Urits I, Olusunmade M et al. Trends of co-morbid depression in hospitalized patients with failed back surgery syndrome: An analysis of the nationwide inpatient sample. *Pain Ther.* 2018;**7**(2):217–226. https://pubmed.ncbi.nlm.nih.gov/30218424/.

29. Chan C, Peng P. Failed back surgery syndrome. *Pain Med.* 2011;**12** (4):577–606. https://pubmed.ncbi.nlm.nih.gov/21463472/.

30. Weinstein JN, Lurie JD, Tosteson TD et al. Surgical versus nonsurgical treatment for lumbar degenerative spondylolisthesis. *N Engl J Med.* 2007;**356** (22):2257–2270. https://pubmed.ncbi.nlm.nih.gov/17538085/.

31. Koc Z, Ozcakir S, Sivrioglu K, Gurbet A, Kucukoglu S. Effectiveness of physical therapy and epidural steroid injections in lumbar spinal stenosis. *Spine (Phila Pa 1976).* 2009;**34**(10):985–989.

32. Bischoff R, Rodriguez R, Gupta K, Righi A, Dalton J. A comparison of computed tomography-myelography, magnetic resonance imaging, and myelography in the diagnosis of herniated nucleus pulposus and spinal stenosis. *Journal of Spinal Disorders.* 1993;**6**(4): 289–295. https://oce-ovid-com.libproxy1.usc.edu/article/00002317-199300040-00002/HTML.

33. Foley BS, Buschbacher RM. Sacroiliac joint pain: Anatomy, biomechanics, diagnosis, and treatment. *Am J Phys Med Rehabil.* 2006;**85**(12):997–1006.

34. Mckenzie-Brown AM, Shah R V, Sehgal N, Everett CR. A systematic review of sacroiliac joint interventions. *Pain Physician.* 2005;**8**(1):115–125.

35. King W, Ahmed SU, Baisden J et al. Spine section original research articles diagnosis and treatment of posterior sacroiliac complex pain: A systematic review with comprehensive analysis of the published data. *Pain Med.* 2015;**16**

(2):257–265. https://academic.oup.com/painmedicine/article/16/2/257/2460376.

36. Roelofs PDDM, Deyo RA, Koes BW, Scholten RJPM, Van Tulder MW. Non-steroidal anti-inflammatory drugs for low back pain. *Cochrane Database Syst Rev.* 2008;**2**(1):CD012087. www-cochranelibrary-com.libproxy2.usc.edu/cds r/doi/10.1002/14651858.CD000396.pub3/full

37. Sills GJ. The mechanisms of action of gabapentin and pregabalin. *Curr Opin Pharmacol.* 2006;**6**(1):108–113. https://pubmed.ncbi.nlm.nih.gov/16376147/.

38. Fariba KA, Saadabadi A. Topiramate. *StatPearls.* 2022. Treasure Island: StatPearls Publishing. PMID: 32119417. https://www.ncbi.nlm.nih.gov/boo ks/NBK554530/.

39. Muehlbacher M, Nickel MK, Kettler C et al. Topiramate in treatment of patients with chronic low back pain: A randomized, double-blind, placebo-controlled study. *Clin J Pain.* 2006;**22**(6):526–531. https://pubmed .ncbi.nlm.nih.gov/16788338/.

40. Vitoula K, Venneri A, Varrassi G et al. Behavioral therapy approaches for the management of low back pain: An up-to-date systematic review. *Pain Ther.* 2018;**7**(1). https://pubmed.ncbi.nlm.nih.gov/29767395/.

41. Manchikanti L, Staats PS, Singh V et al. Evidence-based practice guidelines for interventional techniques in the management of chronic spinal pain practice guidelines. *Pain Physician.* 2003;**6**(1):3–81.

42. Kumar K, Taylor RS, Jacques L et al. Spinal cord stimulation versus conventional medical management for neuropathic pain: a multicentre randomised controlled trial in patients with failed back surgery syndrome. *Pain.* 2007;**132**(1–2):179–188. https://pubmed.ncbi.nlm.nih.gov/17845835/.

43. Berger AA, Liu Y, Possoit H et al. Dorsal root ganglion (DRG) and chronic pain. *Anesthesiol Pain Med.* 2021;**11**(2):e113020. https://pubmed .ncbi.nlm.nih.gov/34336621/.

44. Kaye AD, Ridgell S, Alpaugh ES et al. Peripheral nerve stimulation: A review of techniques and clinical efficacy. *Pain Ther.* 2021;**10**(2):961–972. https:// pubmed.ncbi.nlm.nih.gov/34331668/.

45. Jain S, Deer T, Sayed D et al. Minimally invasive lumbar decompression: A review of indications, techniques, efficacy and safety. *Pain Manag.* 2020;**10** (5):331–348. https://pubmed.ncbi.nlm.nih.gov/32609052/.

| Chapter **16** | # Vertebral Compression Fractures |
| --- | --- |

Karina Charipova, Alan D. Kaye, and Kyle Gress

## Vertebral Compression Fractures (VCFs)

- Osseous fractures affecting the vertebral column of the spine
- Most common type of osteoporotic fracture (PMID: 10692972)
- Also frequently arise from an underlying osteolytic lesion of the spine (2)
- Fracture location usually located on the anterior column of the spine
- Compared to burst fractures that involve the posterior osseous ligamentous complex (1)
- Often causes wide range of symptoms that include pain, disability, progressive kyphosis, and impaired quality of life (3–7)

## Epidemiology and Risk Factors

- 1.5 million adults affected in the US population annually (3)
- Incidence:
  - 10.7 % of all women (3)
  - 5.7% of all men (3)
  - 25% of all postmenopausal women (3)
  - 30% age >80 (4)
  - 5–10% age <80 (4)
- Site of fracture varies
  - Most frequent site: thoracolumbar junction (T12 to L2): 60–75% (1)
  - Second most frequent site: L2 to L5 region: 30% (1)
- Common risk factors for VCFs (2)
  - Osteoporosis (1)
  - Increased age
  - Previous VCF or osteoporotic fracture
  - Female

- ○ Obesity
- ○ Spinal metastasis (32)
- ○ Myeloma (32)
- ○ Radiation exposure (35)
- ○ Hormone dysregulation (38)
- ○ Low-impact trauma (fall from standing)
- ○ Secondary fractures
  - ▪ Prior fracture (40)
  - ▪ Spinal misalignment (40)
  - ▪ Prior vertebroplasty/kyphoplasty (40)

# Pathophysiology

- Characterized by any mechanism that causes bones to weaken and therefore increases an individual's susceptibility to fracture
- Fracture caused by any trauma causing force greater than the existing bone mineral density can handle
- Specifically, weight-bearing bones such as the vertebrae and hips are at highest risk
- Younger individuals (major trauma): (1)
  - ○ Motor vehicle collision (50%)
  - ○ Fall with axial force (25%)
- Older Individuals (Minor Trauma) (1)
  - ○ Fall from standing

## Osteoporosis

- Decreased bone mineral density disrupts the normal microarchitecture of the bone, made of noncollagenous proteins, leading to structural deterioration (1)
- Bone density progressively decreases until nearly half of normal axial bone mass is lost by age 80 (31)

## Low Estrogen Effects

- Estrogen directly inhibits bone resorption and bone remodeling through modulation of osteoblasts, osteocytes, and osteoclasts
- In postmenopausal women, lack of estrogen increases bone resorption through multiple pathways, causing an overall decrease in bone mineral density

## Gestation

- During gestation and lactation, calcium is mobilized from the maternal bone structure to provide nutrients for the developing fetus and child
- An overall decrease in maternal calcium available for bone remodeling is one reason transient bone weakening is seen during pregnancy

## Atypical Light Chain Amyloidosis

- Amyloidosis includes the extracellular deposition of proteins in various locations, including the bony matrix that causes an overall weakening of the bone
- Keeping this disease in the differential for causation is important, because as a treatable disease it is reversible (45)

# Diagnosis

- Diagnosis of vertebral compression fractures is made through a combination of patient history, physical exam maneuvers, radiologic imaging, and even potentially biopsy
- Symptoms (3–7)
  - Often asymptomatic and/or incidental finding on X-ray
  - Localized pain (rarely radiates)
    - Increased with Valsalva maneuver, lifting, changing position
  - Gradual height loss
  - Gradually increasing kyphosis
  - Impaired lung function
  - Spinal cord compression
  - Motors/sensory deficits
- Morbidities (5)
  - Deconditioning
  - Atelectasis / pneumonia
  - Permanent loss of mobility
  - Decreasing quality of life
  - Disability
  - Bed sores
  - Increasing mortality (6,7)
- Physical exam maneuvers should be used when a compression fracture is high on the differential as a gateway to writing for radiologic testing

- ○ Closed fist percussion (44)
  - ▪ Sensitivity 87.5%
  - ▪ Specificity: 90%
- ○ Inability to lay supine due to pain (44)
  - ▪ Sensitivity 81.25%
  - ▪ Specificity 93.3%
- Plain anterior-posterior and lateral radiographs of thoracolumbar spine (1) are usually the first-line formal diagnostic tool
  - ○ Radiologic grades (PMID: 8237484)
    - ▪ Grade 1: 20–25% height deformity
    - ▪ Grade 2: 25–40% height deformity
    - ▪ Grade 3: > 40% height deformity
  - ○ CT and MRI are the current gold standard to distinguish acute versus chronic based on the integrity of posterior ligamentous complex (1)
    - ▪ Able to accurately predict VCF complications such as height loss, induced kyphosis, and progression of osteoporosis (47)
    - ▪ Classifies VCFs by fracture type; concave, dented, swelled-type, bow-shaped, and projecting. These classifications, when used in conjunction with fracture location, have been efficacious in determining when to employ conservative measures and when to intervene with invasive means of stabilization (48)
- Biopsy
  - ○ Imaging and physical exam do not elicit diagnosis; percutaneous core biopsies will distinguish between osteoporosis, metastases, or other nonidentifiable pathologies (46)
- Screening should be performed to look for underlying reasons of a weakened bone matrix and includes:
  - ○ Laboratory workup (43)
    - ▪ CBC
    - ▪ CMP with LFTs
    - ▪ Erythrocyte sedimentation rate
    - ▪ TSH

- 25-OH Vitamin D
- PTH
- C-reactive protein level
  ○ Bone mineral density testing (bone densitometry / DEXA)
    ■ Evaluates absorption of small amounts of dual-energy X-ray radiation by bones
      • T-score $\geq -1$ is normal
      • T-score from $-1.1$ to $-2.4$ is osteopenia
      • T-score $\leq -2.5$ is osteoporosis
    ■ Current National Osteoporosis Foundation Guidelines for individuals who should be screened for osteoporosis (https://www.nof.org/patients/diagnosis-information/bone-density-examtesting/)
      • Women >65 or menopausal with risk factors
      • Men >70 or 50–69 with risk factors
      • Fracture age >50

# Treatment Modalities

- Two main pillars of treatment include nonoperative, conservative treatment versus operative interventions
- Unfortunately, the heterogeneity of research has made it difficult to establish appropriate guidelines (see below)

## Conservative Treatment

- Two thirds of VCFs resolve with conservative management and analgesia
- Multimodal oral analgesics including acetaminophen, calcitonin, lidocaine patches, muscle relaxants, opioid narcotics, and NSAIDs
- Rehabilitative exercise is important as the patient can tolerate it to help strengthen the muscles and rebuild the bone through natural loading
- Osteoporosis treatment including calcitonin, bisphosphonates, and RANK ligand inhibitors is important for prevention of susceptibility to future fractures
- Spinal orthotics are also useful to offload the at-risk area and help promote long-term healing
- Multimodal therapy is recommended to allow the patient the ability to heal optimally (49)

- Risks of conservative treatment mainly focus on opioid dependence – the risk of overuse and dependency in the short term may outweigh the benefits of its analgesic effects, especially in cases necessitating long-term management (50–54)

## Vertebral Augmentation

- Vertebroplasty and kyphoplasty are procedures used to stabilize compressive fractures
  - Vertebroplasty – the simple injection of bone cement into the vertebral body to increase the rate of healing
  - Kyphoplasty – balloon inflated in the vertebral body to create a potential space that bone cement is injected into (42)
- Balloon kyphoplasty tends to have better height restoration than vertebroplasty
- Goals to mitigate the pain and immobility which accompany vertebral compression fractures (41)
- There has been a significant decline in utilization of interventional techniques over the past decade (19–22,55–58)
- Clinicians may at times initially hesitate to recommend intervention; there are data that vertebroplasty and kyphoplasty are safe procedures and can provide utility by achieving pain relief in more severe cases than conservative measures

## Published Research and Guidelines Regarding Treatment Recommendations
## Research Supporting Invasive Procedures

- *2009 (Journal of Neurointerventional Surgery)*: statement developed by five major societies of neurological surgeons and radiologists deem vertebral augmentation as appropriate therapy for treatment of painful vertebral compression fractures (18)
- Multiple systematic reviews, guidelines, clinical trials, cost-effectiveness studies, and quality-of-life studies have demonstrated the effectiveness of vertebral augmentation procedures in the treatment of compression fractures when compared with real-world evidence (4,6,8–10,11–15,22–40)
- Beall et al. (4) "based on 25 Level I and Level II studies, balloon kyphoplasty had significantly better and vertebroplasty tended to have better pain reduction compared with nonsurgical management"

- National Institute for Health and Care Excellence (NICE) technology appraisal guidance (24) also approved augmentation procedures for vertebral compression fractures
- Vertebroplasty for Acute Painful Osteoporotic Fractures (VAPOUR) trial, which is the only blinded trial of vertebroplasty restricted to this patient group, was not appropriately represented

## Research Supporting Conservative Management

- 2015 *Spine*: over a million patients with vertebral compression fractures treated with vertebral augmentation that there is a significant reduction in morbidity and mortality as compared with patients treated with nonsurgical management (11)
- 2009 (*New England Journal of Medicine)* published two randomized trials, each of which demonstrated no beneficial effect of vertebroplasty over sham procedure (17,18)
- 2018 (Cochrane Review): "no demonstrable clinical important benefits of percutaneous vertebroplasty compared with placebo or sham procedure, and sensitivity analysis confirmed that open trials comparing vertebroplasty with usual care are likely to have overestimated any benefit of vertebroplasty"

## Conclusions

- Vertebral compression fractures are characterized by a break in the vertebrae comprising the spinal column, most likely on the anterior side and most commonly occurring when the osseous matrix has been weakened
- There is high morbidity and mortality associated with VCFs that have given rise to an estimated annual medical cost of ₵13.8 billion in the United States alone (31)
- Prevention includes screening at-risk individuals' bone marrow density and augmenting individuals with decreased bone density with bisphosphonates or RANK ligand inhibitors
- The management of VCFs has been heavily debated with argu ments for both conservative management and invasive augmentation through vertebroplasty and kyphoplasty
- Invasive management should be considered in patients with uncontrolled pain, significant vertebral misalignment, and height deformities

# References

1. Donnally II C, Varacallo M. Vertebral compression fractures. *J Community Nurs*. 2018;**25**(6):39–42.

2. Montagu A, Speirs A, Baldock J, Corbett J, Gosney M. A review of vertebroplasty for osteoporotic and malignant vertebral compression fractures. *Age Ageing*. 2012;**41**(4):450–455.

3. Alexandru D, So W. Evaluation and management of vertebral compression fractures. *Perm J*. 2012;**16**(4):46–51.

4. Beall D, Lorio MP, Yun BM et al. Review of vertebral augmentation: An updated meta-analysis of the effectiveness. *Int J Spine Surg*. 2018;**12**(3):295–321.

5. Babayev M, Lachmann E, Nagler W. The controversy surrounding sacral insufficiency fractures: To ambulate or not to ambulate? *Am J Phys Med Rehabil*. 2000;**79**(4):404–409.

6. Lau E, Ong K, Kurtz S, Schmier J, Edidin A. Mortality following the diagnosis of a vertebral compression fracture in the Medicare population. *J Bone Joint Surg Am*. 2008;**90**(7):1479–1486.

7. Cauley JA, Thompson DE, Ensrud KC, Scott JC, Black D. Risk of mortality following clinical fractures. *Osteoporos Int*. 2000;**11**(7):556–561.

8. Chen AT, Cohen DB, Skolasky RL. Impact of nonoperative treatment, vertebroplasty, and kyphoplasty on survival and morbidity after vertebral compression fracture in the Medicare population. *J Bone Joint Surg Am*. 2013;**95**(19):1729–1736.

9. Edidin AA, Ong KL, Lau E, Kurtz SM. Mortality risk for operated and nonoperated vertebral fracture patients in the Medicare population. *J Bone Miner Res*. 2011;**26**(7):617–626.

10. Lange A, Kasperk C, Alvares L, Sauermann S, Braun S. Survival and cost comparison of kyphoplasty and percutaneous vertebroplasty using German claims data. *Spine (Phila Pa 1976)*. 2014;**39**(4):318–326.

11. Edidin AA, Ong KL, Lau E, Kurtz SM. Morbidity and mortality after vertebral fractures: Comparison of vertebral augmentation and nonoperative management in the Medicare population. *Spine (Phila Pa 1976)*. 2015;**40**(15):1228–1241.

12. Clerk-Lamalice O, Beall DP, Ong K, Lorio MP. ISASS policy 2018 –Vertebral augmentation: Coverage indications, limitations, and/or medical necessity. *Int J Spine Surg*. 2019;**13**(1):1–10.

13. Mattie R, Laimi K, Yu S, Saltychev M. Comparing percutaneous vertebroplasty and conservative therapy for treating osteoporotic compression fractures in the thoracic and lumbar spine: A systematic review and meta-analysis. *J Bone Joint Surg Am*. 2016;**98**(12):1041–1051.

14. Xiao H, Yang J, Feng X et al. Comparing complications of vertebroplasty and kyphoplasty for treating osteoporotic vertebral compression fractures: A meta-analysis of the randomized and non-randomized controlled studies. *Eur J Orthop Surg Traumatol.* 2015;**25**(Suppl 1):S77–S85.

15. Zhang H, Xu C, Zhang T, Gao Z, Zhang T. Does percutaneous vertebroplasty or balloon kyphoplasty for osteoporotic vertebral compression fractures increase the incidence of new vertebral fractures? A meta-analysis. *Pain Physician* 2017;**20**(1):E13–E28.

16. Jensen ME, McGraw JK, Cardella JF, Hirsch JA. Position statement on percutaneous vertebral augmentation: A consensus statement developed by the American Society of Interventional and Therapeutic Neuroradiology, Society of Interventional Radiology, American Association of Neurological Surgeons/Congress of Neurological Surgeons, and American Society of Spine Radiology. *J Neurointerv Surg.* 2009;**1**(2):181–185.

17. Buchbinder R, Osborne RH, Ebeling PR et al. A randomized trial of vertebroplasty for painful osteoporotic vertebral fractures. *N Engl J Med.* 2009;**361**(6):557–568.

18. Kallmes DF, Comstock BA, Heagerty PJ et al. A randomized trial of vertebroplasty for osteoporotic spinal fractures. *N Engl J Med.* 2009;**361**(6):569–579.

19. Manchikanti L, Helm S, Benyamin RM, Hirsch JA. A critical analysis of Obamacare: Affordable care or insurance for many and coverage for few? *Pain Physician.* 2017;**20**(3):111–138.

20. Obama B. United States health care reform: Progress to date and next steps. *JAMA.* 2016; **316**:525–532.

21. Manchikanti L, Helm II S, Calodney AK, Hirsch JA. Merit-based incentive payment system: Meaningful changes in the final rule brings cautious optimism. *Pain Physician.* 2017;**20**(1):E1–E12.

22. Medicare Administrative Contractor Multijurisdictional Contractor Advisory Committee (CAC) meeting re Vertebral Augmentation. March 20, 2019. www.ngsmedicare.com/sv/contractor-advisory-committee-cac?lo b=93617%26state=97256%26rgion=93623%26selectedArticleId=446297

23. Beall DP, Chambers MR, Thomas S et al. Prospective and multicenter evaluation of outcomes for quality of life and activities of daily living for balloon kyphoplasty in the treatment of vertebral compression fractures: The EVOLVE trial. *Neurosurg.* 2019;**84**(1):169–178.

24. National Institute for Health and Care Excellence. Percutaneous vertebroplasty and percutaneous balloon kyphoplasty for treating osteoporotic vertebral compression fractures. April 24, 2013. www.nice.org.uk/guidance/ta279.

25. Ong KL, Beall DP, Frohbergh M, Lau E, Hirsch JA. Were VCF patients at higher risk of mortality following the 2009 publication of the vertebroplasty "sham" trials? *Osteoporos Int.* 2018;**29**(2):375–383.

26. Johnell O, Kanis JA, Odén A et al. Mortality after osteoporotic fractures. *Osteoporos Int.* 2004;**15**(3):38–42.

27. Hirsch JA, Beall DP, Chambers MR et al. Management of vertebral fragility fractures: A clinical care pathway developed by a multispecialty panel using the RAND/UCLA Appropriateness Method. *Spine J.* 2018;**18**(11):2152–2161. doi: 10.1016/j.spinee.2018.07.025.

28. Marcia S, Muto M, Hirsch JA et al. What is the role of vertebral augmentation for osteoporotic fractures? A review of the recent literature. *Neuroradiol.* 2018;**60**(8):777–783.

29. Chandra RV, Maingard J, Asadi H et al. Vertebroplasty and kyphoplasty for osteoporotic vertebral fractures: What are the latest data? *AJNR Am J Neuroradiol.* 2018;**39**(5):798–806.

30. Barr JD, Jensen ME, Hirsch JA et al. Position statement on percutaneous vertebral augmentation: A consensus statement developed by the Society of Interventional Radiology (SIR), American Association of Neurological Surgeons (AANS) and the Congress of Neurological Surgeons (CNS), American College of Radiology (ACR), American Society of Neuroradiology (ASNR), American Society of Spine Radiology (ASSR), Canadian Interventional Radiology Association (CIRA), and the Society of NeuroInterventional Surgery (SNIS). *J Vasc Interv Radiol.* 2014;**25**(2):171–181.

31. Wong CC, McGirt MJ. Vertebral compression fractures: A review of current management and multimodal therapy. *J Multidiscip Healthc.* 2013;**6**:205–214.

32. Thibault I, Whyne CM, Zhou S et al. Volume of lytic vertebral body metastatic disease quantified using computed tomography-based image segmentation predicts fracture risk after spine stereotactic body radiation therapy. *Int J Radiat Oncol.* 2017;**97**(1):75–81.

33. Hussain A, Yong C, Tkaczuk KHR et al. Prevalence and risk of skeletal complications and use of radiation therapy in elderly women diagnosed with metastatic breast cancer. *PLoS One.* 2018;**13**(3):e0193661.

34. Jawad MS, Fahim DK, Gerszten PC et al. Vertebral compression fractures after stereotactic body radiation therapy: A large, multi-institutional, multinational evaluation. *J Neurosurg Spine.* 2016;**24**(6):928–936.

35. Boyce-Fappiano D, Elibe E, Schultz L et al. Analysis of the factors contributing to vertebral compression fractures after spine stereotactic radiosurgery. *Int J Radiat Oncol.* 2017;**97**(2):236–245.

36. Matsumoto Y, Shinoto M, Endo M et al. Evaluation of risk factors for vertebral compression fracture after carbon-ion radiotherapy for primary spinal and paraspinal sarcoma. *Biomed Res Int.* 2017;**2017**:9467402.

37. Otani K, Teshima T, Ito Y et al. Risk factors for vertebral compression fractures in preoperative chemoradiotherapy with gemcitabine for pancreatic cancer. *Radiother Oncol.* 2016;**118**(3):424–429.

38. Yun KY, Han SE, Kim SC, Joo JK, Lee KS. Pregnancy-related osteoporosis and spinal fractures. *Obstet Gynecol Sci.* 2017;**60**(1):133.

39. Krishnakumar R, Kumar A, Kuzhimattam M. Spinal compression fractures due to pregnancy-associated osteoporosis. *J Craniovertebr Junction Spine.* 2016;**7**(4):224.

40. Zhang Y-L, Shi L-T, Tang P-F, Sun Z-J, Wang Y-H. Correlation analysis of osteoporotic vertebral compression fractures and spinal sagittal imbalance. *Orthopade.* 2017;**46**(3):249–255.

41. Takahara K, Kamimura M, Moriya H et al. Risk factors of adjacent vertebral collapse after percutaneous vertebroplasty for osteoporotic vertebral fracture in postmenopausal women. *BMC Musculoskelet Disord.* 2016;**17**(1):12.

42. Deibert CP, Gandhoke GS, Paschel EE, Gerszten PC. A longitudinal cohort investigation of the development of symptomatic adjacent level compression fractures following balloon-assisted kyphoplasty in a series of 726 patients. *Pain Physician.* 2016;**19**(8):E1167–1172.

43. Miller PD. Clinical management of vertebral compression fractures. *J Clin Densitom.* 2016;**19**(1):97–101.

44. Langdon J, Way A, Heaton S, Bernard J, Molloy S. Vertebral compression fractures – new clinical signs to aid diagnosis. *Ann R Coll Surg Engl.* 2010;**92**(2):163–166.

45. Wu X, Feng J, Cao X et al. Atypical immunoglobulin light chain amyloidosis. *Medicine (Baltimore).* 2016;**95**(36):e4603.

46. Pagdal SS, Nadkarni S, Hardikar SM, Hardikar MS. Role of transpedicular percutaneous vertebral biopsy for diagnosis of pathology in vertebral compression fractures. *Asian Spine J.* 2016;**10**(5):925.

47. Nguyen HS, Soliman HM, Patel M et al. CT Hounsfield units as a predictor for the worsening of traumatic vertebral compression fractures. *World Neurosurg.* 2016;**93**:50–54.

48. Muratore M, Ferrera A, Masse A, Bistolfi A. Osteoporotic vertebral fractures: predictive factors for conservative treatment failure: A systematic review. *Eur Spine J.* 2018;**27**(10):2565–2576.

49. Ameis A, Randhawa K, Yu H et al. The Global Spine Care Initiative: a review of reviews and recommendations for the non-invasive management of acute osteoporotic vertebral compression fracture pain in low- and middle-income communities. *Eur Spine J.* 2018;**27**(S6):861–869.

50. Manchikanti L, Kaye AM, Knezevic NN et al. Responsible, safe, and effective prescription of opioids for chronic non-cancer pain: American society of

interventional pain physicians (ASIPP) guidelines. *Pain Physician*. 2017: **20** (2S):S3–S92.

51. Manchikanti L, Sanapati J, Benyamin RM et al. Reframing the prevention strategies of the opioid crisis: Focusing on prescription opioids, fentanyl, and heroin epidemic. *Pain Physician*. 2018;**21**(4):309–326.

52. Kaye AD, Jones MR, Kaye AM et al. Prescription opioid abuse in chronic pain: An updated review of opioid abuse predictors and strategies to curb opioid abuse: Part 2. *Pain Physician*. 2017;**20**(2S):S111–S133.

53. Kaye AD, Jones MR, Kaye AM et al. Prescription opioid abuse in chronic pain: An updated review of opioid abuse predictors and strategies to curb opioid abuse: Part 1. *Pain Physician*. 2017;**20**(2S):S93–S109.

54. Chakravarthy K, Manchikanti L, Kaye AD, Christo PJ. Reframing the role of neuromodulation therapy in the chronic pain treatment paradigm. *Pain Physician*. 2018;**21**(6):507–513.

55. Manchikanti L, Pampati V, Benyamin RM, Hirsch JA. Cost calculation methodology exacerbates site-of-service differentials by 10- to 18-fold for soft tissue and joint injections in hospital outpatient departments. *IPM Reports*. 2017;**1**(6):183–189.

56. Manchikanti L, Soin A, Mann DP et al. Reversal of growth of utilization of interventional techniques in managing chronic pain in Medicare population post Affordable Care Act. *Pain Physician*. 2017;**20**(7):551–567.

57. Manchikanti L, Soin A, Mann DP et al. Comparative analysis of utilization of epidural procedures in managing chronic pain in the Medicare population: Pre and post Affordable Care Act. *Spine (Phila Pa 1976)*. 2019;**44**(3):220–232.

58. Manchikanti MV, Manchikanti L, Kaye AD, Pampati V, Hirsch JA. Usage patterns of sacroiliac joint injections – a comparative evaluation of pre and post Affordable Care Act in Medicare population. *IPM Reports*. 2018;**2** (5):157–166.

# Chapter 17

# Sacral Insufficiency Fractures

Karina Charipova, Cyrus Yazdi,
and Kyle Gress

## Sacral Insufficiency Fracture Pain

- Sacral insufficiency fractures (SIF) are a common, often over-looked, source of low back pain (LBP)
  - First described by Lourie in 1982 (1)
  - Defined as a "spontaneous osteoporotic fracture of the sacrum" (1)
  - Can cause severe pain in the back, buttock, hips, groin, and pelvis
  - Have the potential to significantly impact mobility and quality of life
- LBP is associated with significant disability, healthcare expenditure, and treatment risk
  - Nearly 1 in 4 adults suffers from LBP (2,3)
  - The cost of LBP, accounting for lost productivity and wages, exceeds $100 billion (2,3)
  - Prescription of opioids for musculoskeletal conditions, including LBP, has contributed to the rise of US opioid-related deaths (4–7)
  - Nonopioid treatment modalities are being explored but are frequently associated with high costs (8–10)

## Epidemiology and Risk Factors

- Incidence of SIF is estimated to be between 1.0 and 5.0% (11)
- Variability in reported SIF incidence likely due to delay of diagnosis due to nonspecific symptoms and subtle presentation of SIF on X-ray (12)
- The majority of SIF patients are over age 55; predominant age group is 70–75 years
- SIF presents more subtly on X-ray than other types of pelvic fractures (12)

- Risk factors (13–19)
  - Osteoporosis
  - Steroid-induced osteopenia
  - Pregnancy
  - Postmenopause
  - Rheumatoid arthritis
  - Malignancy
  - Pelvic radiation
  - Metabolic bone disorders (e.g., osteomalacia, hyperparathyroidism, Paget's disease, osteodystrophy)
- Osteoporosis is one of the most common conditions linked to SIF (18)
- Metabolic bone disorders are more loosely linked with SIF in the literature (19)

## Pathophysiology

- Sacrum is made up of five fused vertebrae (S1–S5) and three to five small fused bones forming the coccyx
  - Both are weight-bearing structures
  - The alae, lateral projections of the sacrum, articulate with the ilium to form the sacroiliac joint (20,21)
- Sacrum and coccyx are integral for stabilization of the pelvis and functional lumbar support for standing, walking, and sitting (20,21)
  - Sacroiliac joints relieve torsional stress created during the alternating flexion and extension of the lower extremities (20)
  - In patients with sacroiliac pathology (i.e., rheumatoid arthritis) mechanical stress is transferred to the sacrum (20)
  - When sacrum is weakened by conditions like osteoporosis, it cannot withstand stress and can fracture (20)
- SIF results from the interplay of a compromised sacroiliac joint and weakened sacrum (20)

## Diagnosis

### Presentation

- SIF is a challenging diagnosis given its nonspecific symptoms and variable, often subtle findings on X-ray
  - Pain may frequently be endorsed in the back and legs

- ○ Due to nonspecific symptoms, workup may mistakenly focus on lumbar, rather than sacral, region
- ○ Patients with SIF may have concurrent vertebral or iliac fractures, leading to endorsement of hip and thigh pain (22–25)
- Physical exam may be normal (20)
  - ○ Some patients present with diminished ankle reflexes
  - ○ Some may present with back extension restricted by pain

## Approach to Diagnosis

- In a study of 50 SIF patients presenting with nonspecific symptoms, 74% were definitively diagnosed with MRI, 12% diagnosed with CT, 12% diagnosed with X-ray, and 1% diagnosed with bone scintigraphy (18)
- X-ray may be entirely unremarkable
  - ○ X-ray has low sensitivity for SIF
  - ○ Only 28–38% of SIF are visible on X-ray
  - ○ Fracture is most often seen in the sacral ala
  - ○ Fracture lines are estimated to be visible in only 12.5% of cases (20)
  - ○ If using X-ray, anterior-posterior and lateral lumbar spine as well as anterior-posterior pelvis shots are recommended (26)
  - ○ If X-ray is negative but SIF suspicion remains, MRI should be obtained
- MRI may be notable for disc degeneration, lumbar stenosis, or hyper-intensity with foraminal stenosis in the sacral region
  - ○ Recommended imaging modality for SIF diagnosis (18)
  - ○ Advanced SIF has been associated with sacral edema on MRI
  - ○ MRI especially helpful in older patients with LBP and associated osteoporosis or corticosteroid use (18)
- SIF can appear similar to degenerative disc disease, arthritis, and synovitis on bone scintigraphy
  - ○ May be used as supplemental imaging in addition to MRI or CT
  - ○ May be helpful in early stages of SIF when presenting pain is atypical or unspecific
  - ○ Bone scans can help rule in/out concurrent vertebral fractures

## Denis Classification

- The Denis system is a spinal injury classification system based on radiological findings (27)
  - Divides spinal motion segment into 3 columns or "zones" (27)
  - Zone 1: Most lateral sacral fractures, involving sacral ala (27)
    - Most common location of SIF
    - Patients with osteoporosis experience increased trabecular bone loss in the sacral ala, increasing risk for SIF in this region
  - Zone 2: Sacral fracture involving neural foramina (27)
  - Zone 3: Medial sacral fracture involving sacral bodies and transverse central canal (27)
    - Fractures in this region tend to occur vertically
    - Horizontal component may sometimes be seen on MRI as the "H" or "Honda" sign
    - Horizontal tends to occur in more advanced disease when the center of sacrum becomes unable to support the weight of the upper body

## Treatment

### Conservative Management

- Mainstays for SIF treatment have traditionally been conservative: modified bed rest, physical therapy, injection therapy, and traditional analgesics
- Bed rest was traditionally recommended for 3–6 months following a fracture
  - Prolonged bed rest is associated with increased risk of deep vein thrombosis (DVT), muscular atrophy, and cardiac dysfunction (28)
  - Immobility can accelerate osteoclastic bone resorption and diminish bone mineralization
- Recent literature suggests early mobilization may improve outcomes and reduce complication rates (22)
  - Early mobilization stimulates osteoblastic bone formation
  - Weight-bearing exercises (modifiable with assistive devices) and aqua therapy shown to aid in rehabilitation

- A majority of patients with SIF endorse symptom improvement within 1–2 weeks of conservative management (23)
- Significant reduction in pain and increase in mobility seen after 6 months (23)

- Pain control is a focus of SIF treatment
  - Opioids, acetaminophen, and nonsteroidal anti-inflammatory drugs (NSAIDs) are frequently prescribed
  - Recent literature suggests NSAIDs may impair endochondral ossification (29)
  - NSAIDs may reduce bone mineral density and delay fracture healing

- Management of osteoporosis is critical to prevention and treatment of SIF
  - Bone mineralization requires adequate levels of calcium and vitamin D
  - Recommended daily dosages are 1200 mg calcium and 800 IU vitamin D (29,30)
  - Bisphosphonates are approved for treatment of osteoporosis; long-term use is associated with reduced bone remodeling; patients require reassessment after 5 years of use (31)

- Teriparatide is a recombinant form of parathyroid hormone (PTH) proposed to treat SIF
  - Demonstrated to increase bone mineral density and osseous tissue volume; can reduce fracture healing time (32,33,28,34)
  - Retrospective, case-controlled study found that patients with MRI-confirmed SIF receiving 20 micrograms of teriparatide for 3 months had improvement of VAS, reduced analgesic use, reduced time to mobilization, and reduced time to fracture healing (19)
  - Case report of patients with bilateral SIF refractory to traditional management endorsed improvement following 6 months of teriparatide (34)
  - Efficacy of long-term treatment is not yet known (35)

## Minimally Invasive Management

- Sacroplasty and balloon sacroplasty (BSP) are minimally invasive, percutaneous, image-guided techniques for targeted treatment of SIF (36)

- o Both techniques are frequently used in malignancy with primary or metastatic involvement of the sacrum (36)
- o Sacroplasty involves injection of polymethylmethacrylate (PMMA) cement into the compromised bone, improving structural integrity (36)
- o BSP involves the inflation of a balloon catheter within the fracture bone to regain height prior to injection of cement (36)
- o Fluoroscopic guidance may help to improve safety of sacroplasty by enabling full visualization of the needle tip to prevent damage to vital structures (37)

- Sacroplasty has been shown to improve pain scores and participation in activities of daily living (ADLs)
  - o A small study of 16 patients with radiologically confirmed SIF reported significantly improved pain on VAS starting from postoperative day one (38)
  - o Mean initial Oswestry Disability Index (ODI) scores were 59%, improved to 14.8% at three months postop (38)
  - o A prospective study of 15 patients with SIF refractory to conservative treatment also observed pain improvement on VAS both immediately and 1 year following sacroplasty (39)
  - o Pain relief from sacroplasty is believed to be both safe and durable
  - o Larger multicenter studies have supported that CT-guided percutaneous sacroplasty is a safe and effective treatment option for patients with both SIF and pathological sacral lesions (40)

- Long-term outcomes of sacroplasty are promising (41)
  - o A 10-year study compared sacroplasty to conservative management (41)
  - o Sacroplasty group experienced greater pain reduction based on VAS score (41)
  - o All patients in the sacroplasty group ceased use of analgesics at 10-year follow-up (41)
  - o The most common complication was PMMA leakage, found to have little to no clinical implications (41)

- In a comparison of sacroplasty with and without balloon assistance, the balloon-assisted procedure took significantly longer to perform (36)
  - o BSP was associated with less cement leakage (36)

- ○ Both procedures associated with significant improvement of symptoms (36)
- Radiofrequency sacroplasty (RFS) is an alternative to BSP in which a flexible osteotome, rather than a balloon, is used to create space for plaster insertion (42)
  - ○ PMMA cement activated by radiofrequency before delivery into cavity (42)
  - ○ Comparison of RFS and BSP with CT guidance in 40 SIF patients found that both alleviated pain with minimal PMMA leakage, leaving choice to surgeon preference (42)

## Surgical Management
- SIF presents challenges to surgical fixation as it affects osteoporotic bone, making screw fixation difficult
  - ○ Transsacral bar achieves more reliable stabilization and interfragmentary compression than transiliac screw fixation (43)
  - ○ Iliosacral fixation is also used, but may be associated with higher rates of screw loosening (44)
  - ○ Lumbosacral fixation is believed to be a viable option for patients with advanced disease and resulting neurologic symptoms (45)
- Transiliac-transsacral screw stabilization can be offered to patients with refractory pain (46)
  - ○ Small study of forty-one patients comparing transiliac-transsacral screw fixation with nonoperative treatment found that surgical treatment is associated with a greater decrease in VAS pain score (3.9 vs. 0.6) (46)
  - ○ Patient satisfaction with treatment is high (46)
  - ○ Patients are able to maintain mobility and freedom from pain for at least 12 months postoperatively
- Cement augmentation to screw fixation may help to improve structural stability
  - ○ New technique proposes insertion of percutaneous screw and use of screw to introduce aqueous calcium phosphate cement (47)
  - ○ This procedure requires a long-term study

## Conclusion

- SIF is not uncommon, especially in the elderly, and is associated with a significant decrease in quality of life
- SIF is most frequently found in patients with sacroiliac joint pathology in the setting of a sacrum compromised due to conditions such as osteoporosis, rheumatoid arthritis, or radiation therapy
- Nonspecific symptoms of SIF make diagnosis challenging
- MRI is the gold standard for diagnosis of SIF
- Traditional therapies revolved around conservative measures such as bed rest, physical therapy, and analgesia
- Conservative management is safe; minimally invasive treatments such as sacroplasty may provide improved short- and long-term relief
- Surgical management with screw fixation is a viable option for qualifying patients and can be offered in conjunction with cement augmentation

## References

1. Zhiyong C, Yun T, Hui F, Zhongwei Y, Zhaorui L. Unilateral versus bilateral balloon kyphoplasty for osteoporotic vertebral compression fractures: A systematic review of overlapping meta-analyses. *Pain Physician*. 2019;**22**:15–28.

2. Dieleman JL, Baral R, Birger M et al. US spending on personal health care and public health, 1996–2013. *JAMA*. 2016;**316**:2627–2646.

3. Dieleman JL, Squires E, Bui AL et al. Factors associated with increase in US health care spending, 1996–2013. *JAMA*. 2017;**318**:1668–1678.

4. Manchikanti L, Kaye AM, Knezevic NN et al. Responsible, safe, and effective prescription of opioids for chronic non-cancer pain: American Society of Interventional Pain Physicians (ASIPP) guidelines. *Pain Physician*. 2017;**20**: S3–S92.

5. Sanger N, Bhatt M, Singhal N, Ramsden K et al. Adverse outcomes associated with prescription opioids for acute low back pain: a systematic review and meta-analysis. *Pain Physician*. 2019;**22**:119–138.

6. U.S. Department of Health and Human Services. Pain Management Best Practices Inter-Agency Task Force. Final Report on Pain Management Best Practices: Updates, Gaps, Inconsistencies, and Recommendations. May 9, 2019. www.hhs.gov/ash/advisory-committees/pain/reports/index.html.

7. Manchikanti L, Sanapati J, Benyamin RM et al. Reframing the prevention strategies of the opioid crisis: Focusing on prescription opioids, fentanyl, and heroin epidemic. *Pain Physician.* 2018;21:309–326.

8. Manchikanti L, Soin A, Mann DP et al. Reversal of growth of utilization of interventional techniques in managing chronic pain in Medicare population post Affordable Care Act. *Pain Physician.* 2017;20:551–567.

9. Manchikanti L, Soin A, Mann DP et al. Utilization patterns of facet joint interventions in managing spinal pain: a retrospective cohort study in the US fee-for-service Medicare population. *Curr Pain Headache.* Rep 2019;23:73.

10. Manchikanti L, Soin A, Mann DP et al. Comparative analysis of utilization of epidural procedures in managing chronic pain in the Medicare population: Pre and post Affordable Care Act. *Spine (Phila Pa 1976).* 2019;44:220–232.

11. Grasland A. Sacral insufficiency fractures. *Arch Intern Med.* 2011;156:668–674.

12. Tamaki Y, Nagamachi A, Inoue K et al. Incidence and clinical features of sacral insufficiency fracture in the emergency department. *Am J Emerg Med.* 2017;35:1314–1316.

13. Sakaguchi M, Maebayashi T, Aizawa T, Ishibashi N. Risk factors for sacral insufficiency fractures in cervical cancer after whole pelvic radiation therapy. *Anticancer Res.* 2019;39:361–367.

14. Zhang L, He Q, Jiang M et al. Diagnosis of insufficiency fracture after radiotherapy in patients with cervical cancer: Contribution of technetium Tc 99 m-labeled methylene diphosphonate single-photon emission computed tomography/computed tomography. *Int J Gynecol Cancer.* 2018;28:1369–1376.

15. Bostel T, Nicolay NH, Welzel T et al. Sacral insufficiency fractures after high-dose carbon-ion based radiotherapy of sacral chordomas. *Radiat Oncol.* 2018;13:1–7.

16. Kawamoto T, Ito K, Furuya T, Sasai K, Karasawa K. Sacral insufficiency fracture after stereotactic body radiation therapy for sacral metastasis. *Clin Case Reports.* 2018;6:2293–2294.

17. Hmida B, Boudokhane S, Migaou H et al. Postpartum sacral stress fracture associated with mechanical sacroiliac joint disease: A case report. *Medicine (Baltimore).* 2018;97:e11735.

18. Kinoshita H, Miyakoshi N, Kobayashi T et al. Comparison of patients with diagnosed and suspected sacral insufficiency fractures. *J Orthop Sci.* 2019;24:702–707.

19. Yoo JI, Ha YC, Ryu HJ et al. Teriparatide treatment in elderly patients with sacral insufficiency fracture. *J Clin Endocrinol Metab.* 2017;102:560–565.

20. Vleeming A, Schuenke MD, Masi AT et al. The sacroiliac joint: An overview of its anatomy, function and potential clinical implications. *J Anat.* 2012;**221**:537–567.

21. Poiliot AJ, Zwirner J, Doyle T, Hammer N. A systematic review of the normal sacroiliac joint anatomy and adjacent tissues for pain physicians. *Pain Physician.* 2019;**22**:E247–E274.

22. Parry SM, Puthucheary ZA. The impact of extended bed rest on the musculoskeletal system in the critical care environment. *Extrem Physiol Med.* 2015;**4**:16.

23. Lin JT, Lane JM. Sacral Stress Fractures. *J Women's Heal.* 2003;**12**:879–888.

24. Su B, O'Connor JP. NSAID therapy effects on healing of bone, tendon, and the enthesis. *J Appl Physiol.* 2013;**115**:892–899.

25. García-Martínez O, De Luna-Bertos E, Ramos-Torrecillas J, Manzano-Moreno FJ, Ruiz C. Repercussions of NSAIDS drugs on bone tissue: The osteoblast. *Life Sci.* 2015;**123**:72–77.

26. Kim YY, Chung BM, Kim WT. Lumbar spine MRI versus non-lumbar imaging modalities in the diagnosis of sacral insufficiency fracture: A retrospective observational study. *BMC Musculoskelet Disord.* 2018;**19**:257.

27. Denis F. The three column spine and its significance in the classification of acute thoracolumbar spine injuries. *Spine.* 1983;**8**:817–831.

28. Zhang D, Potty A, Vyas P, Lane J. The role of recombinant PTH in human fracture healing: A systematic review. *J Orthop Trauma.* 2014;**28**:57–62.

29. Zadro JR, Shirley D, Ferreira M et al. Is vitamin D supplementation effective for low back pain? A systematic review and meta-analysis. *Pain Physician.* 2018;**21**:121–145.

30. Tang BM, Eslick GD, Nowson C, Smith C, Bensoussan A. Use of calcium or calcium in combination with vitamin D supplementation to prevent fractures and bone loss in people aged 50 years and older: A meta-analysis. *Lancet.* 2007;**370**:657–666.

31. Adler RA, El-Hajj Fuleihan G, Bauer DC et al. Managing osteoporosis in patients on long-term bisphosphonate treatment: Report of a Task Force of the American Society for Bone and Mineral Research. *J Bone Miner Res.* 2016;**31**:16–35.

32. Aspenberg P, Genant HK, Johansson T et al. Teriparatide for acceleration of fracture repair in humans: A prospective, randomized, double-blind study of 102 postmenopausal women with distal radial fractures. *J Bone Miner Res.* 2010;**25**:404–414.

33. Alkhiary Y, Gerstenfeld L, Krall E et al. Enhancement of experimental fracture-healing by systemic administration of recombinant human parathyroid hormone (PTH 1–34). *J Bone Jt Surg Am.* 2005;**87**:731–741.

34. Baillieul S, Guinot M, Dubois C et al. Set the pace of bone healing – Treatment of a bilateral sacral stress fracture using teriparatide in a long-distance runner. *Joint Bone Spine*. 2017;**84**:499–500.

35. Tsai JN, Uihlein AV, Burnett-Bowie SM et al. Effects of two years of teriparatide, denosumab, or both on bone microarchitecture and strength (DATA-HRpQCT study). *J Clin Endocrinol Metab*. 2016;**101**:2023–2030.

36. Yang SC, Tsai TT, Chen HS et al. Comparison of sacroplasty with or without balloon assistance for the treatment of sacral insufficiency fractures. *J Orthop Surg (Hong Kong)*. 2018;**26**:230949901878257.

37. Soo Park H, Cho S, Yeon Kim D et al. Percutaneous sacroplasty under fluoroscopic guidance combined with epidurogram for sacral insufficiency fracture resulting from metastatic tumor and osteoporosis. *Pain Physician*. 2016;**19**:473–480.

38. Choi KC, Shin SH, Lee DC, Shim HK, Park CK. Effects of percutaneous sacroplasty on pain and mobility in sacral insufficiency fracture. *J Korean Neurosurg Soc*. 2017;**60**:60–66.

39. Onen MR, Yuvruk E, Naderi S. Reliability and effectiveness of percutaneous sacroplasty in sacral insufficiency fractures. *J Clin Neurosci*. 2015;**22**:1601–1608.

40. Kortman K, Ortiz O, Miller T et al. Multicenter study to assess the efficacy and safety of sacroplasty in patients with osteoporotic sacral insufficiency fractures or pathologic sacral lesions. *J Neurointerv Surg*. 2013;**5**:461–466.

41. Frey ME, Warner C, Thomas SM et al. Sacroplasty: A ten-year analysis of prospective patients treated with percutaneous sacroplasty: Literature review and technical considerations. *Pain Physician*. 2017;**20**:E1063–E1072.

42. Andresen R, Radmer S, Andresen JR, Schober HC. Comparison of the 18-month outcome after the treatment of osteoporotic insufficiency fractures by means of balloon sacroplasty (BSP) and radiofrequency sacroplasty (RFS) in comparison: A prospective randomised study. *Eur Spine J*. 2017;**26**:3235–3240.

43. Mehling I, Hessmann MH, Rommens PM. Stabilization of fatigue fractures of the dorsal pelvis with a trans-sacral bar: Operative technique and outcome. *Injury*. 2012;**43**:446–451.

44. Oberkircher L, Masaeli A, Bliemel C et al. Primary stability of three different iliosacral screw fixation techniques in osteoporotic cadaver specimens – a biomechanical investigation. *Spine J*. 2016;**16**:226–232.

45. Maki S, Nakamura K, Yamauchi T et al. Lumbopelvic fixation for sacral insufficiency fracture presenting with sphincter dysfunction. *Case Rep Orthop*. 2019;**2019**:1–4.

46. Sanders D, Fox J, Starr A, Sathy A, Chao J. Transsacral-transiliac screw stabilization. *J Orthop Trauma*. 2016;**30**:469–473.

47. Collinge CA, Crist BD. Combined percutaneous iliosacral screw fixation with sacroplasty using resorbable calcium phosphate cement for osteoporotic pelvic fractures requiring surgery. *J Orthop Trauma*. 2016;**30**:e217–e22.

**Chapter 18**

# Carpal Tunnel Syndrome
Vwaire Orhurhu and Kevin Bennett

## Carpal Tunnel Syndrome (CTS)
- Entrapment neuropathy secondary to compression of the median nerve at the wrist
- The tunnel is formed by multiple carpal bones and bordered by the flexor retinaculum anteriorly, and it comprises the median nerve and nine flexor tendons (1)
- Most common entrapment neuropathy accounting for 90% of all cases (1)
- Affects approximately 3% of American adults (2)
- Typically caused by systemic disease or prolonged flexion or extension of the wrist (1)
- Pain and paresthesias are experienced in the first three fingers and the radial half of the fourth finger (3)
- Volar aspect of hand proximal to the first finger overlying thenar eminence is spared (3)
- Motor function of thenar muscles is usually compromised (1)
- Common treatments include wrist immobilization, anti-inflammatory drugs, physical therapy, corticosteroid injection, and, ultimately, surgical decompression of the carpal tunnel (4,5,6)

## Epidemiology and Risk Factors
- Lifetime risk of developing CTS is approximately 10% (1,7)
- Incidence (3,7,8)
  - 0.1% of American adults with peak incidence between ages 40 and 60
  - Female predominance in reported cases per year
    - True incidence is likely even between genders but may develop true female predominance with increasing age >65
- Prevalence of 3% in American adults (2)

- Common systemic risk factors for CTS (1,2,9)
  - Often idiopathic or multifactorial
  - Diabetes mellitus type 1 and type 2
    - Greatest association with prevalence of 30% in patients with coexisting diabetic neuropathy
  - Obesity
  - Advancing age
  - Menopause
  - Hypothyroidism
  - Pregnancy
  - Family history
- Common mechanical risk factors for CTS (1,2,9,10)
  - Occupations or activities involving prolonged or repeated flexion, extension, or direct pressure applied to the volar aspect of the wrist
    - Additionally repeated or prolonged vibration of the hands
  - Arthritis
  - Boney deformities of the wrist
  - Square-shaped wrists
    - Dorsal-volar distance to medial-lateral distance ratio >0.7

## Pathophysiology

- CTS is universally characterized by compression of the medial nerve as it travels through the carpal tunnel (3,10)
- Normal pressure in the carpal tunnel is 2.5–5 mmHg (1,3)
  - Prolonged pressures of 20–30 mmHg or higher cause decreased epineural blood flow, demyelination, and eventual complete peripheral nerve loss
- The extent of damage from compression and increased pressure in the tunnel is positively correlated with the amount of time exposed to the risk factor (3)
- Accumulation of fibrosis in sub-synovial connective tissue within the tunnel is the histologic marker of CTS disease progression (9,11)
  - Other markers include increased expression of TGF-$\beta$ and VEGF leading to downstream increased production of collagen, as well as decreased expression of matrix metalloproteinases

## Diabetes Mellitus

- The mechanism of CTS development in diabetic patients is thought to be similar to that of other diabetic peripheral neuropathy, but is not completely understood (12,13)
  - Hyperglycemia-induced neural edema and inflammation cause direct damage to the median nerve as well as increased hydrostatic pressure
  - The narrow passage of the carpal tunnel extenuates the process as there is little room for tolerable edema before symptoms begin to occur

## Arthritis

- Rheumatoid arthritis, psoriatic arthritis, and osteoarthritis all appear to contribute to the development of CTS (14,15,16)
  - Chronic local inflammation of the carpal bones leads to increased edema, soft tissue thickening, and increased carpal tunnel pressure

## Overuse Injury

- There is a strong correlation between repetitive, forced, angular wrist movements and vibration of the hands and development of CTS (17,18,19,20)
  - Occupations such as seafood-, fruit-, or meat-processing, carpentry, roofing, drywall installation, and other comparable manual labor have been cited as particularly high risk for development of CTS
  - Traumatic movements damage the structures within the carpal tunnel and generate chronic inflammation and soft-tissue proliferation

## Diagnosis

- Diagnosis of CTS is reliant on a combination of patient symptoms, physical examination, and nerve conduction studies (21)
  - Chronic CTS tends to develop over months or years with the patient noticing progressively worsening symptoms by the time they seek diagnosis and treatment
- Symptoms (1,10)
  - Paresthesias in the first 3.5 fingers

- Primarily volar aspect of fingers and volar aspect of corresponding metacarpophalangeal joints
- More proximal volar-radial hand and radial aspect of the flexor crease of the wrist are innervated by the palmar cutaneous branch of the median nerve which runs above the tunnel and is classically spared in CTS
  - Burning pain in fingers relieved by shaking the hand
  - Numbness
  - Weakness
- Physical exam includes several maneuvers designed to compress the median nerve at the carpal tunnel and elicit symptoms, tests of grip strength and thumb adduction, visible thenar atrophy, as well as two-point discrimination tests to evaluate sensory loss (10,22,23)
  - Tinel's sign
    - Sensitivity: 47%
    - Specificity: 56%
  - Phalen's test
    - Sensitivity 50%
    - Specificity 33%
  - Durkan's test
    - Sensitivity: 71%
    - Specificity: 22%
- Nerve conduction studies are widely used as the definitive diagnostic tools of CTS with a sensitivity reported up to 99% (24,25,26)
  - Sensory nerve action potentials
    - Nerve conduction velocities across the carpal tunnel <50 m/s
    - Nerve conduction velocity from wrist-to-finger >10 m/s slower than palm-to-finger
    - Amplitude change of >50% across the carpal tunnel
    - Latency difference of >0.4 m/s across the carpal tunnel
  - Electromyography
    - Tests for the presence of axonal damage of distal median nerve branches by the presence of fibrillation potentials

and positive sharp-waves in the abductor pollicis brevis muscle

- ○ Motor nerve conduction
  - ▪ Compound muscle action potential distal latency >4.2 ms
- ○ There is substantial debate of the value of nerve conduction studies due to more recent studies showing the high potential for false-positives (up to 20%), so they are recommended to be reserved for those with a strong clinical suspicion or severe symptoms

- Ultrasound showing median nerve diameter ≥10 mm at the carpal tunnel measured just proximal to the level of the pisiform elicits comparable sensitivity and specificity to nerve conduction studies in diagnosis of CTS (27,28)
  - ○ Diagnosis
    - ▪ Ultrasound
      - Sensitivity: 89%
      - Specificity: 90%
      - Positive predictive value: 94%
      - Negative predictive value: 82%
      - Accuracy: 89%
    - ▪ Nerve conduction studies
      - Sensitivity: 89%
      - Specificity: 80%
      - Positive predictive value: 89%
      - Negative predictive value: 80%
      - Accuracy: 86%

## Treatments

- Treatment of CTS ranges from multiple noninvasive pharmacologic and physical therapies to the more invasive corticosteroid injections and decompression surgeries

## Wrist Splinting

- 2012 Cochrane review shows nocturnal wrist splinting has moderate benefit vs. placebo in relief of mild to moderate CTS symptoms (29)
  - ○ No significant evidence showing superiority of one splint type

- 2020 randomized controlled trial (RCT) shows symptom severity and median sensory peak latency significantly improved after 6 weeks of neutral wrist splint (30)
  - No significant benefit in extending splinting 6 additional weeks
- 2021 RCT shows improvement in pain and grip/pinch strength with forearm and wrist Kinesio tape application (31)
- 2016 RCT shows significantly greater improvement of pain in wrist splinting with metacarpophalangeal unit vs traditional splint (32)

## Physical Therapy

- 2012 Cochrane review shows minimal benefit vs. placebo for a variety of exercise, stretching, and mobilization techniques (33)
- 2022 RCT shows physical therapy 2×/week for 6 weeks plus neuromobilization of the median nerve results in significant decreases in symptom severity and improvement in functional status (34)
- 2017 RCT shows that neurodynamic techniques, functional massage, and carpal bone mobilizations techniques vs. ultrasound or laser therapy resulted in significant decreases in symptom severity and improvement in functional status (35)
- 2020 RCT shows myofascial stretching of the carpal ligament 4×/day for 6 weeks resulted in statistically significant symptom improvement (36)
- 2021 RCT shows that neuromobilization therapy in addition to home exercise increases long-term symptom improvement and functional status vs. exercise alone (37)
- 2020 RCT of subjects with confirmed CTS awaiting surgery shows that the addition of splinting and neuromobilization exercises decrease the rate of follow-through with surgery and improve subjective perception of symptoms (38)
  - Pain and functional status improved at 6 weeks but no difference between intervention and control groups at 24 weeks
- 2011 RCT shows improvement of functional status in subjects receiving tendon gliding exercises vs. nerve gliding exercises (39)
  - Both groups showed improvement in pain from baseline

- 2021 RCT shows improvement in pre- and post-surgery pain and functional status in subjects receiving neuromobilization therapy preoperatively (40)

## Oral Anti-inflammatory Drugs

- 2010 systematic review of nonsurgical treatment modalities found oral prednisone 20 mg/day for 10–14 days resulted in up to 8 weeks of improvement in pain vs. placebo (41)
  - Nonsteroidal anti-inflammatory drugs were not found to be useful in the treatment of CTS

## Ultrasound and Shock Wave Therapy

- 2013 Cochrane review shows limited evidence to support the value of therapeutic ultrasound in short- and long-term symptom relief (42)
- 2021 RCT shows improved sensory nerve conduction velocity, improved distal motor latency, and subjective improvement of symptoms in participants receiving three sessions of focused extracorporeal shock wave therapy (ESWT) vs. sham procedure (43)
- 2016 RCT shows improved subjective symptoms and median nerve cross-sectional area up to 12 weeks in participants receiving three sessions of radial ESWT plus nightly splinting vs. control group receiving only nightly splinting (44)
- 2015 RCT shows improved pain and functional status in participants receiving radial ESWT vs. participants receiving radial ultrasound therapy (45)
  - Both groups improved from baseline
- 2016 RCT shows dose-dependent improvement in symptoms at 14 weeks with participants receiving 3 weeks of 1×/week ESWT vs. one treatment or sham treatment (46)
- 2018 RCT shows single-dose radial ESWT is as good as, if not superior, in pain reduction and improved functional status to single-dose local corticosteroid injection (LCI) (47,48)
- 2022 RCT shows no difference between ESWT focused on carpal tunnel vs. carpal tunnel and median nerve distal pathways (49)
  - Both groups improved equally from baseline and vs. control

## Local Corticosteroid Injections

- 2007 Cochrane review shows single-dose LCI superior in symptomatic relief to placebo at 1 month and superior to oral corticosteroids at 3 months (50)
- 2013 RCT shows decrease in symptom severity at 10 weeks in participants who received a single 80 mg or 40 mg local methylprednisolone injection vs. placebo (51)
  - Dose-dependent decrease in the percentage of participants undergoing surgery at 1 year post-injection was also observed
- 2012 RCT shows improved clinical and electrophysiological evaluations from baseline at 2 and 6 months in participants receiving either one dose of 40 mg triamcinolone acetonide or one dose of 4 mL of 1% procaine HCl vs. placebo 0.09% saline (52)
  - There was no significant difference in improvement between the two intervention groups
- 2010 RCT shows significant improvement in symptom severity and functional status in the short term with 10 mg triamcinolone acetonide vs. placebo (53)
  - Effect deteriorated over the 12-month follow-up period but never reached pre-injection baseline
- 2018 RCT shows one-dose LCI superior to wrist splinting in decreasing regular over-the-counter pain medication usage and improving finger dexterity at 4 weeks (54)
  - Both methods showed improvement in symptom severity from baseline
- 2017 prospective cohort study shows volume of injectate used in LCI and coexisting rheumatoid arthritis were significant factors in the progression of participants receiving LCI to full carpal tunnel release (CTR) surgery (55)
- 2017 clinical trial shows that ultrasound-guided LCI with a transverse carpal ligament needle release is superior to LCI without needle release (56)
- 2005 study of LCI techniques shows that the median nerve is at the highest risk of injury if LCI is within 1 cm medial or lateral to the palmaris longus, and that the safest technique for LCI is injection through the flexor carpi ulnaris (57)
- 2020 study of LCI technique using anatomic landmarks shows 75.7% accuracy of needle placement in the carpal tunnel, 8.7%

piercing of the median nerve, and 15.6% placement outside the carpal tunnel (58)
- 2018 systematic review of anatomical vs. ultrasound-guided LCI shows that ultrasound guidance during LCI is superior in relief of participants' symptom severity (59)
- 2014 RCT shows improvements of subjective symptoms, electrophysiological studies, and median nerve cross-sectional area at 4 and 12 weeks using an in-plane ultrasound-guided approach to LCI vs. out-of-plane or anatomical techniques (60)

## Platelet-Rich Plasma
- 2018 and 2020 systematic reviews show promising results for the use of platelet-rich plasma (PRP) infusion as a nonsurgical alternative to CTS therapy, but report limited and weak data to recommend it at this time above other accepted therapies (61,62)

## Laser Therapy
- 2017 Cochrane review shows insignificant evidence to support the use of laser therapy in the treatment of CTS (63)

## Surgical Decompression Surgery
- 2007 and 2008 Cochrane reviews show that decompression surgery is the most effective treatment for moderate to severe cases of CTS and that no current alternative therapies perform superior in the management of symptoms in the short or long term (64,65)
- 2014 Cochrane review shows that open and endoscopic techniques of carpal tunnel release surgery are equally effective, with endoscopic having a faster back-to-work time by 8 days (66)

# Conclusions
- CTS is the most common cause of peripheral entrapment neuropathy in the United States
- It is prevalent in approximately 3% of the American adult population and up to 30% in diabetics with coexisting peripheral neuropathy
- Measuring median nerve diameter with ultrasound is a viable alternative to nerve conduction studies when diagnosing CTS
- Wrist-splinting, physical therapy, and shock-wave therapy are all possible first-line treatments for mild to moderate CTS

- LCI benefits pain and functionality in the short term with only a single injection
- Endoscopic decompression surgery is still the gold-standard treatment for patients with moderate to severe CTS that is refractory to other treatments

# References

1. Wang L. Guiding treatment for carpal tunnel syndrome. *Phys Med Rehabil Clin N Am*. 2018;**29**:751–760.

2. Wipperman J, Goerl K. Carpal tunnel syndrome: Diagnosis and management. *Am Fam Physician*. 2016;**94**(12):993–999.

3. Gillig JD, White SD, Rachel JN. Acute carpal tunnel syndrome. *A Review of Current Literature Orthop Clin North Am*. 2016;**47**(3):599–607.

4. Weiss AP, Sachar K, Gendreau M. Conservative management of carpal tunnel syndrome: A reexamination of steroid injection and splinting. *The Journal of Hand Surgery*. 1994;**19**(3):410–415.

5. Huisstede BM, van den Brink J, Randsdorp MS, Geelen SJ, Koes BW. Effectiveness of surgical and postsurgical interventions for carpal tunnel syndrome: A systematic review. *Arch Phys Med Rehabil*. 2018;**99**(8):1660–1680.

6. Ingram J, Mauck BM, Thompson NB, Calandruccio JH. Cost, value, and patient satisfaction in carpal tunnel surgery. *Orthop Clin North Am*. 2018;**49**(4):503–507.

7. Padua L, Coraci D, Erra C et al. Carpal tunnel syndrome: Clinical features, diagnosis, and management. *Lancet Neurol*. 2016;**15**(12):1273–1284.

8. Wipperman J, Goerl K. Carpal tunnel syndrome: Diagnosis and management. *Am Fam Physician*. 2016;**94**(12):993–999.

9. Sharma D, Jaggi AS, Bali A. Clinical evidence and mechanisms of growth factors in idiopathic and diabetes-induced carpal tunnel syndrome. *Eur J Pharmacol*. 2018;**837**:156–163.

10. Minieka MM, Nishida T, Benzon H. Chapter 56 – Entrapment neuropathies. In Honorio T. Benzon, Srinivasa N. Raja, Spencer S. Liu, et al. (eds.). *Essentials of Pain Medicine*, 3rd ed. Elsevier; 2011. pp. 395–402.

11. Festen-Schrier VJMM, Amadio PC. The biomechanics of subsynovial connective tissue in health and its role in carpal tunnel syndrome. *J Electromyogr Kinesiol*. 2018;**38**:232–239.

12. Papanas N, Stamatiou I, Papachristou S. Carpal tunnel syndrome in diabetes mellitus. *Curr Diabetes Rev*. 2022;**18**(4):e010921196025. doi: 10.2174/1573399817666210901114610.

13. Albers JW, Pop-Busui R. Diabetic neuropathy: Mechanisms, emerging treatments, and subtypes. *Curr Neurol Neurosci Rep*. 2014;14(8):473.

14. Shiri R. Arthritis as a risk factor for carpal tunnel syndrome: A meta-analysis. *Scand J Rheumatol*. 2016;45(5):339–346.

15. Hammer HB, Hovden IA, Haavardsholm EA, Kvien TK. Ultrasonography shows increased cross-sectional area of the median nerve in patients with arthritis and carpal tunnel syndrome. *Rheumatology*. 2006;45:584–588.

16. Karadag O, Kalyoncu U, Akdogan A et al. Sonographic assessment of carpal tunnel syndrome in rheumatoid arthritis: Prevalence and correlation with disease activity. *Rheumatol Int*. 2012;32:2313–2319.

17. Luckhaupt SE, Dahlhamer JM, Ward BW et al. Prevalence and work-relatedness of carpal tunnel syndrome in the working population, United States, 2010 national health interview survey. *Am J Ind Med*. 2013;56 (6):615–624.

18. Dale AM, Harris-Adamson C, Rempel D, et al. Prevalence and incidence of carpal tunnel syndrome in US working populations: Pooled analysis of six prospective studies. *Scand J Work Env Hea*. 2013;39(5):495–505.

19. Palmer KT, Harris EC, Coggon D. Carpal tunnel syndrome and its relation to occupation: A systematic literature review. *Occup Med (Lond)*. 2007;57(1):57–66.

20. Franklin GM, Friedman AS. Work-related carpal tunnel syndrome: Diagnosis and treatment guideline. *Phys Med Rehabil Clin N Am*. 2015;26 (3):523–537.

21. Sucher BM, Schreiber AL. Carpal tunnel syndrome diagnosis. *Phys Med Rehabil Clin N Am*. 2014;25(2):229–247.

22. Zhang D, Chruscielski CM, Blazar P, Earp BE. Accuracy of provocative tests for carpal tunnel syndrome. *J Hand Surg Glob Online*. 2020;2(3):121–125.

23. Sasaki T, Makino K, Nimura A et al. Assessment of grip-motion characteristics in carpal tunnel syndrome patients using a novel finger grip dynamometer system. *J Orthop Surg Res*. 2020;15(1):245.

24. Sonoo M, Menkes DL, Bland JDP, Burke D. Nerve conduction studies and EMG in carpal tunnel syndrome: Do they add value? *Clin Neurophysiol Pract*. 2018;3;78–88.

25. Alanazy MH. Clinical and electrophysiological evaluation of carpal tunnel syndrome: Approach and pitfalls. *Neurosciences (Riyadh)*. 2017;22 (3):169–180.

26. Mills KR. The basics of electromyography. *J Neurol Neurosurg Psychiatry*. 2005;76(Suppl 2):ii32–ii35.

27. Duckworth AD, Jenkins PJ, McEachan JE. Diagnosing carpal tunnel syndrome. *J Hand Surg Am*. 2014;39(7):1403–1407.

28. Fowler JR, Munsch M, Tosti R, Hagberg WC, Imbriglia JE. Comparison of ultrasound and electrodiagnostic testing for diagnosis of carpal tunnel syndrome: Study using a validated clinical tool as the reference standard. *J Bone Joint Surg Am*. 2014;**96**(17):e148.

29. Page MJ, Massy-Westropp N, O'Connor D, Pitt V. Splinting for carpal tunnel syndrome. *Cochrane Database Syst Rev*. 2012;7:CD010003.

30. Gatheridge MA, Sholty EA, Inman A et al. Splinting in carpal tunnel syndrome: The optimal duration. *Mil Med*. 2020;**185**(11–12):e2049–e2054.

31. Krause D, Roll SC, Javaherian-Dysinger H, Daher N. Comparative efficacy of the dorsal application of Kinesio tape and splinting for carpal tunnel syndrome: A randomized controlled trial. *J Hand Ther*. 2021;**34**(3):351–361.

32. Golriz B, Ahmadi Bani M, Arazpour M et al. Comparison of the efficacy of a neutral wrist splint and a wrist splint incorporating a lumbrical unit for the treatment of patients with carpal tunnel syndrome. *Prosthet Orthot Int*. 2016;**40**(5):617–623.

33. Page MJ, O'Connor D, Pitt V, Massy-Westropp N. Exercise and mobilisation interventions for carpal tunnel syndrome. *Cochrane Database Syst Rev*. 2012; (6):CD009899.

34. Ijaz MJ, Karimi H, Ahmad A et al. Comparative efficacy of routine physical therapy with and without neuromobilization in the treatment of patients with mild to moderate carpal tunnel syndrome. *Biomed Res Int*. 2022; **2022**:2155765.

35. Wolny T, Saulicz E, Linek P, Shacklock M, Myśliwiec A. Efficacy of manual therapy including neurodynamic techniques for the treatment of carpal tunnel syndrome: A randomized controlled trial. *J Manipulative Physiol Ther*. 2017;**40**(4):263–272.

36. Shem K, Wong J, Dirlikov B. Effective self-stretching of carpal ligament for the treatment of carpal tunnel syndrome: A double-blinded randomized controlled study. *J Hand Ther*. 2020;**33**(3):272–280.

37. Hamzeh H, Madi M, Alghwiri AA, Hawamdeh Z. The long-term effect of neurodynamics vs exercise therapy on pain and function in people with carpal tunnel syndrome: A randomized parallel-group clinical trial. *J Hand Ther*. 2021;**34**(4):521–530.

38. Lewis KJ, Coppieters MW, Ross L et al. Group education, night splinting and home exercises reduce conversion to surgery for carpal tunnel syndrome: A multicentre randomised trial. *J Physiother*. 2020;**66**(2):97–104.

39. Horng YS, Hsieh SF, Tu YK et al. The comparative effectiveness of tendon and nerve gliding exercises in patients with carpal tunnel syndrome: A randomized trial. *Am J Phys Med Rehabil*. 2011;**90**(6):435–442.

40. Paquette P, Higgins J, Danino MA, Harris P, Lamontagne M, Gagnon DH. Effects of a preoperative neuromobilization program offered to individuals

with carpal tunnel syndrome awaiting carpal tunnel decompression surgery: A pilot randomized controlled study. *J Hand Ther* 2021;34(1):37–46.

41. Huisstede BM, Hoogvliet P, Randsdorp MS et al. Carpal tunnel syndrome: Part I: Effectiveness of nonsurgical treatments – a systematic review. *Arch Phys Med Rehabil.* 2010;**91**(7):981–1004.

42. Page MJ, O'Connor D, Pitt V, Massy-Westropp N. Therapeutic ultrasound for carpal tunnel syndrome. *Cochrane Database Syst Rev.* 2013;**2013**(3): CD009601.

43. Gesslbauer C, Mickel M, Schuhfried O et al. Effectiveness of focused extracorporeal shock wave therapy in the treatment of carpal tunnel syndrome: A randomized, placebo-controlled pilot study. *Wien Klin Wochenschr.* 2021;**133**(11–12):568–577.

44. Wu YT, Ke MJ, Chou YC et al. Effect of radial shock wave therapy for carpal tunnel syndrome: A prospective randomized, double-blind, placebo-controlled trial. *J Orthop Res.* 2016;**34**(6):977–984.

45. Paoloni M, Tavernese E, Cacchio A et al. Extracorporeal shock wave therapy and ultrasound therapy improve pain and function in patients with carpal tunnel syndrome: A randomized controlled trial. *Eur J Phys Rehabil Med.* 2015;**51**(5):521–528.

46. Ke MJ, Chen LC, Chou YC et al. The dose-dependent efficiency of radial shock wave therapy for patients with carpal tunnel syndrome: A prospective, randomized, single-blind, placebo-controlled trial. *Sci Rep.* 2016;**6**:38344.

47. Atthakomol P, Manosroi W, Phanphaisarn A et al. Comparison of single-dose radial extracorporeal shock wave and local corticosteroid injection for treatment of carpal tunnel syndrome including mid-term efficacy: A prospective randomized controlled trial. *BMC Musculoskelet Disord.* 2018;**19**(1):32.

48. Seok H, Kim SH. The effectiveness of extracorporeal shock wave therapy vs. local steroid injection for management of carpal tunnel syndrome: A randomized controlled trial. *Am J Phys Med Rehabil.* 2013;**92**(4):327–334.

49. Habibzadeh A, Mousavi-Khatir R, Saadat P, Javadian Y. The effect of radial shockwave on the median nerve pathway in patients with mild-to-moderate carpal tunnel syndrome: A randomized clinical trial. *J Orthop Surg Res.* 2022;**17**(1):46.

50. Marshall S, Tardif G, Ashworth N. Local corticosteroid injection for carpal tunnel syndrome. *Cochrane Database Syst Rev.* 2007;(2):CD001554.

51. Atroshi I, Flondell M, Hofer M, Ranstam J. Methylprednisolone injections for the carpal tunnel syndrome: A randomized, placebo-controlled trial. *Ann Intern Med.* 2013;**159**(5):309–317.

52. Karadaş Ö, Tok F, Akarsu S, Tekin L, Balaban B. Triamcinolone acetonide vs procaine hydrochloride injection in the management of carpal tunnel

syndrome: Randomized placebo-controlled study. *J Rehabil Med.* 2012;**44**(7):601–604.

53. Peters-Veluthamaningal C, Winters JC, Groenier KH, Meyboom-de Jong B. Randomised controlled trial of local corticosteroid injections for carpal tunnel syndrome in general practice. *BMC Fam Pract.* 2010;**11**:54.

54. So H, Chung VCH, Cheng JCK, Yip RML. Local steroid injection versus wrist splinting for carpal tunnel syndrome: A randomized clinical trial. *Int J Rheum Dis.* 2018;**21**(1):102–107.

55. Evers S, Bryan AJ, Sanders TL et al. Corticosteroid injections for carpal tunnel syndrome: Long-term follow-up in a population-based cohort. *Plast Reconstr Surg.* 2017;**140**(2):338–347.

56. Guo XY, Xiong MX, Zhao Y et al. Comparison of the clinical effectiveness of ultrasound-guided corticosteroid injection with and without needle release of the transverse carpal ligament in carpal tunnel syndrome. *Eur Neurol.* 2017;**78**(1–2):33–40.

57. Racasan O, Dubert T. The safest location for steroid injection in the treatment of carpal tunnel syndrome. *J Hand Surg Br.* 2005;**30**(4):412–414.

58. Green DP, MacKay BJ, Seiler SJ, Fry MT. Accuracy of carpal tunnel injection: A prospective evaluation of 756 patients. *Hand (N Y),* 2020;**15**(1):54–58.

59. Babaei-Ghazani A, Roomizadeh P, Forogh B et al. Ultrasound-guided versus landmark-guided local corticosteroid injection for carpal tunnel syndrome: A systematic review and meta-analysis of randomized controlled trials. *Arch Phys Med Rehabil.* 2018;**99**(4):766–775.

60. Lee JY, Park Y, Park KD, Lee JK, Lim OK. Effectiveness of ultrasound-guided carpal tunnel injection using in-plane ulnar approach: A prospective, randomized, single-blinded study. *Medicine (Baltimore).* 2014;**93**(29):e350.

61. Malahias MA, Chytas D, Mavrogenis AF et al. Platelet-rich plasma injections for carpal tunnel syndrome: A systematic and comprehensive review. *Eur J Orthop Surg Traumatol.* 2019;**29**(1):1–8.

62. Catapano M, Catapano J, Borschel G et al. Effectiveness of platelet-rich plasma injections for nonsurgical management of carpal tunnel syndrome: A systematic review and meta-analysis of randomized controlled trials. *Arch Phys Med Rehabil.* 2020;**101**(5):897–906.

63. Rankin IA, Sargeant H, Rehman H, Gurusamy KS. Low-level laser therapy for carpal tunnel syndrome. *Cochrane Database Syst. Rev.* 2017;8(8):CD012765.

64. Scholten RJPM, Mink van der Molen A, Uitdehaag BMJ, Bouter LM, de Vet HCW. Surgical treatment options for carpal tunnel syndrome. *Cochrane Database Syst. Rev.* 2007;(4):CD003905. doi: 10.1002/14651858.CD003905.pub3.

65. Verdugo RJ, Salinas RA, Castillo JL, Cea G. Surgical versus non-surgical treatment for carpal tunnel syndrome. *Cochrane Database Syst. Rev.* 2008;(4): CD001552. doi: 10.1002/14651858.CD001552.pub2.

66. Vasiliadis HS, Georgoulas P, Shrier I, Salanti G, Scholten RJ. Endoscopic release for carpal tunnel syndrome. *Cochrane Database Syst Rev.* 2014;(1): CD008265.

# Adhesive Capsulitis of the Shoulder

Kevin Bennett and Riki Patel

## Adhesive Capsulitis of the Shoulder (AC)

- Inflammation within the glenohumeral joint capsule leading to pain and decreased range-of-motion (1)
- Prevalent in 2% of the general population (2)
- Most significant risk factors include diabetes, hypothyroidism, and female gender (2,3)
- There is generally no attributable trauma to the shoulder before onset of symptoms (4)
- Pain is generally noticed early in disease, whereas range-of-motion deficit tends to develop over several months (5)
- Preserved strength and neurological function are present in AC, and occasionally imaging is required to rule out other causes of pain or decreased range-of-motion (5,6)
- Conservative treatment with physical therapy, oral anti-inflammatories, and local glucocorticoid injections (LCI) is usually effective in reversing the disease course within a few years, but more invasive procedures are available for refractory cases (7,8)

## Epidemiology and Risk Factors

- Prevalence of at least 2% in the general population (2)
  - Diabetic patients are particularly affected with a 20% prevalence
  - Prevalence of diabetes in those found to have AC: approximately 39%
  - Prevalence of prediabetes in those found to have AC: approximately 33%
- Other common risk factors for AC (9–13)
  - Hyperthyroidism
  - Hyperlipidemia

○ Chronic liver disease
○ Dupuytren's disease
○ Obesity
○ Age <50 years
○ Female sex
○ African-American or Hispanic race
○ Mastectomy for breast cancer treatment

## Pathophysiology

- The exact cause of AC is not clear; however, the known cellular pathophysiology includes synovitis within the glenohumeral joint, reactive fibrosis of the surrounding connective tissue, and eventual formation of adhesions causing contracture of the glenohumeral joint capsule (14)

  ○ Immunohistochemical studies reveal high levels of inflammatory cytokines in the subacromial bursa (15)
  ○ Varying proteomic patterns retrieved from different loci of AC within the glenohumeral joint may elucidate specific etiologies of the disease depending on its focus (16)
  ○ Classic arthroscopic findings include thickened coracohumeral ligament, decreased glenohumeral joint volume, contracted axillary fold, and obliteration of the sub-coracoid fat triangle (17)

- The course of AC generally follows three well-described phases over the course of approximately 2 years (18,19)

  ○ Painful synovitis in the glenohumeral joint with normal range-of-motion
  ○ Progressive decrease in active and passive flexion, abduction, and external/internal rotation while pain appears to improve
  ○ Gradual improvement of range-of-motion over 6 months to 1 year

## Diagnosis

- Diagnosis of AC is reliably based on a classic clinical presentation alone; however, occasionally blood tests and imaging could be used to rule out systemic disease or non-AC causes of shoulder pain
- Common patient complaints (4,6)
  ○ Earlier disease
    ▪ Insidious onset of diffuse pain and stiffening of the shoulder

- No history of trauma
- Pain worse in the evening
  - Later disease
    - Difficulty raising arm above head
    - Pain relatively subsided
    - Strength and sensation intact
- Physical exam (4,5,6)
  - Diffuse tenderness (point tenderness could indicate different pathology)
  - Primarily decreased shoulder external rotation and abduction
  - Loss of arm swing while walking
  - Normal strength in rotator cuff, biceps brachii, brachialis, and deltoid
    - Special tests all negative with baseline decreased range-of-motion
  - Normal neurologic assessment
- Lidocaine injection test can differentiate AC from rotator cuff tear or bursitis (20,21)
  - Inject 2 mL of 1% lidocaine into subacromial bursa
    - AC patients will have continued pain with decreased range-of-motion
    - Rotator cuff tear and bursitis patients will have relief of symptoms and improved range-of-motion
    - Reduced pain and improved active/passive range-of-motion after subacromial bursa injection implies an extra-glenohumeral joint pathology
- Ultrasound of the coracohumeral ligament revealing >0.7 mm thickness is also suggestive of AC, although it is infrequently used in diagnostics (22)

## Treatments

- The typical AC treatment course is a conservative approach of physical therapy, nonsteroidal anti-inflammatory drugs (NSAIDs), oral glucocorticoids, and local corticosteroid injections (LCIs) before proceeding to surgery (7)
  - Most cases spontaneously resolve within 1–3 years (8)

## Physical Therapy

- 2014 Cochrane review shows no evidence to support the use of physical therapy as a sole or adjunct therapy for AC (23)
- 2021 systematic review shows improvements from baseline pain, functionality, and range-of-motion in multiple physical therapy modalities but limited evidence to suggest one method is superior to another (24)
- 2016 and two 2022 systematic reviews show improvements in pain and range-of-motion with joint mobilization, stretching, and general exercise therapy (25,26,27)
- 2019 systematic review shows superior improvements to pain, range-of-motion, and functionality with proprioceptive neuro-muscular facilitation vs. conventional physical therapy (28)

## Oral Anti-inflammatory Drugs

- 2006 Cochrane review shows evidence to support oral corticosteroids for pain control in AC for up to 6 weeks (29)
- Multiple reviews report a possible role for NSAIDs in the relief of pain during the early stage of AC, but the ultimate consensus is that they are not useful (30–33)

## Local Corticosteroid Injection

- Four systematic reviews and one meta-analysis show significant evidence supporting the use of intraarticular corticosteroids (often 20 mg or 40 mg triamcinolone) for short-term symptom relief (6–12 weeks) (34–38)
  - It is noted that LCIs lose their efficacy in the long term and will not have statistically significant benefit over placebo
- 2016 prospective cohort study with matched controls shows that intraarticular corticosteroid injections decrease fibrosis, vascular hyperplasia, and recruitment of fibroblasts to the damaged area of the joint (39)
- 2019 systematic review found that there is no difference in pain relief, range-of-motion, or functionality of the affected arm in AC patients receiving either intraarticular or subacromial corticosteroid injections (40)
- 2010 systematic review shows LCIs superior to physiotherapy in pain relief, external rotation, and shoulder disability at 6 weeks, and marginally superior at 12, 16, and 26 weeks (41)

- 2004 clinical trial shows 40 mg triamcinolone injected intraarticularly is 5.8× superior to triamcinolone orally in relief of pain at 1 week (42)
- 2021 Cochrane review shows no benefit to using ultrasound guidance when performing corticosteroid injections in the shoulder (43)

## Sodium Hyaluronate Injection
- 2014 randomized controlled trial (RCT) and 2011 and 2017 systematic reviews show intraarticular hyaluronate injection to be safe and as effective as LCIs in short-term symptom relief from AC (44,45,46)

## Botulinum Toxin-A Injection
- 2010 and 2015 systematic reviews report weak evidence to suggest significant symptom improvement in AC patients given botulinum toxin-A injections due to poor quality of data, small number of studies, and too few participants (47,48)

## Suprascapular Nerve Block
- 2012 prospective cohort study of AC patients with comorbid diabetes mellitus who were refractory to intraarticular corticosteroids shows significant improvement in pain and range-of-motion after intervention with a suprascapular nerve block (SSNB) (49)
  - Participants assessed at 1, 4, and 12 weeks post block
  - Block performed with 40 mg methylprednisolone acetate and 5 mL 1% lidocaine
- 2015 RCT shows that, while SSNB and physical therapy independently improve symptoms of AC, they have an even superior effect of reducing pain severity and functional disability when combined (50)
- 2016 study shows SSNB provides quicker pain relief, range-of-motion gains, and fewer side effects than LCIs (51)
- 2019 retrospective cohort study shows that SSNB plus intraarticular corticosteroid injection provided superior pain relief and functional improvement to either one individually (52)

## Manipulation under Anesthesia
- 2019 systematic review shows significant pain reduction, return of range-of-motion, and high patient satisfaction from 3 weeks postop to 15 years (53)

- 2015 cohort study shows that the best circumstance in which to consider manipulation under anesthesia in an AC patient refractory to other treatments from 6 to 9 months after the first onset of symptoms (54)
- 2009 RCT shows no difference in clinical outcomes between LCI and manipulation under anesthesia (55)

## Arthroscopic Capsulotomy

- Five recent trials showed significant improvement in pain and range-of-motion as well as quicker adoption of physical therapy regimens in patients receiving anteroinferior capsule release for refractory AC (56–60)

## Conclusions

- AC is a common cause of shoulder pain and disability, affecting nearly 2% of the general population
- It is present in approximately 20% of all diabetics, highly correlated with several other systemic conditions and predispositions, yet is still idiopathic in etiology
- Diffuse, insidious onset of shoulder pain with no known trauma is seen in early disease, while symptoms of later disease are dominated by a progressive stiffening that restricts multiple planes of movement
- AC is primarily managed conservatively with oral anti-inflammatories, local injections, and physical therapy, and the majority of patients achieve spontaneous resolution of symptoms within 1–3 years
- While not conclusively superior to less invasive measures, manipulation under anesthesia and arthroscopic capsulotomy are viable alternatives to patients refractory to conservative therapies

## References

1. Neviaser AS, Neviaser RJ. Adhesive capsulitis of the shoulder. J Am Acad Orthop Surg. 2011;19(9):536–542.

2. Tighe CB, Oakley WS Jr. The prevalence of a diabetic condition and adhesive capsulitis of the shoulder. South Med J. 2008;101(6):591–595.

3. Milgrom C, Novack V, Weil Y et al. Risk factors for idiopathic frozen shoulder. Isr Med Assoc J. 2008;10(5):361–364.

4. Kelley MJ, Shaffer MA, Kuhn JE et al. Shoulder pain and mobility deficits: Adhesive capsulitis. J Orthop Sports Phys Ther. 2013;43(5):A1–31.

5.  Rundquist PJ, Anderson DD, Guanche CA, Ludewig PM. Shoulder kinematics in subjects with frozen shoulder. *Arch Phys Med Rehabil.* 2003;**84** (10):1473–1479.

6.  Ewald A. Adhesive capsulitis: A review. *Am Fam Physician.* 2011;**83** (4):417–422.

7.  Rangan A, Hanchard N, McDaid C. What is the most effective treatment for frozen shoulder? *BMJ.* 2016;**354**:i4162.

8.  Dias R, Cutts S, Massoud S. Frozen shoulder. *BMJ* 2005;**331** (7530):1453–1456.

9.  Kingston K, Curry EJ, Galvin JW, Li X. Shoulder adhesive capsulitis: Epidemiology and predictors of surgery. *J Shoulder Elbow Surg.* 2018;**27** (8):1437–1443.

10. Huang SW, Lin JW, Wang WT et al. Hyperthyroidism is a risk factor for developing adhesive capsulitis of the shoulder: A nationwide longitudinal population-based study. *Sci Rep.* 2014;**4**:4183.

11. Smith SP, Devaraj VS, Bunker TD. The association between frozen shoulder and Dupuytren's disease. *J Shoulder Elbow Surg.* 2001;**10**(2):149–151.

12. Yang S, Park DH, Ahn SH et al. Prevalence and risk factors of adhesive capsulitis of the shoulder after breast cancer treatment. *Support Care Cancer.* 2017;**25**(4):1317–1322.

13. Lo SF, Chu SW, Muo CH et al. Diabetes mellitus and accompanying hyperlipidemia are independent risk factors for adhesive capsulitis: A nationwide population-based cohort study (version 2). *Rheumatol Int.* 2014;**34**(1):67–74.

14. Ryan V, Brown H, Minns Lowe CJ, Lewis JS. The pathophysiology associated with primary (idiopathic) frozen shoulder: A systematic review. *BMC Musculoskelet Disord.* 2016;**17**(1):340.

15. Lho YM, Ha E, Cho CH et al. Inflammatory cytokines are overexpressed in the subacromial bursa of frozen shoulder. *J Shoulder Elbow Surg.* 2013;**22** (5):666–672.

16. Hagiwara Y, Mori M, Kanazawa K et al. Comparative proteome analysis of the capsule from patients with frozen shoulder. *J Shoulder Elbow Surg.* 2018;**27**(10):1770–1778.

17. Fields BKK, Skalski MR, Patel DB et al. Adhesive capsulitis: Review of imaging findings, pathophysiology, clinical presentation, and treatment options. *Skeletal Radiol.* 2019;**48**(8):1171–1184.

18. Whelton C, Peach CA. Review of diabetic frozen shoulder. *Eur J Orthop Surg Traumatol.* 2018;**28**(3):363–371.

19. Wong CK, Levine WN, Deo K et al. Natural history of frozen shoulder: Fact or fiction? A systematic review. *Physio.* 2017;**103**(1):40–47.

20. Kim SJ, Gee AO, Hwang JM, Kwon JY. Determination of steroid injection sites using lidocaine test in adhesive capsulitis: A prospective randomized clinical trial. *J Clin Ultrasound.* 2015;**43**(6):353–360.

21. Bak K, Sørensen AK, Jørgensen U et al. The value of clinical tests in acute full-thickness tears of the supraspinatus tendon: Does a subacromial lidocaine injection help in the clinical diagnosis? A prospective study. *Arthrosc.* 2010;**26**(6):734–742.

22. Tandon A, Dewan S, Bhatt S, Jain AK, Kumari R. Sonography in diagnosis of adhesive capsulitis of the shoulder: A case-control study. *J Ultrasound.* 2017;**20**(3):227–236.

23. Page MJ, Green S, Kramer S et al. Manual therapy and exercise for adhesive capsulitis (frozen shoulder). *Cochrane Database Syst. Rev.* 2014;**8**: CD011275.

24. Nakandala P, Nanayakkara I, Wadugodapitiya S, Gawarammana I. The efficacy of physiotherapy interventions in the treatment of adhesive capsulitis: A systematic review. *J Back Musculoskelet Rehabil.* 2021;**34**(2):195–205.

25. Noten S, Meeus M, Stassijns G et al. Efficacy of different types of mobilization techniques in patients with primary adhesive capsulitis of the shoulder: A systematic review. *Arch Phys Med Rehabil.* 2016;**97**(5):815–825.

26. Mertens MG, Meert L, Struyf F, Schwank A, Meeus M. Exercise therapy is effective for improvement in range of motion, function, and pain in patients with Frozen shoulder: A systematic review and meta-analysis. *Arch Phys Med Rehabil.* 2022;**103**(5):998–1012.

27. Costantino C, Nuresi C, Ammendolia A, Ape L, Frizziero A. Rehabilitative treatments in adhesive capsulitis: A systematic review. *J Sports Med Phys Fitness.* 2022;**62**(11):1505–1511. doi: 10.23736/S0022-4707.22.13054-9.

28. Tedla JS, Sangadala DR. Proprioceptive neuromuscular facilitation techniques in adhesive capsulitis: A systematic review and meta-analysis. *J Musculoskelet Neuronal Interact.* 2019;**19**(4):482–491.

29. Buchbinder R, Green S, Youd JM, Johnston RV. Oral steroids for adhesive capsulitis. *Cochrane Database Syst Rev.* 2006;(**4**):CD006189.

30. van der Windt DA, van der Heijden GJ, Scholten RJ, Koes BW, Bouter LM. The efficacy of non-steroidal anti inflammatory drugs (NSAIDS) for shoulder complaints. A systematic review. *J Clin Epidemiol.* 1995;**48** (5):691–704.

31. Hsu JE, Anakwenze OA, Warrender WJ, Abboud JA. Current review of adhesive capsulitis. *J Shoulder Elbow Surg.* 2011;**20**(3):502–514.

32. Neviaser AS, Hannafin JA. Adhesive capsulitis: A review of current treatment. *Am J Sports Med.* 2010;**38**(11):2346–2356.

33. Georgiannos D, Markopoulos G, Devetzi E, Bisbinas I. Adhesive capsulitis of the shoulder: Is there consensus regarding the treatment? A comprehensive review. *Open Orthop J.* 2017;**11**:65–76.

34. Song A, Higgins LD, Newman J, Jain NB. Glenohumeral corticosteroid injections in adhesive capsulitis: A systematic search and review. *PM R.* 2014;**6**(12):1143–1156.

35. Griesser MJ, Harris JD, Campbell JE, Jones GL. Adhesive capsulitis of the shoulder: A systematic review of the effectiveness of intra-articular corticosteroid injections. *J Bone Joint Surg Am* 2011;**93**(18):1727–1733.

36. Wang W, Shi M, Zhou C et al. Effectiveness of corticosteroid injections in adhesive capsulitis of shoulder: A meta-analysis. *Medicine (Baltimore)* 2017;**96**(28):e7529.

37. Xiao RC, Walley KC, DeAngelis JP, Ramappa AJ. Corticosteroid injections for adhesive capsulitis: A review. *Clin J Sport Med.* 2017;**27**(3):308–320.

38. Koh KH. Corticosteroid injection for adhesive capsulitis in primary care: A systematic review of randomised clinical trials. *Singapore Med J* 2016;**57**(12):646–657.

39. Hettrich CM, DiCarlo EF, Faryniarz D et al. The effect of myofibroblasts and corticosteroid injections in adhesive capsulitis. *J Shoulder Elbow Surg.* 2016;**25**(8):1274–1279.

40. Shang X, Zhang Z, Pan X, Li J, Li Q. Intra-articular versus subacromial corticosteroid injection for the treatment of adhesive capsulitis: A meta-analysis and systematic review. *Biomed Res Int.* 2019;1274790. doi: 10.1155/2019/1274790. PMID: 31737653

41. Blanchard V, Barr S, Cerisola FL. The effectiveness of corticosteroid injections compared with physiotherapeutic interventions for adhesive capsulitis: A systematic review. *Physiotherapy* 2010;**96**(2):95–107.

42. Widiastuti-Samekto M, Sianturi GP. Frozen shoulder syndrome: Comparison of oral route corticosteroid and intra-articular corticosteroid injection. *Med J Malaysia.* 2004;**59**(3):312–316.

43. Zadro J, Rischin A, Johnston RV, Buchbinder R. Image-guided glucocorticoid injection versus injection without image guidance for shoulder pain. *Cochrane Database Syst Rev.* 2021;**8**(8):CD009147.

44. Harris JD, Griesser MJ, Copelan A, Jones GL. Treatment of adhesive capsulitis with intra-articular hyaluronate: A systematic review. *Int J Shoulder Surg.* 2011;**5**(2):31–37.

45. Papalia R, Tecame A, Vadalà G et al. The use of hyaluronic acid in the treatment of shoulder capsulitis: A systematic review. *J Biol Regul Homeost Agents.* 2017;**31**(4 Suppl 2):23–32.

46. Lim TK, Koh KH, Shon MS et al. Intra-articular injection of hyaluronate versus corticosteroid in adhesive capsulitis. *Orthopedics*. 2014;**37**(10):860–865.

47. Khenioui H, Houvenagel E, Catanzariti JF et al. Usefulness of intra-articular botulinum toxin injections: A systematic review. *Jt Bone Spine*. 2016;**83**(2):149–154.

48. Singh JA, Fitzgerald PM. Botulinum toxin for shoulder pain. *Cochrane Database Syst Rev*. 2010;(**9**):CD008271.

49. Ozkan K, Ozcekic AN, Sarar S et al. Suprascapular nerve block for the treatment of frozen shoulder. *Saudi J Anaesth*. 2012;**6**(1):52–55.

50. Klç Z, Filiz MB, Çakr T, Toraman NF. Addition of suprascapular nerve block to a physical therapy program produces an extra benefit to adhesive capsulitis: A randomized controlled trial. *Am J Phys Med Rehabil*. 2015;**94**(10 Suppl 1):912–920.

51. Sonune SP, Gaur AK, Gupta S. Comparative study of ultrasound guided supra-scapular nerve block versus intra-articular steroid injection in frozen shoulder. *Int J Res Orthop*. 2016;**2**(4):387.

52. Jung TW, Lee SY, Min SK, Lee SM, Yoo JC. Does Combining a Suprascapular Nerve Block With an Intra-articular Corticosteroid Injection Have an Additive Effect in the Treatment of Adhesive Capsulitis? A Comparison of Functional Outcomes After Short-term and Minimum 1-Year Follow-up. *Orthop J Sports Med*. 2019;**7**(7):2325967119859277.

53. Kraal T, Beimers L, The B et al. Manipulation under anaesthesia for frozen shoulders: Outdated technique or well-established quick fix? *EFORT Open Rev*. 2019;**4**(3):98–109.

54. Vastamäki H, Varjonen L, Vastamäki M. Optimal time for manipulation of frozen shoulder may be between 6 and 9 months. *Scand J Surg*. 2015;**104**(4):260–266.

55. Jacobs LG, Smith MG, Khan SA, Smith K, Joshi M. Manipulation or intra-articular steroids in the management of adhesive capsulitis of the shoulder? A prospective randomized trial. *J Shoulder Elbow Surg*. 2009;**18**(3):348–353.

56. Ranalletta M, Rossi LA, Zaidenberg EE et al. Midterm outcomes after arthroscopic anteroinferior capsular release for the treatment of Idiophatic Adhesive Capsulitis. *Arthrosc*. 2017;**33**(3):503–508.

57. Barnes CP, Lam PH, Murrell GA. Short-term outcomes after arthroscopic capsular release for adhesive capsulitis. *J Shoulder Elbow Surg*. 2016;**25**(9):256–264.

58. Tsai MJ, Ho WP, Chen CH, Leu TH, Chuang TY. Arthroscopic extended rotator interval release for treating refractory adhesive capsulitis. *J Orthop Surg (Hong Kong)*. 2017;**25**(1):2309499017692717.

59. Mubark IM, Ragab AH, Nagi AA, Motawea BA. Evaluation of the results of management of frozen shoulder using the arthroscopic capsular release. *Ortop Traumatol Rehabil.* 2015;**17**(1):21–28.

60. Smith CD, Hamer P, Bunker TD. Arthroscopic capsular release for idiopathic frozen shoulder with intra-articular injection and a controlled manipulation. *Ann R Coll Surg Engl.* 2014;**96**(1):55–60.

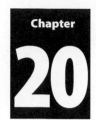

# Chapter 20

# Thoracic Outlet Syndrome

Nazir Noor and Alan D. Kaye

- Thoracic outlet syndrome (TOS) is a syndrome that results from compression of neurovascular bundle, specifically the brachial plexus (BP), exiting the thoracic outlet (1,2)
- Symptoms include upper extremity pallor, paresthesia, weakness, muscle atrophy, and pain (3)
- Causes can be neurogenic, venous, or arterial; each of these can be congenital, traumatic, or functionally acquired causes (4)
- >90% of TOS is neurogenic in origin (4)
- Symptom onset between the ages of 20 and 50 (5)
- More prevalent in women (5)
- Management involves conservative lifestyle modifications, medications, anticoagulation, physical therapy, minimally invasive procedures, and surgical interventions (6)

## Epidemiology

- 95% neurogenic TOS, most common in women (4)
- 3–5% venous TOS (involving subclavian and axillary veins), more common in men (4)
- 1–2% arterial TOS (involving subclavian and axillary arteries), affects men and women equally (4)

## Anatomy and Etiology

- Subcategorized into neurogenic, venous, or arterial
- Neurogenic TOS involves BP trunks or cords from nerve roots C5–T1
- Thoracic outlet is the space from the supraclavicular fossa to the axilla
- TOS results from compression of BP nerves, subclavian artery and vein, and axillary artery and vein
- Anatomic spaces of TOS
  - Interscalene triangle (7,8)

- Borders:
  - Anteriorly – anterior scalene muscle (BP)
  - Posteriorly – middle scalene muscle (subclavian artery)
  - Inferiorly – first rib
- Costoclavicular space (8,9)
  - Borders:
    - Anteriorly – subclavius muscle (BP)
    - Inferoposteriorly – first rib and anterior scalene muscle (subclavian artery)
    - Superiorly – clavicle (subclavian vein)
- Subcoracoid (retropectoralis) space (8,9)
  - Borders:
    - Anteriorly – pectoralis minor muscle (BP)
    - Posteriorly – ribs 2–4 (axillary artery)
    - Superiorly – coracoid (axillary vein)
- Mechanisms eliciting TOS characteristic pathology
  - Trauma, repetitive motion, anatomic variation, tumor (9)
  - Trauma (9)
    - High velocity, often in setting of motor vehicle accident
    - Hemorrhage, hematoma, or displaced fracture may compress nerves or vasculature of thoracic outlet (9)
      - Midshaft clavicular fracture is a well-recognized cause
    - Fibrosis after initial insult may produce TOS symptoms (7)
    - Whiplash injuries are associated with neurogenic TOS, especially in patients with a cervical rib (10)
  - Repetitive motion
    - Repetitive motions lead to muscle hypertrophy, contributing to compression (11)
    - Overuse injury in setting of repetitive motions can lead to swelling, small hemorrhages, subsequent fibrosis (11)
    - Venous TOS possible with repetitive motions (11)
    - Paget-Schroetter disease or "effort thrombosis" involves axially or subclavian venous thrombosis following strenuous repetitive activity of upper extremities (11)
  - Anatomic variation
    - Presence of cervical rib, especially in whiplash patients (7)

- 1–2% of general population has cervical rib (7)
- 20% of neurogenic TOS cases solely attributable to presence of cervical rib (7)
- Presence of cervical rib also predisposes one to development of arterial TOS (10)
  - May compress subclavian artery and causes stenosis or aneurysm (10)
- Congenital variations in musculature (7)
  - Supernumerary scalene muscle $\rightarrow$ compression within interscalene triangle (7)
- Tumor (benign or malignant) (12,13)
  - Mass effect causing compression (12)
  - Pancoast tumors, also known as superior pulmonary sulcus tumors, may invade and compress BP
  - Benign tumors (13)
    - Multiple hereditary exostosis $\rightarrow$ combined venous, arterial, and neurogenic TOS secondary to large osteosarcomas (13)

# Clinical Presentation

- Neurogenic TOS
  - Often seen in young patients who participate in athletic activities involving repetitive overhead upper extremity motions and heavy lifting (10)
  - Symptoms: upper extremity paresthesia, neck pain, trapezius pain, shoulder/arm pain, supraclavicular pain, chest pain, occipital headache, paresthesia in all fingers
- Venous TOS (also known as Paget-von Schroetter syndrome)
  - Mechanical compression and repetitive injury of the subclavian vein between the clavicle and the first rib can abrupt blood flow stagnation and subsequent effort thrombosis (11)
  - Symptoms: acute upper extremity swelling, cyanosis, heaviness, ultimately pain, unilateral Raynaud's-like symptoms (14)
    - Unlike neurogenic TOS, venous TOS pain does not worsen with overhead upper arm positioning
  - Arterial TOS (rarest type)

○ Often seen in physically active patients, athletes in whom arterial entrapment may occur at the level of pectoralis minor tendon and humeral head (15)

○ Arterial compression results in intimal damage → turbulent blood flow → vessel dilation → arterial thrombosis and distal embolization → acute distal upper extremity ischemia (1)

## Diagnosis

- Physical Exam
  - ○ Include shoulders, upper extremities, and cervical spine (1)
  - ○ Compare affected and contralateral sides (1)
    - Muscle atrophy, weakness, skin color changes, temperature, hair distribution differences, supraclavicular fullness, aneurysmal pulsations (1)
  - ○ Physical exam tests (16)
    - Adson test, Roos test, upper limb tension test (16)
  - ○ Neurogenic TOS
    - Muscular atrophy, weakness (17)
      - Gilliatt-Sumner hand – constellation of atrophic abductor pollicis brevis, hypothenar, interossei muscles (17)
    - Electromyography abnormality (18)
    - Diagnostic injections with local anesthetic into anterior scalene and pectoralis minor muscles of affected side → suggestive of up to 94% positive outcome for surgical decompression (1)
  - ○ Vascular TOS
    - Large differences in BP readings between arms (>20 mmHg) (19)
    - Venous TOS
      - Shoulder and chest edematous (19)
    - Arterial TOS
      - Upper extremity pale/cyanotic (19)
- MRI, CT, ultrasound for anatomical abnormalities (prominent cervical ribs, fracture calluses, compressive tumors, etc.) (20)

# Management

- Conservative
  - Patient education (17)
  - Physical therapy and rehabilitation – postural mechanics, weight control, relaxation techniques, activity modification, target muscle stretching and strengthening (17)
  - Pharmacologic – NSAIDs, opioids, muscle relaxants, anticonvulsants, antidepressants (6)
  - Interventional – local anesthetic injection of anterior scalene and pectoralis minor muscles, botulinum toxin type A injection of anterior scalene and pectoralis minor muscles (21)

- Surgical – reserved for patients who failed conservative management (1)

  - For patients with arterial or venous TOS, initial interventional is often surgical (22)
  - Procedure – first rib resection with scalenectomy or scalenotomy (23)
  - 95% of surgical patients for neurogenic TOS reported "excellent" results (24)

# References

1. Jones MR, Prabhakar A, Viswanath O et al. Thoracic outlet syndrome: A comprehensive review of pathophysiology, diagnosis, and treatment. *Pain Ther*. 2022;**8**:5–18. https://doi.org/10.6084/.

2. Aljabri B, Al-Omran M. Surgical management of vascular thoracic outlet syndrome: A teaching hospital experience. *Ann Vasc Dis*. 2013;**6**(1):74–79. https://pubmed.ncbi.nlm.nih.gov/23641288/.

3. Laulan J, Fouquet B, Rodaix C et al. Thoracic outlet syndrome: Definition, aetiological factors, diagnosis, management and occupational impact. *J Occup Rehabil*. 2011;**21**(3):366–373. https://pubmed.ncbi.nlm.nih.gov/21193950/.

4. Freischlag J, Orion K. Understanding thoracic outlet syndrome. *Scientifica (Cairo)*. 2014;**2014**:1–6. https://pubmed.ncbi.nlm.nih.gov/25140278/.

5. Maru S, Dosluoglu H, Dryjski M et al. Thoracic outlet syndrome in children and young adults. *Eur J Vasc Endovasc Surg*. 2009;**38**(5):560–564. https://pubmed.ncbi.nlm.nih.gov/19703780/.

6. Brooke BS, Freischlag JA. Contemporary management of thoracic outlet syndrome. *Curr Opin Cardiol*. 2010;**25**(6):535–540. https://pubmed.ncbi.nlm.nih.gov/20838336/.

7.  Stewman C, Vitanzo PC, Harwood MI. Neurologic thoracic outlet syndrome: Summarizing a complex history and evolution. *Curr Sports Med Rep*. 2014;**13** (2):100–106. https://pubmed.ncbi.nlm.nih.gov/24614423/.

8.  Raptis CA, Sridhar S, Thompson RW, Fowler KJ, Bhalla S. Imaging of the patient with thoracic outlet syndrome. *Radiographics*. 2016;**36**(4):984–1000. https://pubmed.ncbi.nlm.nih.gov/27257767/.

9.  Ferrante MA. The thoracic outlet syndromes. *Muscle Nerve*. 2012;**45** (6):780–795. https://pubmed.ncbi.nlm.nih.gov/22581530/.

10. Sanders RJ, Hammond SL, Rao NM. Diagnosis of thoracic outlet syndrome. *J Vasc Surg*. 2007;**46**(3):601–604. https://pubmed.ncbi.nlm.nih.gov/17826254/.

11. Ibrahim R, Dashkova I, Williams M et al. Paget-Schroetter syndrome in the absence of common predisposing factors: A case report. *Thromb J*. 2017;**15** (1):20. https://pubmed.ncbi.nlm.nih.gov/28781584/.

12. Davis GA, Knight SR. Pancoast tumors. *Neurosurg Clin N Am*. 2008;**19** (4):545–557. https://pubmed.ncbi.nlm.nih.gov/19010280/.

13. Abdolrazaghi H, Riyahi A, Taghavi M, Farshidmehr P, Mohammadbeigi A. Concomitant neurogenic and vascular thoracic outlet syndrome due to multiple exostoses. *Ann Card Anaesth*. 2018;**21**(1):71–73. https://pubmed .ncbi.nlm.nih.gov/29336398/.

14. Cooke RA. Thoracic outlet syndrome–aspects of diagnosis in the differential diagnosis of hand-arm vibration syndrome. *Occup Med (Lond)*. 2003;**53** (5):331–336. https://pubmed.ncbi.nlm.nih.gov/12890833/.

15. Duwayri YM, Emery VB, Driskill MR et al. Positional compression of the axillary artery causing upper extremity thrombosis and embolism in the elite overhead throwing athlete. *J Vasc Surg*. 2011;**53**(5):1329–1340. https://pub med.ncbi.nlm.nih.gov/21276687/.

16. Povlsen S, Povlsen B. Diagnosing thoracic outlet syndrome: Current approaches and future directions. *Diagnostics (Basel, Switzerland)*. 2018;**8** (1):21. https://pubmed.ncbi.nlm.nih.gov/29558408/.

17. Huang JH, Zager EL, McGillicuddy JE et al. Thoracic outlet syndrome. *Neurosurg*. 2004;**55**(4):897–903. https://pubmed.ncbi.nlm.nih.gov/15458598/.

18. Tsao BE, Ferrante MA, Wilbourn AJ, Shields RW. Electrodiagnostic features of true neurogenic thoracic outlet syndrome. *Muscle Nerve*. 2014;**49** (5):724–727. https://pubmed.ncbi.nlm.nih.gov/24006176/.

19. Kuhn JE, Lebus V GF, Bible JE. Thoracic outlet syndrome. *J Am Acad Orthop Surg*. 2015;**23**(4):222–232. https://pubmed.ncbi.nlm.nih.gov/25808686/.

20. Demondion X, Herbinet P, Van Sint Jan S et al. Imaging assessment of thoracic outlet syndrome. *Radiographics*. 2006;**26**(6):1735–1750. https://pub med.ncbi.nlm.nih.gov/17102047/.

21. Foley JM, Finlayson H, Travlos A. A review of thoracic outlet syndrome and the possible role of botulinum toxin in the treatment of this syndrome. *Toxins (Basel)*. 2012;4(11):1223–1235. https://pubmed.ncbi.nlm.nih.gov/23202313/.

22. Vemuri C, McLaughlin LN, Abuirqeba AA, Thompson RW. Clinical presentation and management of arterial thoracic outlet syndrome. *J Vasc Surg*. 2017;**65**(5):1429–1439. https://pubmed.ncbi.nlm.nih.gov/28189360/.

23. Burt BM. Thoracic outlet syndrome for thoracic surgeons. *J Thorac Cardiovasc Surg*. 2018;**156**(3):1318–1323.e1. https://pubmed .ncbi.nlm.nih.gov/29628349/.

24. Urschel HC, Razzuk MA. Upper plexus thoracic outlet syndrome: Optimal therapy. *Ann Thorac Surg*. 1997;**63**(4):935–939. https://pubmed .ncbi.nlm.nih.gov/9124966/.

# Osteoarthritic Hip Pain

Kevin Bennett, Elyse M. Cornett, and Jamal Hasoon

- Osteoarthritis (OA) is a common cause of hip pain, especially in the ageing population >45 years (1)
- Incidence of OA in the hip as well as associated disability is increasing significantly across the world over the past 30 years (2)
- Most significant risk factors include increasing age, female gender, genetics, obesity, and lifestyle/occupations with significant impact to the hip joint (3,5)
- The process is initiated by a loss of the protein:water ratio and local damage which leads to a positive feedback loop of inflammation to continue the process (4,5)
- Pain is localized to the affected joint, achy in quality, worse at night or after use, and associated with stiffness and swelling (4,5)
- A presumptive diagnosis and initial treatment regimen can be made based on clinical presentation, but imaging can help to clarify uncertainties (5)
- Conservative treatment of physical therapy, oral anti-inflammatories, and intraarticular injections is effective in managing symptoms and slowing disease progression, but more invasive procedures, including hip replacement, are available for severe cases (5)

## Epidemiology and Risk Factors

- Since 1990, global incidence has increased 115.4% (2)
  - From 740,000 new cases per year in 1990 to 1,580,000 per year in 2019
  - Disability-adjusted life years also increased by 126.97% during this time
  - Incidence is highest between 60 and 64 years
- Estimated prevalence in American adults >50 years is 18.5% (6)

- ○ Radiographic OA of the hip seen in 24.7% of males and 13.6% of females
- ○ Symptomatic OA of the hip seen in 5.2% of males and 3.0% of females
- Common risk factors for OA of the hip (3)
  - ○ Genetics (7)
    - ▪ Genetic contribution in approximately 60% of hip OA
  - ○ Increasing age
  - ○ Female
  - ○ Obesity
  - ○ Poor diet
  - ○ High-impact/-stress activities or occupation

## Pathophysiology

- The general pathophysiology of OA in the hip is the result of a cascade of similar injuries, extracellular matrix (ECM) degradation, and dysfunctional repair of joint space to that of OA (8)
  - ○ Ageing disrupts articular chondrocytes to have baseline increased levels of oxidative stress and an altered repair response with a shift toward matrix metalloproteinase (MMP) catabolism
  - ○ Obesity causes increased mechanical load and injury to the hip joint, as well as low-level systemic inflammation that triggers MMP activation in chondrocytes via release of adipokines and multiple pro-inflammatory interleukins
  - ○ Acute traumatic injury to the hip has also been shown to lead to chronically elevated inflammatory markers and higher rates of OA in the affected joint
  - ○ Genetic factors linked to OA of the hip include a variety of systemic inflammatory abnormalities, dysfunctional ECM breakdown, and ECM structural abnormalities

## Diagnosis

- Presumptive diagnosis of OA of the hip can be made with a classic history, physical exam, and pertinent risk factors, but often anteroposterior and lateral hip radiographs are helpful in confirming diagnosis, establishing disease severity, and guiding therapy
- Common patient complaints (5)

- Pain in affected joint
  - Use-dependent early in disease
  - More constant later in disease
- Stiffness/painful range-of-motion
  - Prominent on waking up in the morning, but alleviates with light use
  - Not to be confused with similar complaint in rheumatoid arthritis which tends to last longer
- Chronic onset (typically months to years before presentation)
- Physical exam (5)
  - Internal rotation <15°
    - Sensitivity: 66%
    - Specificity: 72%
    - Likelihood ratio: 2.4
  - Pain with internal rotation
    - Sensitivity: 82%
    - Specificity: 39%
    - Likelihood ratio: 1.3
  - Decreased hip adduction
    - Sensitivity: 80%
    - Specificity: 81%
    - Likelihood ratio: 4.2
- Hip radiographs (5)
  - Femoral or acetabular osteophytes
    - Sensitivity: 89%
    - Specificity: 90%
    - Likelihood ratio: 8.9
  - Superior joint space narrowing
    - Sensitivity: 85%
    - Specificity: 66%
    - Likelihood ratio: 2.5
  - Osteophytes with hip pain on physical exam
    - Sensitivity: 89%

- Specificity: 90%
- Likelihood ratio: 8.9
  ○ Symptoms of hip OA can present with normal radiographs, so initiation of conservative treatment with a presumptive diagnosis is appropriate with a strong clinical suspicion

# Treatments

- Treatment of hip OA primarily involves mitigation of disease progression with conservative therapy; however, many patients will fail conservative treatment after a number of years and require surgical intervention (5,9,10)

## Weight Loss

- Three recent systematic reviews reveal weak evidence to support weight loss or bariatric surgery as a treatment for symptomatic OA of the hip (11,12,13)

## Exercise

- Three Cochrane reviews show good evidence to support the implementation of a land- or water-based exercise regimen to reduce pain, improve the range-of-motion, and improve the overall quality of life (14,15,16)

## Oral Medications

- 2017 Cochrane review shows that celecoxib improves pain and physical function in hip OA patients vs. placebo with no risk for withdrawal side effects (17)
  ○ There was no significant difference reported between celecoxib and traditional cox-1-inhibiting nonsteroidal anti-inflammatory drugs (NSAIDs)
- 2006 Cochrane review shows that acetaminophen is superior to placebo but inferior to traditional NSAIDs in relief of hip pain in patients with OA (18)
- 2019 Cochrane review shows that tramadol is ineffective in treating pain from OA alone or in conjunction with acetaminophen (19)
  ○ Moderate quality evidence showed increased nausea, dizziness, and fatigue in those taking tramadol
- 2014 Cochrane review shows that non-tramadol opioids given orally or transdermally improve pain and function slightly better than placebo (20)

- ○ Risk of side effects and withdrawal from opioids was significant and outweighs any potential benefits
- ○ Not recommended
- 2005 Cochrane review shows that glucosamine has a moderate effect on pain and functionality associated with hip OA (21)
  - ○ Radiologic evidence showed additional slowing of OA structural changes
- 2015 Cochrane review shows chondroitin to be superior to placebo in control of mild OA symptoms (22)

## Intraarticular Glucocorticoids

- 2020 systematic review shows that local corticosteroid injection (LCI) is efficacious in pain relief as an immediate intervention and up to 12 weeks post-injection (23)
  - ○ 2016 systematic review also shows short-term efficacy in pain control peaking at 1 week and maintaining through 8 weeks post-injection (24)
- 2021 cohort study shows that, while there is limited evidence for LCI in less severe cases, patients who are older, with more severe pain, and with radiographic evidence of osteoarthritis benefit significantly more from LCI (25)
- 2008 review of injection techniques reports that ultrasound guidance during intraarticular injection improves the efficacy of the steroid and improves the safety of the procedure (26)
- 2015 review of LCI safety before total hip arthroplasty shows that there is no increased risk of postoperative infection if the injection is given 1–5 years prior to surgery (27)
  - ○ Slight increased risk of postoperative infection if given within the year preceding surgery
  - ○ 2016 review shows that the most significant risk is 0–3 months prior to surgery (28)
  - ○ Multiple injections are shown to increase risk regardless of timing (29)

## Other Intraarticular Injections

- 2021 systematic review shows immediate improvements in functionality and pain relief with no added harm following injection with hyaluronic acid (30)

- ○ Concurrently, another 2021 systematic review shows that intraarticular saline injection relieves pain and improves mobility at 2, 4, and 6 months post-injection the same as hyaluronic acid (31)
- 2022 systematic review shows similar improvements in pain and mobility up to 1 year post-injection in patients receiving either hyaluronic acid or platelet-rich plasma (32)
- 2020 systematic review shows that, while hyaluronic acid results in some improvement, glucocorticoid injection appears to be superior in short-term pain relief (33)
- 2017 cohort shows mesenchymal stem cell therapy improves pain, stiffness, and mobility while also slowing the radiographic progression of osteoarthritis up to 30 months post-injection (34)
  - ○ 2018 systematic review confirms these findings but reports that more studies are needed to provide sufficient power to back further recommendations (35)
- 2018 cohort shows bone marrow aspirate concentrate injections provide significant pain relief and improved function in patients with no additional harm (36)
  - ○ 2018 case series recommends multiple injections in succession to optimize anti-inflammatory effect (37)

## Conclusions

- OA of the hip is a common source of pain and disability associated with aging
- Radiographic evidence of hip OA is present in approximately 24.7% of males and 13.6% of females over 50 years old, with symptoms seen in 5.2% of males and 3.0% of females
- "Wear and tear" damage to hip joint leading to dysfunctional ECM reorganization leads to chronic onset of pain that is worse with use and associated with decreased hip mobility
- Years of conservative treatment with exercise, weight loss, and oral anti-inflammatories can mitigate the disease progression, but severe cases may require intraarticular injections or hip arthroplasty
- Some promising injections hope to better manage chronic symptoms by reversing the course of the disease; however, total hip arthroplasty remains a gold-standard treatment for severe hip OA

# References

1. Jordan JM, Helmick CG, Renner JB et al. Prevalence of hip symptoms and radiographic and symptomatic hip osteoarthritis in African Americans and Caucasians: The Johnston County osteoarthritis project. *J Rheumatol.* 2009;**36**(4):809–815.

2. Long H, Liu Q, Yin H, et al. Prevalence trends of site-specific osteoarthritis from 1990 to 2019: Findings from the global burden of disease study 2019. *Arthritis Rheumatol.* 2022;**74**(7):1172–1183. doi: 10.1002/art.42089.

3. Johnson VL, Hunter DJ. The epidemiology of osteoarthritis. *Best Pract Res Clin Rheumatol.* 2014;**28**(1):5–15.

4. Loeser RF. The role of aging in the development of osteoarthritis. *Trans Am Clin Climatol Assoc.* 2017;**128**:44–54.

5. Katz JN, Arant KR, Loeser RF. Diagnosis and treatment of hip and knee osteoarthritis: A review. *JAMA.* 2021;**325**(6):568–578.

6. Kim C, Linsenmeyer KD, Vlad SC et al. Prevalence of radiographic and symptomatic hip osteoarthritis in an urban United States community: The Framingham osteoarthritis study. *Arthritis Rheumatol.* 2014;**66** (11):3013–3017.

7. Spector TD, MacGregor AJ. Risk factors for osteoarthritis: Genetics. *Osteoarthritis Cartilage.* 2004;**12**(Suppl A):S39–S44.

8. Chen D, Shen J, Zhao W et al. Osteoarthritis: Toward a comprehensive understanding of pathological mechanism. *Bone Res.* 2017;**5**:16044. doi: 10.1038/boneres.2016.44.

9. Urits I, Orhurhu V, Powell J et al. Minimally invasive therapies for osteoarthritic hip pain: A comprehensive review. *Curr Pain Headache Rep.* 2020;**24**(7):37. doi: 10.1007/s11916-020-00874-8.

10. Bannuru RR, Osani MC, Vaysbrot EE et al. OARSI guidelines for the non-surgical management of knee, hip, and polyarticular osteoarthritis. *Osteoarthritis Cartilage.* 2019;**27**(11):1578–1589.

11. Robson EK, Hodder RK, Kamper SJ et al. Effectiveness of weight-loss interventions for reducing pain and disability in people with common musculoskeletal disorders: A systematic review with meta-analysis. *J Orthop Sports Phys Ther.* 2020;**50**(6):319–333.

12. Daugaard CL, Hangaard S, Bartels EM et al. The effects of weight loss on imaging outcomes in osteoarthritis of the hip or knee in people who are overweight or obese: A systematic review. *Osteoarthritis Cartilage.* 2020;**28** (1):10–21.

13. Gill RS, Al-Adra DP, Shi X et al. The benefits of bariatric surgery in obese patients with hip and knee osteoarthritis: A systematic review. *Obes Rev.* 2011;**12**(12):1083–1089.

14. Hurley M, Dickson K, Hallett R et al. Exercise interventions and patient beliefs for people with hip, knee or hip and knee osteoarthritis: A mixed methods review. *Cochrane Database Syst Rev.* 2018;4(4):CD010842.

15. Bartels EM, Juhl CB, Christensen R et al. Aquatic exercise for the treatment of knee and hip osteoarthritis. *Cochrane Database Syst Rev.* 2016;3:CD005523.

16. Fransen M, McConnell S, Hernandez-Molina G, Reichenbach S. Exercise for osteoarthritis of the hip. *Cochrane Database Syst Rev.* 2014;(4):CD007912. doi: 10.1002/14651858.CD007912.pub2.

17. Puljak L, Marin A, Vrdoljak D et al. Celecoxib for osteoarthritis. *Cochrane Database Syst Rev.* 2017;5(5):CD009865.

18. Towheed TE, Maxwell L, Judd MG et al. Acetaminophen for osteoarthritis. *Cochrane Database Syst Rev.* 2006;(1):CD004257. doi: 10.1002/14651858. CD004257.pub2.

19. Toupin April K, Bisaillon J, Welch V et al. Tramadol for osteoarthritis. *Cochrane Database Syst Rev.* 2019;5(5):CD005522.

20. da Costa BR, Nüesch E, Kasteler R et al. Oral or transdermal opioids for osteoarthritis of the knee or hip. *Cochrane Database Syst Rev.* 2014;(9): CD003115. doi: 10.1002/14651858.CD003115.pub4.

21. Towheed TE, Maxwell L, Anastassiades TP et al. Glucosamine therapy for treating osteoarthritis. *Cochrane Database Syst Rev.* 2005;(2):CD002946. doi: 10.1002/14651858.CD002946.pub2.

22. Singh JA, Noorbaloochi S, MacDonald R, Maxwell LJ. Chondroitin for osteoarthritis. *Cochrane Database Syst Rev.* 2015;1:CD005614.

23. Zhong HM, Zhao GF, Lin T et al. Intra-articular steroid injection for patients with hip osteoarthritis: A systematic review and meta-analysis. *Biomed Res Int.* 2020;2020:6320154. doi: 10.1155/2020/6320154.

24. McCabe PS, Maricar N, Parkes MJ, Felson DT, O'Neill TW. The efficacy of intra-articular steroids in hip osteoarthritis: A systematic review. *Osteoarthritis Cartilage.* 2016;24(9):1509–1517.

25. Kanthawang T, Lee A, Baal JD et al. Predicting outcomes in patients undergoing intra-articular corticosteroid hip injections. *Skeletal Radiol.* 2021;50(7):1349–1357.

26. Kruse DW. Intraarticular cortisone injection for osteoarthritis of the hip. Is it effective? Is it safe? *Curr Rev Musculoskelet Med.* 2008;1(3–4):227–233.

27. Ravi B, Escott BG, Wasserstein D et al. Intraarticular hip injection and early revision surgery following total hip arthroplasty: A retrospective cohort study. *Arthritis Rheumatol.* 2015;67(1):162–168.

28. Schairer WW, Nwachukwu BU, Mayman DJ, Lyman S, Jerabek SA. Preoperative hip injections increase the rate of periprosthetic infection after total hip arthroplasty. *J Arthroplasty.* 2016;31(Suppl 9):166–169.

29. Chambers AW, Lacy KW, Liow MHL et al. Multiple hip intra-articular steroid injections increase risk of periprosthetic joint infection compared with single injections. *J Arthroplast*. 2017;**32**(6):1980–1983.

30. Ebad Ali SM, Farooqui SF, Sahito B et al. Clinical outcomes of intra-articular high molecular weight hyaluronic acid injection for hip osteoarthritis: A systematic review and meta-analysis. *J Ayub Med Coll Abbottabad*. 2021;**33**(2):315–321.

31. Gazendam A, Ekhtiari S, Bozzo A, Phillips M, Bhandari M. Intra-articular saline injection is as effective as corticosteroids, platelet-rich plasma and hyaluronic acid for hip osteoarthritis pain: A systematic review and network meta-analysis of randomised controlled trials. *Br J Sports Med*. 2021;**55**(5):256–261.

32. Belk JW, Houck DA, Littlefield CP et al. Platelet-rich plasma versus hyaluronic acid for hip osteoarthritis yields similarly beneficial short-term clinical outcomes: A systematic review and meta-analysis of level I and II randomized controlled trials. *Arthroscopy*. 2022;**38**(6):2035–2046.

33. Vilabril F, Rocha-Melo J, Gonçalves JV, Vilaça-Costa J, Brito I. Hip osteoarthritis treatment with intra-articular injections: Hyaluronic acid versus glucocorticoid: A systematic review. *Acta Reumatol Port*. 2020;**45**(2):127–136.

34. Mardones R, Jofré CM, Tobar L, Minguell JJ. Mesenchymal stem cell therapy in the treatment of hip osteoarthritis. *J Hip Preserv Surg*. 2017;**4**(2):159–163.

35. McIntyre JA, Jones IA, Han B, Vangsness CT. Intra-articular Mesenchymal stem cell therapy for the human joint: A systematic review. *Am J Sports Med*. 2018;**46**(14):3550–3563.

36. Rodriguez-Fontan F, Piuzzi NS, Kraeutler MJ, Pascual-Garrido C. Early clinical outcomes of intra-articular injections of bone marrow aspirate concentrate for the treatment of early osteoarthritis of the hip and knee: A cohort study. *PM&R*. 2018;**10**(12):1353–1359.

37. Darrow M, Shaw B, Darrow B, Wisz S. Short-term outcomes of treatment of hip osteoarthritis with 4 bone marrow concentrate injections: A case series. *Clin Med Insights Case Rep*. 2018;**11**:1–4.

# Osteoarthritic Knee Pain

Jamal Hasoon and Kevin Bennett

- Knee osteoarthritis (OA) is a leading cause of chronic knee pain, disability, and healthcare expense affecting >12% of the US population over 60 years old (1)
- By 2030, people over 60 years old will comprise 21% of the US population and double in total size compared to the population in the year 2000 (2)
- Most significant risk factors include increasing age, female gender, genetics, obesity, previous knee injury, and occupations with significant impact to the knee joint (3,4)
- A loss of the protein:water ratio and local damage to the knee lead to a chronic inflammatory process that remodels the joint and surrounding connective tissue (5)
- Pain is typically localized to the unilateral affected joint, worse at night or after use, and associated with morning stiffness and decreased range-of-motion (6)
- Early diagnosis and prevention are encouraged to slow disease progression as symptoms do not typically arise until irreversible damage has been done (6)
- Aerobic exercise, strength exercise, weight reduction, and range-of-motion exercises are all recommended as first-line treatment or prevention (5,6)
- Acetaminophen and oral nonsteroidal anti-inflammatory drugs (NSAIDs) are recommended for prn pain relief as well as local corticosteroid injections (LCIs) for more severe cases (5,6)
- Ultimately, knee replacement is a gold-standard treatment for severe knee osteoarthritis refractory to more conservative management (5,6)

## Epidemiology and Risk Factors

- Global incidence in those >20 years old is 203 per 10,000 person-years (7)
  - 86.7 million individuals yearly

- ○ 130 per 10,000 person-years in the United States
- ○ Incidence peaks from 70 to 79 years old
- Global prevalence of knee OA in those >40 years old is 22.9% (7)
  - ○ Asian countries reported higher overall prevalence than non-Asian
  - ○ Global prevalence of radiographic evidence is 28.7%
  - ○ Global prevalence of symptomatic OA is 12.4%
- Common risk factors for OA of the hip (7)
  - ○ Increasing age
  - ○ Female gender
    - ▪ Ratio of prevalence and incidence is 1.69 in females and 1.39 in males
  - ○ Obesity
  - ○ Poor diet
  - ○ Low physical activity
  - ○ High-impact/-stress occupation
  - ○ Lower educational attainment

## Pathophysiology

- OA of the knee, much like OA in other parts of the body, is a combination of repetitive traumatic injury/biomechanical stress, extracellular matrix (ECM) degradation, and dysfunctional repair of the joint space (5,8)
  - ○ Ageing disrupts articular chondrocytes to have baseline increased levels of oxidative stress and an altered repair response with a shift toward matrix metalloproteinase (MMP) catabolism
  - ○ Obesity causes increased mechanical load and injury to the hip joint, as well as low-level systemic inflammation that triggers MMP activation in chondrocytes via release of adipokines and multiple pro-inflammatory interleukins
  - ○ Acute traumatic injury to the hip has also been shown to lead to chronically elevated inflammatory markers and higher rates of OA in the affected joint

## Diagnosis

- Early-stage detection of knee OA is encouraged through a classic pattern of history, physical exam, and lifestyle risk factors, but often anteroposterior and lateral knee radiographs are used to confirm the diagnosis, monitor disease progression, and better inform decisions on therapy

- Common patient complaints (6,9)
  - Pain in affected joint
    - Use-dependent early in disease (95% sensitivity, 19% specificity)
    - More constant later in disease (53% sensitivity, 71% specificity)
  - Stiffness/painful range-of-motion
    - Prominent on waking up in the morning, but alleviates with light use (88% sensitivity, 52% specificity)
    - Not to be confused with similar complaints in rheumatoid arthritis which tends to last longer through the morning
  - Functional limitations
    - Disturbed gait and overall decreased mobility/use of the affected knee (56% sensitivity, 63% specificity)
  - Chronic onset (typically months to years of insidious pain before presentation)
- Physical exam (9)
  - Crepitus
    - Sensitivity: 89%
    - Specificity: 60%
    - Likelihood ratio: 2.3
  - Bony enlargement
    - Sensitivity: 55%
    - Specificity: 95%
    - Likelihood ratio: 11.81
  - Decreased passive/active range-of-motion
    - Sensitivity: 17%
    - Specificity: 96%
    - Likelihood ratio: 4.4
  - Palpable effusion
    - Sensitivity: 43%
    - Specificity: 41%
    - Likelihood ratio: 0.73

- Knee radiographs (9)
  - Joint space narrowing
    - Sensitivity: 44%
    - Specificity: 79%
    - Likelihood ratio: 2.19
  - Osteophytes
    - Sensitivity: 51%
    - Specificity: 83%
    - Likelihood ratio: 3.29
  - Sclerosis
    - Sensitivity: 33%
    - Specificity: 89%
    - Likelihood ratio: 2.56

## Treatments

- Treatment of knee OA primarily involves mitigation of disease progression with lifestyle intervention for everyone and conservative therapy prn for pain episodes; however, many patients will fail conservative treatment after a number of years and require surgical intervention

### Weight Loss

- 2022 and 2020 systematic reviews show that weight loss with increased protein intake and increased percentage of lean muscle mass have a moderate effect on pain control in patients with knee osteoarthritis (10,11)
- 2018 systematic review shows that weight gain increases synovitis compared to a stable weight group (12)

### Exercise

- 2021 and 2019 systematic reviews show that multiple exercise regimens provide significant pain relief and increased functionality for several months before diminishing returns (13,14)
- 2015 Cochrane review shows 3,913 participants, most with mild to moderate symptomatic knee OA, completing several months of standard aerobic, functional, and strength exercises report: (15)
  - Absolute pain improvement of 12%

- Absolute physical function improvement of 10%
- Absolute quality-of-life improvement of 4%

## Oral Medications

- 2017 Cochrane review shows that celecoxib improves pain and physical function in knee OA patients vs. placebo with no risk for withdrawal side effects (16)
  - There was no significant difference reported between celecoxib and traditional cox-1 inhibiting NSAIDs
- 2006 Cochrane review shows that acetaminophen is superior to placebo but inferior to traditional NSAIDs in relief of knee pain in patients with OA (17)
- 2019 Cochrane review shows that tramadol is ineffective in treating pain from OA alone or in conjunction with acetaminophen (18)
  - Moderate quality evidence showed increase nausea, dizziness, and fatigue in those taking tramadol
- 2014 Cochrane review shows that non-tramadol opioids given orally or transdermal improve pain and function slightly better than placebo (19)
  - Risk of side effects and withdrawal from opioids was significant and outweighs any potential benefits
  - Not recommended
- 2005 Cochrane review shows that glucosamine has a moderate effect on pain and functionality associated with knee OA (20)
  - Radiologic evidence showed additional slowing of OA structural changes
- 2015 Cochrane review shows chondroitin to be superior to placebo in controlling mild OA symptoms (21)

## Intraarticular Glucocorticoids

- 2015 Cochrane review shows absolute improvement in pain of 13% in a single-dose LCI vs. placebo, absolute improvement in physical function of 10%, and absolute reduction in side effects of 2% (22)
  - Repeat injections every 3 months for 2 years result in greater cartilage loss than saline injection (23)

## Other Intraarticular Injections

- 2021 and 2016 systematic reviews show that intraarticular platelet-rich plasma (PRP) injections every other week provided superior pain relief at 12 months to a single LCI (24,25)
- Three systematic reviews show efficacy of viscosupplementation in relief of pain vs. placebo with a longer duration of effect compared to LCIs up to 13 weeks (26–28)
  - 2021 systematic review shows Hylan G-F 20, sodium hyaluronate preparations, and hyaluronan exhibit good safety profiles, minimal side effects, and some degree of benefit over placebo at least (29)
- 2019 systematic review of bone marrow-derived, adipose tissue-derived, and amnion-derived mesenchymal stem cells shows minimal, but sufficient, evidence to support the use of mesenchymal stem cell intraarticular injection in knee OA (30)

## Conclusions

- OA is a common etiology of chronic knee pain and disability associated with aging, weight, and physical inactivity
- Global radiographic evidence of knee OA is present in 28.7% of people over 40 years old
- Global symptomatic evidence of knee OA is present in 12.4% of people over 40 years old
- "Wear and tear" damage to hip joint leading to dysfunctional ECM reorganization leads to chronic onset of pain that is worse with use and associated with decreased knee mobility
- Years of conservative treatment with exercise, weight loss, and oral anti-inflammatories can mitigate the disease progression, but severe cases may require intraarticular injections or knee arthroplasty
- Some promising injections hope to better manage chronic symptoms by reversing the course of the disease; however, knee arthroplasty remains a gold-standard treatment for severe knee OA

## References

1. Dillon CF, Rasch EK, Gu Q, Hirsch R. Prevalence of knee osteoarthritis in the United States: Arthritis data from the Third National Health and Nutrition Examination Survey 1991–94. *J Rheumatol.* 2006;**33**(11):2271–2279.

2. Federal Interagency Forum on Aging-Related Statistics. *Older Americans 2016: Key indicators of well-being.* US Government Printing Office; 2016.

3. Felson DT, Niu J, Clancy M et al. Effect of recreational physical activities on the development of knee osteoarthritis in older adults of different weights: The Framingham study. *Arthritis Rheum.* 2007;**57**:6–12.

4. Barbour KE, Hootman JM, Helmick CG et al. Meeting physical activity guidelines and the risk of incident knee osteoarthritis: A population-based prospective cohort study. *Arthritis Care Res (Hoboken).* 2014;**66**:139–146.

5. Mora JC, Przkora R, Cruz-Almeida Y. Knee osteoarthritis: Pathophysiology and current treatment modalities. *J Pain Res.* 2018;**11**:2189–2196.

6. Heidari B. Knee osteoarthritis diagnosis, treatment and associated factors of progression: Part II. *Caspian J Intern Med.* 2011;**2**(3):249–255.

7. Cui A, Li H, Wang D et al. Global, regional prevalence, incidence and risk factors of knee osteoarthritis in population-based studies. *EClinicalMedicine.* 2020;**29–30**:100587. doi: 10.1016/j.eclinm.2020.100587.

8. Chen D, Shen J, Zhao W et al. Osteoarthritis: Toward a comprehensive understanding of pathological mechanism. *Bone Res.* 2017;**5**:16044. doi: 10.1038/boneres.2016.44.

9. Zhang W, Doherty M, Peat G et al. EULAR evidence-based recommendations for the diagnosis of knee osteoarthritis. *Ann Rheum Dis.* 2010;**69**(3):483–489.

10. Webb EJ, Osmotherly PG, Baines SK. Effect of dietary weight loss and macronutrient intake on body composition and physical function in adults with knee osteoarthritis: A systematic review. *J Nutr Gerontol Geriatr.* 2022;**41**(2):103–125.

11. Robson EK, Hodder RK, Kamper SJ et al. Effectiveness of weight-loss interventions for reducing pain and disability in people with common musculoskeletal disorders: A systematic review with meta-analysis. *J Orthop Sports Phys Ther.* 2020;**50**(6):319–333.

12. Landsmeer MLA, de Vos BC, van der Plas P et al. Effect of weight change on progression of knee OA structural features assessed by MRI in overweight and obese women. *Osteoarthritis Cartilage.* 2018;**26**(12):1666–1674.

13. Goh SL, Persson MSM, Stocks J et al. Efficacy and potential determinants of exercise therapy in knee and hip osteoarthritis: A systematic review and meta-analysis. *Ann Phys Rehabil Med.* 2019;**62**(5):356–365.

14. Raposo F, Ramos M, Lúcia Cruz A. Effects of exercise on knee osteoarthritis: A systematic review. *Musculoskeletal Care.* 2021;**19**(4):399–435.

15. Fransen M, McConnell S, Harmer AR et al. Exercise for osteoarthritis of the knee. *Cochrane Database Syst Rev.* 2015;**1**:CD004376.

16. Puljak L, Marin A, Vrdoljak D et al. Celecoxib for osteoarthritis. *Cochrane Database Syst Rev.* 2017;**5**(5):CD009865.

17. Towheed TE, Maxwell L, Judd MG et al. Acetaminophen for osteoarthritis. *Cochrane Database Syst Rev.* 2006;(1):CD004257. doi: 10.1002/14651858 .CD004257.pub2.

18. Toupin April K, Bisaillon J, Welch V et al. Tramadol for osteoarthritis. *Cochrane Database Syst Rev.* 2019;**5**(5):CD005522.

19. da Costa BR, Nüesch E, Kasteler R et al. Oral or transdermal opioids for osteoarthritis of the knee or hip. *Cochrane Database Syst Rev.* 2014;(9): CD003115. doi: 10.1002/14651858.CD003115.pub4.

20. Towheed TE, Maxwell L, Anastassiades TP et al. Glucosamine therapy for treating osteoarthritis. *Cochrane Database Syst Rev.* 2005;(2):CD002946. doi: 10.1002/14651858.CD002946.pub2.

21. Singh JA, Noorbaloochi S, MacDonald R, Maxwell LJ. Chondroitin for osteoarthritis. *Cochrane Database Syst Rev.* 2015;**1**(1):CD005614.

22. Jüni P, Hari R, Rutjes AW et al. Intra-articular corticosteroid for knee osteoarthritis. *Cochrane Database Syst Rev.* 2015;(10):CD005328. doi: 10.1002/14651858.CD005328.pub3.

23. McAlindon TE, LaValley MP, Harvey WF et al. Effect of intra-articular triamcinolone vs saline on knee cartilage volume and pain in patients with knee osteoarthritis: A randomized clinical trial. *JAMA.* 2017;**317**:1967–1975.

24. McLarnon M, Heron N. Intra-articular platelet-rich plasma injections versus intra-articular corticosteroid injections for symptomatic management of knee osteoarthritis: Systematic review and meta-analysis. *BMC Musculoskelet Disord.* 2021;**22**(1):550. doi: 10.1186/s12891-021-04308-3.

25. Meheux CJ, McCulloch PC, Lintner DM, Varner KE, Harris JD. Efficacy of intra-articular platelet-rich plasma injections in knee osteoarthritis: A systematic review. *Arthroscopy.* 2016;**32**(3):495–505.

26. Bellamy N, Campbell J, Robinson V et al. Viscosupplementation for the treatment of osteoarthritis of the knee. *Cochrane Database Syst Rev.* 2006;(2): CD005321. doi: 10.1002/14651858.CD005321.pub2.

27. Richette P, Chevalier X, Ea HK et al. Hyaluronan for knee osteoarthritis: An updated meta-analysis of trials with low risk of bias. *RMD Open.* 2015;**1**(1): e000071.

28. Xing D, Wang B, Liu Q et al. Intra-articular hyaluronic acid in treating knee osteoarthritis: A PRISMA-compliant systematic review of overlapping meta-analysis. *Sci Rep.* 2016;**6**:32790. doi: 10.1038/srep32790.

29. Peck J, Slovek A, Miro P et al. A comprehensive review of viscosupplementation in osteoarthritis of the knee. *Orthop Rev (Pavia).* 2021;**13**(2):25549. doi: 10.52965/001c.25549.

30. Di Matteo B, Vandenbulcke F, Vitale ND et al. Minimally manipulated mesenchymal stem cells for the treatment of knee osteoarthritis: A systematic review of clinical evidence. *Stem Cells Int.* 2019;2019:1735242. doi: 10.1155/ 2019/1735242.

# Chapter 23

# Chronic Ankle and Foot Pain

Kevin Bennett and Jamal Hasoon

- The complexity of the ankle/foot mechanism and its role in locomotion makes the associated structures highly susceptible to repetitive trauma and chronic pain
- An average of 20% of adults >45 years old will experience frequent foot or ankle pain that has a significant impact on mobility (1,2)
- Foot and ankle surgery accounted for $11 billion of Medicare spending in 2011, with most of the cost being in dislocations, fractures, and reconstructive surgery (3)
- Common risk factors for ankle and foot pain include increased metatarsal pressure during gait, increased walking during the day, increased BMI, increased age, and history of osteo- or rheumatoid-arthritis (4–6)
- Chronic ankle instability (CAI) is a common source of chronic pain secondary to repetitive trauma of ligamentous structures in the ankle joint (7–9)
- Other common causes of chronic ankle or foot pain include Morton's neuroma, Achilles tendinopathy, tarsal tunnel syndrome, plantar fasciitis (discussed in Chapter 24), gout, ankle osteoarthritis, rheumatoid arthritis, and posterior tibial tendon dysfunction (10)
- Early treatment and prevention of many of these conditions relies on weight loss, foot biomechanics correction, and foot/ankle-strengthening exercises (11)
- Acetaminophen and oral nonsteroidal anti-inflammatory drugs (NSAIDs) are recommended for prn pain relief as well as local corticosteroid injections (LCIs) for more severe cases (10,12)
- Surgery is often reserved for severe cases of any given condition, but is sometimes considered as an earlier treatment based on the patient's specific clinical picture (13–15)

# Epidemiology and Risk Factors

- Prevalence of foot pain in adults age >45 years is 24% (1)
  - Most common location is forefoot
- Prevalence of ankle pain in adults age >45 years is 15% (1)
  - CAI among the most common diagnoses associated with ageing (7–9)
- Common risk factors for chronic foot and ankle pain secondary to CAI (4–6,10)
  - Increasing age
  - Female gender
  - Obesity
  - History of osteoarthritis
  - History of rheumatoid arthritis
  - Low physical activity
  - High-impact/-stress occupation
  - Poor foot biomechanics
- Morton's neuroma risk factors include female gender, shoes/ activities that put prolonged pressure on the metatarsal transverse ligament, dancing, running, walking (16)
- Achilles tendinopathy risk factors include excessive heel strike while running, repetitive exertion to the tendon, vascularization of the tendon, increasing age, female gender, increasing BMI, and poor ankle stability/strength (17)
- Tarsal tunnel syndrome risk factors include increasing age, female gender, competitive athletes, and occupations that require prolonged standing or walking (18)
- Gout risk factors include increasing age, meat and alcohol in diet, increasing BMI, hypertension, diabetes, genetic predispositions, and other systemic conditions leading to a hyperuricemic state (19,20)

# Pathophysiology

- CAI (21)
  - Failure of the ankle joint integrity after repetitive injury to the ligamentous complex
  - Combination of mechanical instability and functional compromise from neuromuscular weakness
- Morton's neuroma (22)
  - Irritation and inflammation of the interdigital nerve (most commonly between the third and fourth metatarsal heads)

- ○ Secondary to increased pressure on the nerve from chronic hyperpronation, narrowing of the toe box in shoes, or other foot deformities
- Achilles tendinopathy (17,23)
  - ○ Chronic overexertion of the Achilles tendon coupled with inflammation and degenerative changes
  - ○ Related to poor foot mechanics with excessive heel-strike while running
- Tarsal tunnel syndrome (18)
  - ○ Compressive entrapment neuropathy of the posterior tibial nerve and distal branches at the tarsal tunnel
  - ○ Related to trauma, mechanical compressive stress (external or anatomical), mass effect from a tumor or other bone growth, inflammatory changes to the tarsal tunnel, or increased tunnel pressure from obesity and edema
- Gout (24)
  - ○ Inflammatory arthritis caused by deposition of monosodium urate crystals in joints
  - ○ Caused by either increased uric acid production, decreased uric acid excretion, or an altered step in purine metabolism, all leading to hyperuricemia
- Osteoarthritis (25)
  - ○ Chronic mechanical damage to a joint space with inflammatory infiltrates, altered extracellular matrix reconstruction, and a gradual loss of cartilage and flexibility in the joint
- Rheumatoid arthritis (26)
  - ○ Autoimmune synovitis targeting symmetric synovial joints
  - ○ Chronic inflammation causes structural changes in joint space, extracellular matrix, and nearby bony structures

# Diagnosis

- CAI (21,27)
  - ○ Patient history will typically include chronic pain with use, previous sprains, fractures, or surgeries, and ankle weakness with gait
  - ○ Physical exam includes assessment of passive laxity of ligamentous structures, inspection of bilateral ankle, hindfoot,

and midfoot structures for abnormalities, and full gait and strength tests of the lower leg

- Morton's neuroma (16,22)
  - Patient history will include a sharp mass-like pain in the forefoot that is worse with pronation or wearing narrow shoes
  - The Mulder test puts pressure on the metatarsals, resulting in pain at the lesion and a clicking sensation as the structures compress
  - Ultrasound will reveal a hypoechoic lesion in the interdigital space

- Achilles tendinopathy (28,29)
  - Patients will report pain in the posterior heel that is aggravated by walking, jumping, and tight-fitting shoes
  - Physical exam will show tenderness to palpation of the posterior calcaneus where the Achilles tendon inserts
  - Ultrasound and MRI are used to grade the severity of the disease by pathological changes in the tendon, but not necessary to diagnose

- Tarsal tunnel syndrome (30,31)
  - Patient history is the best diagnostic tool with the description of paresthesia and hyperesthesia along the distribution of the tibial nerve distal to the tarsal tunnel
  - Tinel's sign is also suggestive of tarsal tunnel syndrome if tapping over the tunnel results in distal paresthesias
  - Nerve conduction studies are also used to confirm diagnosis

- Gout (24)
  - Most patients present initially with an acute episode of painful monoarthritis
  - Physical exam will elicit exquisite tenderness to palpation and swelling of the affected joint
  - The presence of monosodium urate crystals in the synovial fluid can confirm the diagnosis while blood levels of uric acid help to monitor risk of flare-ups

- Osteoarthritis (25,32)
  - While less common than other forms of osteoarthritis, a patient will complain of similar symptoms of dull, aching, chronic pain that is asymmetric and worse with use throughout the day
  - Painful and altered gait, bony enlargement of the ankle joint, and decreased active and passive range of motion

- X-ray will show osteophytic changes, joint space narrowing, and sclerosis
- Rheumatoid arthritis (33,34)
  - Many patients will exhibit other sequelae of rheumatoid arthritis, but classically the pain will be symmetric with no swelling and no tenderness to palpation
  - Physical exam may look similar to other diseases with swelling, redness, tenderness, warmth, painful range of motion, and deformity in later disease
  - Elevated ESR and CRP are indicative of rheumatoid arthritis and RF and anti-CCP antibodies can help confirm a diagnosis

# Treatments

- Treatment of chronic foot and ankle pain usually begins with prevention, mitigation of disease progression, and as-needed symptomatic treatment with physical therapy, exercise, and over-the-counter pain medication; however, several minimally invasive nonsurgical treatment methods have been discovered for the various ailments (10,12)
- *CAI*
  - Corticosteroid injections have been studied in a number of cases of chronic ankle pain and instability and are generally found to be no better than placebo (12,35)
  - 2022 systematic review shows that hyaluronic acid injection is effective in pain relief and return of functionality in soft tissue injuries; however, only one article on CAI was included in the study (36)
  - 2009 randomized controlled trial (RCT) reports hyaluronic acid injection resulted in fewer recurrent ankle sprains and better baseline pain relief over 2 years when compared to placebo injections plus standard conservative treatment (37)
  - 2015 systematic review shows that platelet-rich plasma (PRP) injection was more effective in controlling pain and restoring function in various cartilaginous ankle pathologies vs. placebo (38)
  - Joint mobilization and strength/proprioceptive exercises are effective therapies for regaining function (39–41)
  - While many surgeries are effective in restoring function to a severe CAI case, there is insufficient evidence to support a consensus on surgical approach (42)

- *Morton's neuroma*
  - 2019 systematic review of nonsurgical approaches to Morton's neuroma treatment shows effective pain control up to 6 months with direct corticosteroid injections (43)
  - 2018 systematic review of alcohol plus local anesthetic reports promising results for pain control but extreme heterogeneity of methods and follow-up period (44)
    - 4–50% alcohol solutions were used with a variety of local anesthetic formulations and concentrations
    - Frequency and number of injections was also nonstandardized
  - 2016 RCT of 0.1 mg capsaicin injected directly into a Morton's neuroma shows significant pain relief vs. placebo for at least 12 weeks post-injection (45)
  - 2018 case series of 83 patients receiving hyaluronic acid injection shows functional improvement and pain control up to 12 months (46)
  - The traditional surgical approach of neurectomy is becoming less popular as effective noninvasive treatments become available (22)

- *Achilles tendinopathy*
  - 2018 systematic review of PRP injection for Achilles tendinopathy shows no clear benefit over normal saline injection (47)
    - Authors report small sample size and insufficient number of RCTs to come to an accurate conclusion
    - Call for more trials is based on success of PRP therapy with other tendon pathologies (48)
  - 2011 RCT of prolotherapy injections vs. eccentric loading exercise shows a significant decrease in pain and improvement in function for 12 months in favor of prolotherapy (49)

- *Tarsal tunnel syndrome*
  - Corticosteroid injections into the tarsal tunnel are recommended along with oral anti-inflammatory drugs as conservative first-line treatment despite little-to-no recorded evidence to support its use (50–52)
  - 2022 systematic review reports that, while surgical intervention by means of endoscopic tarsal tunnel release is only required in select patients who fail conservative management with physical therapy, orthotics, and pharmaceutical pain relief, it is an effective method of management in refractory cases (53)

- *Gout*
  - Two RCTs on the use of steroid injections for acute gout attacks show that it is effective in acute pain relief vs. placebo (54,55)
  - Despite lack of RCTs on the topic, several guidelines and systematic reviews recommend the use of local corticosteroid injections for patients with gout-related pain, especially those with a contraindication to oral therapy, due to the safety profile of the treatment (56–58)

- *Osteoarthritis*
  - The majority of foot and ankle osteoarthritis (OA) is controlled with NSAIDs, orthotics, physical therapy, and exercise; however, local injections are also a hallmark of conservative treatment (59)
  - Several clinical trials have shown pain relief following intraarticular corticosteroid injection for at least 3 months (60–62)
    - One study found that participants with BMI<30 experienced pain relief for 12 months
  - 2007 RCT comparing corticosteroid injection to hyaluronic acid injection shows improvement from baseline in both groups up to 56 days following injection with hyaluronic acid yielding superior results during the follow-up period (63)
  - 2018 systematic review of intraarticular injections for ankle arthritis shows that hyaluronic acid provides significant pain relief at 6 months post-injection with some studies reporting relief up to 18 months (64)
  - Two 2017 trials of PRP injection for ankle OA show significant pain control from 5 to 17 months post-injection (65,66)
  - A small 2015 trial of mesenchymal stem cells shows significant pain relief and function improvement for at least 30 months post-injection (67)
    - WOMAC pain score maintained from 40 to 8.3 at 30 months
    - Tolerable walking distance from 1,010 m pre-injection was improved to 2,333 m at 30 months

- *Rheumatoid Arthritis*
  - Three trials of intraarticular corticosteroid injection for rheumatoid arthritis show significant pain relief from 1 to 12 weeks post-injection (68–70)

- ○ One 2018 study compared intraarticular corticosteroids to intraarticular methotrexate in 58 ankles showing significant pain relief up to 20 weeks (71)

  - ▪ Methotrexate additionally resulted in significantly decreased synovitis evidenced by ultrasound

## Conclusions

- Chronic foot and ankle pain is a common symptom of a wide variety of conditions
- Nationwide burden of substantial foot or ankle pain is 24% and 15%, respectively, resulting in a significant healthcare burden
- While certain conditions have more specific etiologies or risk factors, many origins of chronic pain lie in obesity, lack of exercise/foot strength, and poor foot biomechanics
- Chronic repetitive damage to the surrounding ligaments of the ankle joint structure or repetitive damage to the synovial joint itself can lead to CAI and osteoarthritis, respectively
- Systemic disease, acute and overuse injuries, and anatomical deformities must also be considered when evaluating for the origin of pain
- For many conditions, conservative treatment with oral anti-inflammatory drugs, orthotics, and physical therapy are first-line treatment and mitigate symptoms effectively in a majority of compliant patients
- There is good evidence for the use of various modalities of pharmaceutical injections before recommending a patient to a more invasive surgical procedure

## References

1. Thomas MJ, Roddy E, Zhang W et al. The population prevalence of foot and ankle pain in middle and old age: A systematic review. *Pain.* 2011;**152** (12):2870–2880.

2. Menz HB, Dufour AB, Casey VA et al. Foot pain and mobility limitations in older adults: The Framingham foot study. *J Gerontol A Biol Sci Med Sci.* 2013;**68**(10):1281–1285.

3. Belatti DA, Phisitkul P. Economic burden of foot and ankle surgery in the US Medicare population. *Foot Ankle Int.* 2014;**35**(4):334–340.

4. Werner RA, Gell N, Hartigan A, Wiggermann N, Keyserling WM. Risk factors for foot and ankle disorders among assembly plant workers. *Am J Ind Med*. 2010;**53**(12):1233–1239.

5. Oh-Park M, Kirschner J, Abdelshahed D, Kim DDJ. Painful foot disorders in the geriatric population: A narrative review. *Am J Phys Med Rehabil*. 2019;**98** (9):811–819.

6. Yong RJ, Mullins PM, Bhattacharyya N. Prevalence of chronic pain among adults in the United States. *Pain*. 2022;**163**(2):e328–e332.

7. Gribble PA. Evaluating and differentiating ankle instability. *J Athl Train*. 2019;**54**(6):617–627.

8. Miklovic TM, Donovan L, Protzuk OA, Kang MS, Feger MA. Acute lateral ankle sprain to chronic ankle instability: A pathway of dysfunction. *Phys Sportsmed*. 2018;**46**(1):116–122.

9. Czajka CM, Tran E, Cai AN, DiPreta JA. Ankle sprains and instability. *Med Clin North Am*. 2014;**98**(2):313–329.

10. Urits I, Smoots D, Franscioni H et al. Injection techniques for common chronic pain conditions of the foot: A comprehensive review. *Pain Ther*. 2020;**9**(1):145–160.

11. van der Merwe C, Shultz SP, Colborne GR, Fink PW. Foot muscle strengthening and lower limb injury prevention. *Res Q Exerc Sport*. 2021;**92** (3):380–387.

12. Urits I, Hasegawa M, Orhurhu V et al. Minimally invasive treatment of chronic ankle instability: A comprehensive review. *Curr Pain Headache Rep*. 2020;**24**(3): 1040–1048. doi: 10.1007/s00167-016-4041-1.

13. Khlopas H, Khlopas A, Samuel LT et al. Current concepts in osteoarthritis of the ankle: Review. *Surg Technol Int*. 2019;**35**:280–294.

14. Pietramaggiori G, Sapino G, De Santis G, Bassetto F, Scherer S. Chronic knee and ankle pain treatment through selective microsurgical approaches: A minimally invasive option in the treatment algorithm for refractory lower limb pain. *J Reconstr Microsurg*. 2021;**37**(3):234–241.

15. Arroyo-Hernández M, Mellado-Romero M, Páramo-Díaz P, García-Lamas L, Vilà-Rico J. Chronic ankle instability: Arthroscopic anatomical repair. *Rev Esp Cir Ortop Traumatol*. 2017;**61**(2):104–110.

16. Di Caprio F, Meringolo R, Shehab Eddine M, Ponziani L. Morton's interdigital neuroma of the foot: A literature review. *Foot Ankle Surg*. 2018;**24** (2):92–98.

17. Longo UG, Ronga M, Maffulli N. Achilles tendinopathy. *Sports Med Arthrosc Rev*. 2018;**26**(1):16–30.

18. McSweeney SC, Cichero M. Tarsal tunnel syndrome: A narrative literature review. *Foot (Edinb)*. 2015;**25**(4):244–250.

19. Kuo CF, Grainge MJ, Zhang W, Doherty M. Global epidemiology of gout: Prevalence, incidence and risk factors. *Nat Rev Rheumatol.* 2015;**11**(11):649–662.

20. Evans PL, Prior JA, Belcher J et al. Obesity, hypertension and diuretic use as risk factors for incident gout: A systematic review and meta-analysis of cohort studies. *Arthritis Res Ther.* 2018;**20**(1):136. doi: 10.1186/s13075-018-1612-1.

21. Al-Mohrej OA, Al-Kenani NS. Chronic ankle instability: Current perspectives. *Avicenna J Med.* 2016;**6**(4):103–108.

22. Gougoulias N, Lampridis V, Sakellariou A. Morton's interdigital neuroma: Instructional review. *EFORT Open Rev.* 2019;**4**(1):14–24.

23. Kader D, Saxena A, Movin T, Maffulli N. Achilles tendinopathy: Some aspects of basic science and clinical management. *Br J Sports Med.* 2002;**36**(4):239–249.

24. Ragab G, Elshahaly M, Bardin T. Gout: An old disease in new perspective: A review. *J Adv Res.* 2017;**8**(5):495–511.

25. Paterson KL, Gates L. Clinical assessment and management of foot and ankle osteoarthritis: A review of current evidence and focus on pharmacological treatment. *Drugs Aging.* 2019;**36**(3):203–211.

26. Aletaha D, Neogi T, Silman AJ et al. Rheumatoid arthritis classification criteria: An American College of Rheumatology/European League Against Rheumatism collaborative initiative. *Arthritis Rheum.* 2010;**62**(9):2569–2581.

27. Gribble PA, Delahunt E, Bleakley CM et al. Selection criteria for patients with chronic ankle instability in controlled research: A position statement of the International Ankle Consortium. *J Athl Train.* 2014;**49**(1):121–127.

28. Weinfeld SB. Achilles tendon disorders. *Med Clin North Am.* 2014;**98**(2):331–338.

29. Zellers JA, Bley BC, Pohlig RT, Alghamdi NH, Silbernagel KG. Frequency of pathology on diagnostic ultrasound and relationship to patient demographics in individuals with insertional Achilles tendinopathy. *Int J Sports Phys Ther.* 2019;**14**(5):761–769.

30. Antoniadis G, Scheglmann K. Posterior tarsal tunnel syndrome diagnosis and treatment. *Dtsch Arztebl.* 2008;**105**(45):776–781.

31. Rinkel WD, Cabezas MC, Van Neck JW et al. Validity of the Tinel sign and prevalence of tibial nerve entrapment at the tarsal tunnel in both diabetic and nondiabetic subjects: A cross-sectional study. *Plast Reconstr Surg.* 2018;**142**(5):1258–1266.

32. Roddy E, Thomas MJ, Marshall M et al. The population prevalence of symptomatic radiographic foot osteoarthritis in community-dwelling older adults: Cross-sectional findings from the clinical assessment study of the foot. *Ann Rheum Dis.* 2015;**74**(1):156–163.

33. Simonsen MB, Hørslev-Petersen K, Cöster MC, Jensen C, Bremander A. Foot and ankle problems in patients with rheumatoid arthritis in 2019: Still an important issue. *ACR Open Rheumatol.* 2021;3(6):396–402.

34. Heidari B. Rheumatoid arthritis: Early diagnosis and treatment outcomes. *Caspian J Intern Med.* 2011;2(1):161–170.

35. Gerstner Garces JB. Chronic ankle instability. *Foot Ankle Clin.* 2012;17 (3):389–398.

36. Khan M, Shanmugaraj A, Prada C et al. The role of hyaluronic acid for soft tissue indications: A systematic review and meta-analysis. *Sports Health.* 2022;15(1):86–96. doi: 10.1177/19417381211073316. .

37. Petrella MJ, Cogliano A, Petrella RJ. Original research: Long-term efficacy and safety of periarticular hyaluronic acid in acute ankle sprain. *Phys Sportsmed.* 2009;37:64–70.

38. Vannini F, Di Matteo B, Filardo G. Platelet-rich plasma to treat ankle cartilage pathology – from translational potential to clinical evidence: A systematic review. *J Exp Orthop.* 2015;2(1):2. doi: 10.1186/s40634-015-0019-z.

39. Cruz-Díaz D, Lomas Vega R, Osuna-Pérez MC, Hita-Contreras F, Martínez-Amat A. Effects of joint mobilization on chronic ankle instability: A randomized controlled trial. *Disabil Rehabil.* 2015;37(7):601–610.

40. Cain MS, Ban RJ, Chen YP et al. Four-week ankle-rehabilitation programs in adolescent athletes with chronic ankle instability. *J Athl Train.* 2020;55 (8):801–810.

41. Anguish B, Sandrey MA. Two 4-week balance training programs for chronic ankle instability. *J Athl Train.* 2018;53(7):662–671.

42. Chang SH, Morris BL, Saengsin J et al. Diagnosis and treatment of chronic lateral ankle instability: Review of our biomechanical evidence. *J Am Acad Orthop Surg.* 2021;29(1):3–16.

43. Matthews BG, Hurn SE, Harding MP, Henry RA, Ware RS. The effectiveness of non-surgical interventions for common plantar digital compressive neuropathy (Morton's neuroma): A systematic review and meta-analysis. *J Foot Ankle Res.* 2019;12.12 doi; 10.1186/s13047-019-0320-7.

44. Santos D, Morrison G, Coda A. Sclerosing alcohol injections for the management of intermetatarsal neuromas: A systematic review. *Foot (Edinb).* 2018;35:36–47.

45. Campbell CM, Diamond E, Schmidt WK et al. A randomized, double-blind, placebo-controlled trial of injected capsaicin for pain in Morton's neuroma. *Pain.* 2016;157(6):1297–1304.

46. Lee K, Hwang IY, Ryu CH, Lee JW, Kang SW. Ultrasound-guided hyaluronic acid injection for the management of Morton's neuroma. *Foot Ankle Int.* 2018;39(2):201–204.

47. Zhang YJ, Xu SZ, Gu PC et al. Is platelet-rich plasma injection effective for chronic Achilles tendinopathy? A meta-analysis. *Clin Orthop Relat Res.* 2018;**476**(8):1633–1641.

48. Chen X, Jones IA, Park C, Vangsness CT Jr. The efficacy of platelet-rich plasma on tendon and ligament healing: A systematic review and meta-analysis with bias assessment. *Am J Sports Med.* 2018;**46**(8):2020–2032.

49. Yelland MJ, Sweeting KR, Lyftogt JA et al. Prolotherapy injections and eccentric loading exercises for painful Achilles tendinosis: A randomised trial. *Br J Sports Med.* 2011;**45**(5):421–428.

50. Ferkel E, Davis WH, Ellington JK. Entrapment neuropathies of the foot and ankle. *Clin Sports Med.* 2015;**34**(4):791–801.

51. Tu P. Heel pain: Diagnosis and management. *Am Fam Physician.* 2018;**97**(2):86–93.

52. Choo YJ, Park CH, Chang MC. Rearfoot disorders and conservative treatment: A narrative review. *Ann Palliat Med.* 2020;**9**(5):3546–3552.

53. Vij N, Kaley HN, Robinson CL et al. Clinical results following conservative management of tarsal tunnel syndrome compared with surgical treatment: A systematic review. *Orthop Rev (Pavia).* 2022;**14**(3):37539. doi: 10.52965/001c.37539.

54. Kang MH, Moon KW, Jeon YH, Cho SW. Sonography of the first metatarsophalangeal joint and sonographically guided intraarticular injection of corticosteroid in acute gout attack. *J Clin Ultrasound.* 2015;**43**(3):179–186.

55. Fernández C, Noguera R, González JA, Pascual E. Treatment of acute attacks of gout with a small dose of intraarticular triamcinolone acetonide. *J Rheumatol.* 1999;**26**(10):2285–2286.

56. Wechalekar MD, Vinik O, Moi JH et al. The efficacy and safety of treatments for acute gout: Results from a series of systematic literature reviews including Cochrane reviews on intraarticular glucocorticoids, colchicine, nonsteroidal antiinflammatory drugs, and interleukin-1 inhibitors. *J Rheumatol Suppl.* 2014;**92**:15–25.

57. Richette P, Doherty M, Pascual E et al. 2016 updated EULAR evidence-based recommendations for the management of gout. *Ann Rheum Dis.* 2017;**76**(1):29–42.

58. Wechalekar MD, Vinik O, Schlesinger N, Buchbinder R. Intra-articular glucocorticoids for acute gout. *Cochrane Database Syst Rev.* 2013;(4):CD009920. doi: 10.1002/14651858.CD009920.pub2.

59. Roddy E, Menz HB. Foot osteoarthritis: Latest evidence and developments. *Therap Adv Musculoskelet Dis.* 2018;**10**:91–103.

60. Drakonaki EE, Kho JSB, Sharp RJ, Ostlere SJ. Efficacy of ultrasound-guided steroid injections for pain management of midfoot joint degenerative disease. *Skelet Radiol.* 2011;**40**(8):1001–1006.

61. Protheroe D, Gadgil A. Guided intra-articular corticosteroid injections in the midfoot. *Foot Ankle Int.* 2018;**39**(8):1001–1004.

62. Grice J, Marsland D, Smith G, Calder J. Efficacy of foot and ankle corticosteroid injections. *Foot Ankle Int.* 2017;**38**(1):8–13.

63. Pons M, Alvarez F, Solana J, Viladot R, Varela L. Sodium hyaluronate in the treatment of hallux rigidus. A single-blind, randomized study. *Foot ankle Int.* 2007;**28**(1):38–42.

64. Vannabouathong C, Del Fabbro G, Sales B et al. Intra-articular injections in the treatment of symptoms from ankle arthritis: A systematic review. *Foot Ankle Int.* 2018;**39**(10):1141–1150.

65. Fukawa T, Yamaguchi S, Akatsu Y et al. Safety and efficacy of intra-articular injection of platelet-rich plasma in patients with ankle osteoarthritis. *Foot Ankle Int.* 2017;**38**(6):596–604.

66. Repetto I, Biti B, Cerruti P, Trentini R, Felli L. Conservative treatment of ankle osteoarthritis: Can platelet-rich plasma effectively postpone surgery? *J Foot Ankle Surg.* 2017;**56**(2):362–365.

67. Emadedin M, Ghorbani Liastani M, Fazeli R et al. Long-term follow-up of intra-articular injection of autologous mesenchymal stem cells in patients with knee, ankle, or hip osteoarthritis. *Arch Iran Med.* 2015;**18**(6):336–344.

68. Lopes RV, Furtado RNV, Parmigiani L et al. Accuracy of intra-articular injections in peripheral joints performed blindly in patients with rheumatoid arthritis. *Rheumatology.* 2008;**47**(12):1792–1794.

69. Cunnington J, Marshall N, Hide G et al. A randomized, double-blind, controlled study of ultrasound-guided corticosteroid injection into the joint of patients with inflammatory arthritis. *Arthritis Rheum.* 2010;**62** (7);1862–1869.

70. Furtado RNV, Machado FS, da Luz KR et al. Intra-articular injection with triamcinolone hexacetonide in patients with rheumatoid arthritis: Prospective assessment of goniometry and joint inflammation parameters. *Rev Bras Reumatol (English Ed.).* 2017;**57**(2):115–121.

71. Mortada MA, Abdelwhab SM, Elgawish MH. Intra-articular methotrexate versus corticosteroid injections in medium-sized joints of rheumatoid arthritis patients: An intervention study. *Clin Rheumatol.* 2018;**37** (2):331–337.

# Chapter 24

# Plantar Fasciitis

Kevin Bennett and Morgan Hasegawa

- Inflammation of plantar fascia secondary to chronic, repetitive microtrauma and a number of contributing risk factors (1)
- The fascia is formed by three bands of connective tissue emerging from the medial aspect of the calcaneus and coursing distally along the plantar aspect of the foot to the proximal phalanx of each toe (1)
- Cause of approximately one million patient visits per year (2)
- Estimated healthcare spending burden of up to $376 million per year (3)
- Typically caused by repetitive trauma to the heel, obesity, and poor foot/ankle biomechanics (2,4,5)
- Pain experienced primarily in the inferior aspect of the calcaneus with radiation along the plantar aspect of the foot (6)
- Pain is reproducible by direct palpation of the inferior heel or extension of the toes on a dorsiflexed ankle (4)
- Classic presentation is pain in the morning while stepping out of bed and improving throughout the day (6)
- Common treatments include stretching, anti-inflammatory drugs, physical therapy, local corticosteroid injections (LCI), and surgical intervention (4,6)

## Epidemiology and Risk Factors

- Lifetime prevalence of approximately 10% in American adults (2)
- 2013 U.S. National Health and Wellness Survey of 75,000 individuals (7)
  - PF present in 0.85% of the entire population
  - 1.19% of women and 0.47% of men affected
  - 1.33% prevalence in those aged 45–64 years
    - 0.53% prevalence in those aged 18–44 years
  - 1.48% prevalence in obese participants

- 0.29% prevalence in those with BMI <25
- Common risk factors for PF (2,4,5,8)
  - Occupations or recreational activities requiring repetitive micro-trauma to the inferior heel
    - Long-distance running
    - Jobs involving prolonged standing
    - Military
  - Obesity
  - Flat or high arches
  - Poor foot and ankle biomechanics, strength, and flexibility
  - Sedentary lifestyle

# Pathophysiology

- The plantar fascia is actually an aponeurosis of three bands of connective tissue on the plantar aspect of the foot (1)
  - Bands originate at the medial tuberosity of the calcaneus and insert at the base of the proximal phalanx of each metatarsal head
- It helps to structure the foot's arch and aids heavily in the biomechanics of the foot during walking and running (1)
  - The tissue stores potential energy generated by pronation and weight-loading on the distal metatarsals at the beginning of a stride and releases kinetic energy back through to the distal foot as the foot plantarflexes and continues motion forward
- PF's name implies an inflammatory process; however, histological findings of the plantar fascia imply more of a chronic degenerative condition possibly secondary to chronic inflammation (1,9)
  - Repetitive inflammatory responses lead to fibrosis, local elastic tissue degeneration, thickening of the plantar fascia, and, ultimately, a reduction of elasticity
  - Stretching of the new, inelastic tissue is thought to be the source of the symptoms of PF (8,9)

# Diagnosis

- Diagnosis of PF is highly sensitive and specific to a group of classic symptoms and physical exam findings, but can be confirmed with ultrasound imaging
- Common patient presentation (4,6,8,10)

- ○ Sharp, burning pain in the inferior heel with radiation to the arch
- ○ Pain worse in the morning, while walking, and after standing for a long period of time
- ○ Both sedentary and active lifestyles and risk factors
- Physical exam will show point tenderness at the origin of the plantar fascia, decreased dorsiflexion of ankle <10°, and exacerbation of pain with dorsiflexion of the ankle and extension of the toes (the Windlass test) (11,12)
  - ○ Windlass test
    - Sensitivity: 31.8%
    - Specificity: 100%
- Ultrasound, MRI, and X-ray imaging can be used in confirmation of PF diagnosis, but are rarely implemented in practice (13,14)
  - ○ Ultrasound of the inferior heel will show increased heel-pad thickness and plantar fascia thickness >4 mm with hypoechoic fascia
    - Sensitivity: 80%
    - Specificity: 88.5%
  - ○ Lateral X-ray of the foot will show increased plantar fascial thickness and heel fat pad abnormalities
    - Sensitivity: 85%
    - Specificity: 95%
    - Calcaneal spurs were also present in 85% of PF and 46% of controls

## Treatments

- PF treatment is heavily geared toward noninvasive and conservative management, with nonsteroidal anti-inflammatory drugs, physical therapy, strengthening exercises, weight loss, and local injections being the successful mainstay of therapy

## Weight Loss

- 2018 retrospective cohort observed 163 obese patients (average BMI of 45) of the Cleveland Clinic Bariatric and Metabolic Institute who had a known diagnosis of PF and underwent bariatric surgery for weight loss (15)

- 90% of patients experienced resolution of PF symptoms after the weight loss effects of the surgery
- Postoperative mean BMI of 34.8 and mean excess weight loss of 51.0%
- Mean number of treatment methods used for PF per patient fell from 1.9 per patient preoperatively to 0.3 per patient postoperatively

## Stretching

- 2010 RCT shows that static progressive stretch braces as well as static stretching exercises improve pain and mobility in patients with plantar fasciitis (16)
- 2020 clinical trial shows that a 3-week gastrocnemius stretching program significantly reduced plantar fascial pain and improved ankle and foot muscle strength (17)
- 2020 systematic review shows that plantar fascia–specific stretching is superior to gastrocnemius stretching in relief of PF symptoms (18)
- 2016 RCT shows that 8 weeks of extrinsic and intrinsic foot muscle strengthening exercise, abductor and lateral rotator muscle strengthening exercise, or self-stretching of hamstrings, calf, and plantar fascia all had equal benefits in reducing pain in PF patients (19)
- 2006 RCT shows significant improvement in pain and functionality at 2 years after implementation of either plantar fascial stretching alone or plantar fascial stretching with previous calf stretching (20)
  - 77% of participants reported no functional limitations at 2 years
  - 94% of participants reported decrease in pain from baseline
  - Only 24% of participants still sought any level of treatment from a clinician

## Strengthening

- 2017 systematic review shows that intrinsic foot muscle strengthening exercise improves pain and functionality in PF patients without affecting the plantar fascial thickness (21)
- 2014 RCT shows that high-load foot strengthening exercise performed every second day outperformed plantar-specific stretching at 3 months with respect to self-reported pain and foot function (22)

## Orthotics

- 2008 Cochrane review shows unclear and insufficient evidence to support the use of orthotics in plantar fasciitis pain (23)
- 2018 RCT shows decreased pain and decreased plantar fascial thickness in PF patients wearing custom foot orthoses at 4 and 12 weeks (24)
- 2015 RCT shows custom foot orthoses superior in restoring functional mobility with a 5.6-fold greater improvement to pre-fabricated orthoses or sham orthoses (25)

## Oral Anti-inflammatory Drugs

- 2018 National Health and Wellness Survey reports that 70% of patients with PF take nonsteroidal anti-inflammatory drugs (NSAIDs) or acetaminophen regularly for control of their symptoms (7)
- 2011 literature review and 2007 RCT show some moderate evidence for the benefit of NSAIDs or oral corticosteroids when used in conjunction with a multimodal conservative treatment program (26,27)

## Local Anesthetic and Corticosteroid Injections

- 2017 Cochrane review shows weak evidence to support the use of LCI for pain relief up to 1 month in PF (28)
- Approximately 10% of patients receiving repeated corticosteroid injections will experience fascial rupture (29,30)
- While evidence is limited, many comparative studies have shown that LCIs improve PF symptoms from baseline for 1 to 3 months (29,31,32,33,34)

## Platelet-rich Plasma Injections

- 2019, 2018, 2017, and 2015 RCTs show that platelet-rich plasma (PRP) injections provide similar or inferior pain relief in the short term (1 to 6 months post-injection) but superior pain relief to LCIs at 18 months post-injection (35,36,37,38)
  - Despite inferior pain relief in the long term, LCIs experienced no drop-off of efficacy at 18 months

## Botulinum Toxin Injections

- 2022 systematic review shows that botulinum toxin-A injections are effective in treating PF pain and improving functionality (39)

- 2022 and 2012 RCTs show that botulinum toxin-A injections have equal short-term and superior long-term symptom improvement to LCI (40,41)
- 2020 and 2010 RCTs show that injection of the medial head of the gastrocnemius or injection of the plantar fascia directly results in effective control of pain and improved foot mobility (42,43)

## Extracorporeal Shockwave Therapy

- 2017 meta-analysis shows that extracorporeal shockwave therapy (ESWT) significantly improves first-step pain in the morning and pain throughout the day by at least 60% (44)
- 2017 systematic review showed that ESWT is a safe procedure with few side effects other than transient pain and skin redness at the therapy site (45)
  - Average follow-up time was 14 months post-therapy
- 2016 and 2017 RCTs and 2020 meta-analysis shows that ESWT is a superior treatment in short- and long-term reduction of pain and improvement of foot mobility over botulinum toxin-A or LCIs (46,47,48)

## Radiofrequency Ablation Therapy

- 2016 study of radiofrequency ablation of the first branch of the lateral plantar nerve and the medial calcaneal nerve sensory branches showed significant improvement of plantar heel pain in patients refractory to LCIs or ESWT (49)
- 2014 study shows radiofrequency ablation of the calcaneal branches of the inferior calcaneal nerve improved pain refractory to other treatments (50)
  - 85.7% of patients reported continued symptom relief up to 2 years post-therapy
- 2017 study shows ultrasound-guided ablation of the posterior tibial nerve resulted in relief of plantar heel pain in recalcitrant PF patients (51)

# Conclusions

- PF is a common cause of chronic foot and heel pain in active and sedentary adults
- It is present in approximately 0.85% of the population and is more common in the obese, women, and those aged 45–64 years

- Point tenderness at the inferior calcaneus, radiation of pain to plantar fascia on dorsiflexion of ankle and extension of toes, and thickening of the plantar fascia on imaging are strong diagnostic indications of PF
- Most cases of PF can be managed with conservative therapy, including weight loss stretching, foot strengthening, and NSAIDs
- LCI, PRP, and botulinum toxin-A injections at the plantar fascia are all effective in relief of symptoms and return of functionality in the foot
- Treatments such as radiofrequency ablation of local nerves and ESWT are even superior to local injections and effective in many patients refractory to all other treatment

# References

1. Cutts S, Obi N, Pasapula C, Chan W. Plantar fasciitis. *Ann R Coll Surg Engl.* 2012;**94**(8):539–542.

2. Riddle DL, Schappert SM. Volume of ambulatory care visits and patterns of care for patients diagnosed with plantar fasciitis: A national study of medical doctors. *Foot Ankle Int.* 2004;**25**(5):303–310.

3. Tong KB, Furia J. Economic burden of plantar fasciitis treatment in the United States. *Am J Orthop (Belle Mead NJ).* 2010;**39**(5):227–231.

4. Thompson JV, Saini SS, Reb CW, Daniel JN. Diagnosis and management of plantar fasciitis. *J Am Osteopath Assoc.* 2014;**114**(12):900–906.

5. Muth CC. Plantar fasciitis. *JAMA.* 2017;**318**(4):400. doi: 10.1001/jama.2017.5806.

6. Carek PJ, Edenfield KM, Michaudet C, Nicolette GW. Foot and ankle conditions: Plantar fasciitis. *FP Essent.* 2018;**465**:11–17.

7. Nahin RL. Prevalence and pharmaceutical treatment of plantar fasciitis in United States adults. *J Pain.* 2018;**19**(8):885–896.

8. Thing J, Maruthappu M, Rogers J. Diagnosis and management of plantar fasciitis in primary care. *Br J Gen Pract.* 2012;**62**(601):443–444. doi: 10.3399/bjgp12X653769.

9. Miller LE, Latt DL. Chronic plantar fasciitis is mediated by local hemodynamics: Implications for emerging therapies. *North Am J Med Sci.* 2015;**7**(1):1–5.

10. Johnson RE, Haas K, Lindow K, Shields R. Plantar fasciitis: What is the diagnosis and treatment? *Orthop Nurs.* 2014;**33**(4):198–204.

11. Bolgla LA, Malone TR. Plantar fasciitis and the Windlass mechanism: A biomechanical link to clinical practice. *J Athl Train.* 2004;**39**(1):77–82.

12. De Garceau D, Dean D, Requejo SM, Thordarson DB. The association between diagnosis of plantar fasciitis and Windlass test results. *Foot Ankle Int.* 2003;**24**(3):251–255.

13. Sabir N, Demirlenk S, Yagci B, Karabulut N, Cubukcu S. Clinical utility of sonography in diagnosing plantar fasciitis. *J Ultrasound Med.* 2005;**24** (8):1041–1048.

14. Osborne HR, Breidahl WH, Allison GT. Critical differences in lateral X-rays with and without a diagnosis of plantar fasciitis. *J Sci Med Sport.* 2006;**9** (3):231–237.

15. Boules M, Batayyah E, Froylich D et al. Effect of surgical weight loss on plantar fasciitis and health-care use. *J Am Podiatr Med Assoc.* 2018;**108** (6):442–448.

16. Sharma NK, Loudon JK. Static progressive stretch brace as a treatment of pain and functional limitations associated with plantar fasciitis: A pilot study. *Foot Ankle Spec.* 2010;**3**(3):117–124.

17. Boonchum H, Bovonsunthonchai S, Sinsurin K, Kunanusornchai W. Effect of a home-based stretching exercise on multi-segmental foot motion and clinical outcomes in patients with plantar fasciitis. *J Musculoskelet Neuronal Interact.* 2020;**20**(3):411–420.

18. Siriphorn A, Eksakulkla S. Calf stretching and plantar fascia-specific stretching for plantar fasciitis: A systematic review and meta-analysis. *J Bodyw Mov Ther.* 2020;**24**(4):222–232.

19. Kamonseki DH, Gonçalves GA, Yi LC, Júnior IL. Effect of stretching with and without muscle strengthening exercises for the foot and hip in patients with plantar fasciitis: A randomized controlled single-blind clinical trial. *Man Ther.* 2016;**23**:76–82.

20. Digiovanni BF, Nawoczenski DA, Malay DP et al. Plantar fascia-specific stretching exercise improves outcomes in patients with chronic plantar fasciitis: A prospective clinical trial with two-year follow-up. *J Bone Joint Surg Am.* 2006;**88**(8):1775–1781.

21. Huffer D, Hing W, Newton R, Clair M. Strength training for plantar fasciitis and the intrinsic foot musculature: A systematic review. *Phys Ther Sport.* 2017;**24**:44–52.

22. Rathleff MS, Mølgaard CM, Fredberg U et al. High-load strength training improves outcome in patients with plantar fasciitis: A randomized controlled trial with 12-month follow-up. *Scand J Med Sci Sports.* 2015;**25**(3):292–300.

23. Hawke F, Burns J, Radford JA, du Toit V. Custom-made foot orthoses for the treatment of foot pain. *Cochrane Database Syst Rev.* 2008;(3):CD006801. doi: 10.1002/14651858.CD006801.pub2.

24. Bishop C, Thewlis D, Hillier S. Custom foot orthoses improve first-step pain in individuals with unilateral plantar fasciopathy: A pragmatic randomised

controlled trial. *BMC Musculoskelet Disord.* 2018;**19**(1):222. doi: 10.1186/s12891-018-2131-6.

25. Wrobel JS, Fleischer AE, Crews RT, Jarrett B, Najafi B. A randomized controlled trial of custom foot orthoses for the treatment of plantar heel pain. *J Am Podiatr Med Assoc.* 2015;**105**(4):281–294.

26. Goff JD, Crawford R. Diagnosis and treatment of plantar fasciitis. *Am Fam Physician.* 2011;**84**(6):676–682.

27. Donley BG, Moore T, Sferra J, Gozdanovic J, Smith R. The efficacy of oral nonsteroidal anti-inflammatory medication (NSAID) in the treatment of plantar fasciitis: A randomized, prospective, placebo-controlled study. *Foot Ankle Int.* 2007;**28**(1):20–23.

28. David JA, Sankarapandian V, Christopher PR, Chatterjee A, Macaden AS. Injected corticosteroids for treating plantar heel pain in adults. *Cochrane Database Syst Rev.* 2017;**6**(6):CD009348.

29. Tsai WC, Hsu CC, Chen CP et al. Plantar fasciitis treated with local steroid injection: Comparison between sonographic and palpation guidance. *J Clin Ultrasound.* 2006;**34**(1):12–16.

30. Sellman JR. Plantar fascia rupture associated with corticosteroid injection. *Foot Ankle Int.* 1994;**15**(7):376–381.

31. Mahindra P, Yamin M, Selhi HS, Singla S, Soni A. Chronic plantar fasciitis: Effect of platelet-rich plasma, corticosteroid, and placebo. *Orthopedics.* 2016;**39**(2):285–289.

32. Singh P, Madanipour S, Bhamra JS, Gill I. A systematic review and meta-analysis of platelet-rich plasma versus corticosteroid injections for plantar fasciopathy. *Int Orthop.* 2017;**41**(6):1169–1181.

33. Kamel M, Kotob H. High frequency ultrasonographic findings in plantar fasciitis and assessment of local steroid injection. *J Rheumatol.* 2000;**27**(9):2139–2141.

34. Monto RR. Platelet-rich plasma efficacy versus corticosteroid injection treatment for chronic severe plantar fasciitis. *Foot Ankle Int.* 2014;**35**(4):313–318.

35. Shetty SH, Dhond A, Arora M, Deore S. Platelet-rich plasma has better long-term results than corticosteroids or placebo for chronic plantar fasciitis: Randomized control trial. *J Foot Ankle Surg.* 2019;**58**(1):42–46.

36. Jain K, Murphy PN, Clough TM. Platelet rich plasma versus corticosteroid injection for plantar fasciitis: A comparative study. *Foot (Edinb).* 2015;**25**(4):235–237.

37. Acosta-Olivo C, Elizondo-Rodriguez J, Lopez-Cavazos R et al. Plantar fasciitis: A comparison of treatment with intralesional steroids versus

platelet-rich plasma a randomized, blinded study. *J Am Podiatr Med Assoc.* 2017;**107**(6):490–496.

38. Jain SK, Suprashant K, Kumar S, Yadav A, Kearns SR. Comparison of plantar fasciitis injected with platelet-rich plasma vs corticosteroids. *Foot Ankle Int.* 2018;**39**(7):780–786.

39. Acosta-Olivo C, Simental-Mendía LE, Vilchez-Cavazos F, Peña-Martínez VM et al. Clinical efficacy of botulinum toxin in the treatment of plantar fasciitis: A systematic review and meta-analysis of randomized controlled trials. *Arch Phys Med Rehabil.* 2022;**103**(2):364–371.

40. Ahadi T, Nik SS, Forogh B, Madani SP, Raissi GR. Comparison of the effect of ultrasound-guided injection of botulinum toxin type A and corticosteroid in the treatment of chronic plantar fasciitis: A randomized controlled trial. *Am J Phys Med Rehabil.* 2022;**101**(8):733–737.

41. Díaz-Llopis IV, Rodríguez-Ruíz CM, Mulet-Perry S et al. Randomized controlled study of the efficacy of the injection of botulinum toxin type A versus corticosteroids in chronic plantar fasciitis: Results at one and six months. *Clin Rehabil.* 2012;**26**(7):594–606.

42. Abbasian M, Baghbani S, Barangi S et al. Outcomes of ultrasound-guided gastrocnemius injection with botulinum toxin for chronic plantar fasciitis. *Foot Ankle Int.* 2020;**41**(1):63–68.

43. Huang YC, Wei SH, Wang HK, Lieu FK. Ultrasonographic guided botulinum toxin type A treatment for plantar fasciitis: An outcome-based investigation for treating pain and gait changes. *J Rehabil Med.* 2010;**42**(2):136–140.

44. Lou J, Wang S, Liu S, Xing G. Effectiveness of extracorporeal shock wave therapy without local anesthesia in patients with recalcitrant plantar fasciitis: A meta-analysis of randomized controlled trials. *Am J Phys Med Rehabil.* 2017;**96**(8):529–534.

45. Roerdink RL, Dietvorst M, van der Zwaard B, van der Worp H, Zwerver J. Complications of extracorporeal shockwave therapy in plantar fasciitis: Systematic review. *Int J Surg.* 2017;**46**:133–145.

46. Roca B, Mendoza MA, Roca M. Comparison of extracorporeal shock wave therapy with botulinum toxin type A in the treatment of plantar fasciitis. *Disabil Rehabil.* 2016;**38**(21):2114–2121.

47. Hocaoglu S, Vurdem UE, Cebicci MA et al. Comparative effectiveness of radial extracorporeal shockwave therapy and ultrasound-guided local corticosteroid injection treatment for plantar fasciitis. *J Am Podiatr Med Assoc.* 2017;**107**(3):192–199.

48. Sun K, Zhou H, Jiang W. Extracorporeal shock wave therapy versus other therapeutic methods for chronic plantar fasciitis. *Foot Ankle Surg.* 2020;**26**(1):33–38.

49. Arslan A, Koca TT, Utkan A, Sevimli R, Akel İ. Treatment of chronic plantar heel pain with radiofrequency neural ablation of the first branch of the lateral plantar nerve and medial calcaneal nerve branches. *J Foot Ankle Surg.* 2016;**55**(4):767–771.

50. Erken HY, Ayanoglu S, Akmaz I, Erler K, Kiral A. Prospective study of percutaneous radiofrequency nerve ablation for chronic plantar fasciitis. *Foot Ankle Int.* 2014;**35**(2):95–103.

51. Wu YT, Chang CY, Chou YC et al. Ultrasound-guided pulsed radiofrequency stimulation of posterior tibial nerve: A potential novel intervention for recalcitrant plantar fasciitis. *Arch Phys Med Rehabil.* 2017;**98**(5):964–970.

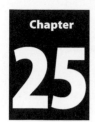

**Chapter 25**

# Phantom Limb Pain

Vwaire Orhurhu and Kevin Bennett

- The phenomenon of post-amputation pain and sensation in the lost limb is a common occurrence in amputees that leads to significant pain (1)
- In 2008, it was estimated that more than 1 in 200 individuals in the United States was an amputee to some degree and that this prevalence was expected to double to 1 in 100 by 2050 (2)
- The majority of amputations are in the lower extremities, involve at least more than one toe, and are due to vascular disease (2)
- Approximately 50% of amputees will experience phantom limb pain (PLP) in the first 24 hours post-amputation and up to 85% in the first week (3)
- The pain of PLP is described inconsistently from patient to patient; however, many develop chronic pain (3)
- While the pain itself is not necessarily indicative of a pathology, the psychological sequalae of long-term PLP lead to significant impacts on the quality of life (4)
- Treatment often requires a multidisciplinary approach including cognitive therapy, oral neuropathic pain medications, local anesthetics, and selective nerve stimulation (3)

## Epidemiology and Risk Factors

- Total number of amputees in the United States predicted to rise from 1.6 million in 2005 to 3.6 million in 2050 (2)
- Prevalence of PLP at any point post-amputation is estimated between 50 and 85% in amputees, with one 2020 systematic review reporting an average of 64% (3,5)
- Common risk factors for PLP include (5)
  - Significant chronic pain in the limb pre-amputation
  - Use of a cosmetic prosthetic leg
    - As opposed to a prosthesis that provided proprioceptive sensory input

- ○ More proximal amputations
- ○ Other non-painful phantom limb sensations
- ○ Lack of psychological counseling prior to amputation

## Pathophysiology

- The pathophysiology of PLP is not completely understood, and at this time several major theories are debated among experts as to the true mechanism of the pain
- Cortical remapping theory (6)
  - ○ This theory states that the process of "remapping" the somatosensory cortex following the brain's awareness that a limb is missing causes phantom limb sensations and pain
  - ○ It has been shown that the amount of cortical reorganization after arm amputation in adult monkeys is positively correlated to the severity of the PLP
- Neuromatrix theory (7,8)
  - ○ This theory proposes an origin of pain linked to a communication error between peripheral and central nervous systems
  - ○ Lack of visual feedback and body perception in dreams have been positively correlated with increased PLP (9)
- Proprioceptive memory theory (10)
  - ○ This theory purports that there is a proprioceptive memory in limbs that is useful in triggering pain based on the limb's position and movements, and that post-amputation movements trigger the memory that there should be pain based on the position of the remaining portion of the limb

## Diagnosis

- The presence of sensations or pain in the area of an amputated limb is consistent with phantom limb; however, there are a few diagnostic concerns to take note of when a patient presents with this syndrome
- PLP is extremely variable diagnostically but easily identified by its etiology (1,11,12)
  - ○ Onset can be immediate (24 hours to 1 week post-amputation) or years later
  - ○ It can present as an acute episode of pain or develop into a chronic issue

- It can be described as sharp, dull, stabbing, burning, pressure, electric, etc.
- Pain can be worse with stress and during sleep
- Phantom limb sensations can be broken down into (1)
  - Kinetic – perceived voluntary movements of missing limb
  - Kinesthetic – perceived change in size or position of the limb
  - Exteroceptive – perceived sensation of temperature, pressure, or vibrations
- Patients may also complain of "telescoping" where they perceive the sensation of the distal portion of the amputated limb retracting into the stump (1,11)

## Treatments

- Treatment of chronic foot and ankle pain usually begins with prevention, mitigation of disease progression, and as-needed symptomatic treatment with physical therapy, exercise, and over-the-counter pain medication; however, several minimally invasive non-surgical treatment methods have been discovered for various ailments (10,12)

## Psychiatric

- It should be noted first that there appears to be a large psychiatric component to the mechanism, treatment, and prevention of PLP that should not be underestimated for the safety of the patient and the holistic treatment of pain (13)
- One study of amputees found the prevalence of major depressive disorder at 71.2%, suicidality at 30.5%, and posttraumatic stress disorder at 20.3% (14)
- It has also been observed that higher psychiatric comorbidity correlates with worse perception of PLP (15)

## Mirror Therapy

- 2021 and 2017 systematic reviews on the use of mirror therapy and visual feedback in treatment of PLP show that pain scores are significantly reduced up to 12 months with therapy and that those with PLP for over 1 year benefited the most (16,17)
  - Reviews did report that there was significant heterogeneity among methods

## Opioids

- 2001 and 2002 crossover studies of oral and IV morphine showed significant pain relief and treatment satisfaction vs. placebo (18,19)

## Ketamine

- 2008 study of ketamine infusion for PLP pain shows that a one-time infusion of ketamine at 0.5 mg/kg significantly reduced reported pain >50% (20)

## Gabapentin

- 2016 Cochrane review pooled results from 2 RCTs studying the effect of 2.4 g/day of gabapentin for 6 weeks on PLP and shows a significant decrease in pain vs. placebo (21)

## Spinal Cord Stimulation

- 2013 case series of twelve patients undergoing cervical or thoracic spinal cord stimulation for upper or lower PLP shows eleven out of twelve patients confirming significant pain relief and five reporting relief for an average of 11 years post-stimulation (22)
- 2018 study of spinal cord stimulation plus anterior cingulotomy shows an average of 90% reduction in PLP and 80.6% improvement in depression at 2 years post-procedure (23)

## Dorsal Root Ganglion Stimulation

- 2015 case series shows a 52% reduction in PLP when electrical nodes were placed at the dorsal root ganglions proximal to the missing limb (24)

## Peripheral Cutaneous Electrical Stimulation

- 2015 case report shows rapid reduction in pain when electrical leads were placed subcutaneously on either side of a patient's missing limb for 10 days (25)
  - Relief was consistent at 6-month follow-up

## Transcranial Magnetic Stimulation

- 2016 RCT of transcranial magnetic stimulation (TMS) vs. sham procedure shows that TMS for 20 minutes a day over 10 days resulted in significantly decreased PLP for at least 2 weeks post-intervention (26)

# Conclusions

- PLP is a common source of distress and discomfort post-amputation
- Up to 85% of amputees will experience PLP at some point, and many cases become chronic pain conditions
- While the pain has been well documented for decades, the exact pathophysiology is still unclear, thus hindering a more accurate means of treatment
- Patients with significant pain in the limb pre-amputation, lack of psychological counseling, and more proximal amputations in general seem to be more prone to pain; however, the presentation of PLP varies greatly from case to case
- There are many noninvasive therapies, exercises, and medications that are recommended as first-line treatment, but the most effective and best evidenced treatments involve electrical stimulation of peripheral nerves
- Despite this lead on a promising treatment, the quality of evidence supporting or refuting any given modality is overall weak and requires much more homogenous study to truly be analyzed for efficacy

# References

1. Hsu E, Cohen SP. Postamputation pain: Epidemiology, mechanisms, and treatment. *J Pain Res.* 2013;**6**:121–136.

2. Ziegler-Graham K, MacKenzie EJ, Ephraim PL, Travison TG, Brookmeyer R. Estimating the prevalence of limb loss in the United States: 2005 to 2050. *Arch Phys Med Rehabil.* 2008;**89**:422–429.

3. Flahaut M, Laurent NL, Michetti M et al. Patient care for postamputation pain and the complexity of therapies: Living experiences. *Pain Manag.* 2018;**8**:441–453.

4. Padovani MT, Martins MRI, Venâncio A, Forni JEN. Anxiety, depression and quality of life in individuals with phantom limb pain. *Acta Ortop Bras.* 2015;**23**:107–110.

5. Limakatso K, Bedwell GJ, Madden VJ, Parker R. The prevalence and risk factors for phantom limb pain in people with amputations: A systematic review and meta-analysis. *PLoS One.* 2020;**15**(10):e0240431.

6. Flor H, Elbert T, Knecht S et al. Phantom-limb pain as a perceptual correlate of cortical reorganization following arm amputation. *Nature.* 1995;**375**(6531):482–484.

7.  Melzack R. Pain and the neuromatrix in the brain. *J Dent Educ*. 2001;**65**(12):1378–1382.

8.  Flor H. Phantom-limb pain: Characteristics, causes, and treatment. *Lancet Neurol*. 2002;**1**(3):182–189.

9.  Bekrater-Bodmann R, Schredl M, Diers M et al. Post-amputation pain is associated with the recall of an impaired body representation in dreams – results from a nation-wide survey on limb amputees. *PLoS One*. 2015;**10**(3):e0119552.

10. Anderson-Barnes VC, McAuliffe C, Swanberg KM, Tsao JW. Phantom limb pain: A phenomenon of proprioceptive memory? *Med Hypotheses*. 2009;**73**(4):555–558.

11. Anderson ML. What phantom limbs are. *Conscious Cogn*. 2018;**64**:216–226.

12. Lendaro E, Hermansson L, Burger H et al. Phantom motor execution as a treatment for phantom limb pain: Protocol of an international, double-blind, randomised controlled clinical trial. *BMJ Open*. 2018;**8**: e021039.

13. Padovani MT, Martins MRI, Venâncio A, Forni JEN. Anxiety, depression and quality of life in individuals with phantom limb pain. *Acta Ortop Bras*. 2015;**23**:107–110.

14. Sahu A, Gupta R, Sagar S, Kumar M, Sagar R. A study of psychiatric comorbidity after traumatic limb amputation: A neglected entity. *Ind Psychiatry J*. 2017;**26**:228–232.

15. Vase L, Egsgaard LL, Nikolajsen L et al. Pain catastrophizing and cortical responses in amputees with varying levels of phantom limb pain: A high-density EEG brain-mapping study. *Exp Brain Res Springer-Verlag*. 2012;**218**:407–417.

16. Herrador Colmenero L, Perez Marmol JM, Martí-García C et al. Effectiveness of mirror therapy, motor imagery, and virtual feedback on phantom limb pain following amputation: A systematic review. *Prosthet Orthot Int*. 2018;**42**(3):288–298.

17. Xie HM, Zhang KX, Wang S et al. Effectiveness of mirror therapy for phantom limb pain: A systematic review and meta-analysis. *Arch Phys Med Rehabil*. 2022;**103**(5):988–997.

18. Wu C, Tella P, Staats P et al. Analgesic effects of intravenous lidocaine and morphine on postamputation pain. *Anesthesiology*. 2002;**96**(2):841–848.

19. Huse E, Larbig W, Flor H, Birbaumer N. The effect of opioids on phantom limb pain and cortical reorganization. *Pain*. 2001;**90**(1–2):47–55.

20. Eichenberger U, Neff F, Sveticic G et al. Chronic phantom limb pain: The effects of calcitonin, ketamine, and their combination on pain and sensory thresholds. *Anesthesia & Analgesia*. 2008;**106**(4):1265–1273.

21. Alviar MJ, Hale T, Dungca M. Pharmacologic interventions for treating phantom limb pain. *Cochrane Database Syst Rev.* 2016;**10**(10):CD006380.

22. McAuley J, van Gröningen R, Green C. Spinal cord stimulation for intractable pain following limb amputation. *Neuromodulation Technol Neural Interface.* 2013;**16**:530–536.

23. Deng Z, Li D, Zhan S et al. Spinal cord stimulation combined with anterior cingulotomy to manage refractory phantom limb pain. *Stereotact Funct Neurosurg.* 2018;**96**:204–208.

24. Eldabe S, Burger K, Moser H et al. Dorsal root ganglion (DRG) stimulation in the treatment of phantom limb pain (PLP). *Neuromodulation.* 2015;**18**:610–617.

25. Cornish P, Wall C. Successful peripheral neuromodulation for phantom limb pain. *Pain Med.* 2015;**16**:761–764.

26. Malavera A, Silva FA, Fregni F, Carrillo S, Garcia RG. Repetitive transcranial magnetic stimulation for phantom limb pain in land mine victims: A double-blinded, randomized, sham-controlled trial. *J Pain.* 2016;**17**:911–918.

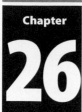

Chapter

# 26

# Post-herpetic Neuralgia (PHN)

Nazir Noor and Nolan Weinstein

- Most common complication of herpes zoster (HZ, shingles)
- Infection resulting from reactivated dormant varicella zoster virus (VZV)
- Occurs in sensory ganglia following primary infection (1)
- HZ: blistering, painful rash in dermatomal distribution
- PHN: pain lingering longer than 90 days after HZ rash
- Significantly reduces the quality of life (1,2)

## Epidemiology and Risk Factors

- Approximately 1 million cases of HZ in the United States annually (3)
- PHN occurs in about 20% of HZ patients (1,4)
- Over 50% of PHN are > 60 years old (1,4)
- Effective vaccine developed in 2006
  - Incidence has remained the same (5)
- Risk factors:
  - Increasing age, especially after 50 (6)
  - Female gender (3)
  - Severe immunosuppression (6)
  - Diabetes mellitus (6)
  - Severity of HZ infection – severe rash, acute pain
  - Prodromal pain (6)
  - Ophthalmic distribution (6)

## Pathophysiology

- Pathophysiology not clearly understood
- Reactivation of VZV infection
  - Spreads from dorsal root ganglia to periphery (7,8)

- Viral propagation causes immune response and peripheral nerve destruction
  ○ Damage results in lower threshold of neuron for pain (8,9)
  ○ Sensation of pain to nonpainful stimulus called allodynia (9)
- Alteration in voltage-gated ion channels in damaged nerves (10)
  ○ Increases hyperexcitability and nociception (8)
  ○ Elevated pain signals, sensation can be intact or altered (9)
- Viral damage also weakens descending pain inhibition pathways (8,9)
  ○ Results in prolonged activation of second-order neurons in dorsal horn (8,9)
  ○ Also loss of GABA inhibitory neurons (8,11)
- All leads to amplified afferent pain signaling, called central sensitization
- Aβ-fibers, normally relaying harmless tactile stimuli, reorganized to connect to chronically activated second-order neurons resulting in allodynia (8,12)

## Diagnosis
- PHN more difficult to diagnose than HZ
- Greater than 90 days of pain following shingles rash in the dermatomal region where the rash occurred (13)
- Quality of pain can be: sharp, intermittent, burning, stabbing, or throbbing (14)
- Severity of pain varies widely
- Patients exhibit allodynia with or without intact sensation (9)
- Diagnosis made based on history of HZ and clinical suspicion
- Can be supported by HZ antibody testing and viral cultures (13)

## Treatment
- Prevention: Two current vaccination options
  ○ Live attenuated (ZVL/Zostavax) and recombinant vaccines (RZV/Shingrix)
  ○ Both approved by the FDA for use in patients > 50 years old (15)
  ○ Vaccines not indicated in acute infection and should be withheld until resolution
- Pharmacologic options (16,17):

- ○ Tricyclic antidepressants (TCAs) first line
  - Amitriptyline, nortriptyline, and desipramine (16)
    - Inhibit sensory perceptions in the central nervous system (18–20)
  - Common side effects: anticholinergic, cardiac toxicity, and sedation (21)
  - Secondary amines have reduced side effect profile and are often used first (22)
- ○ Calcium channel $\alpha_2\delta$ ligands (anticonvulsants), also first-line therapy (16)
  - Includes gabapentin and pregabalin
  - Increased GABA availability and decrease glutamate (21)
- ○ Opioids (21,23,24)
  - Limited evidence and support of efficacy (25,26)
  - Tramadol less risk for abuse but less efficacious
  - Third-line medication, not often used (27)
- ○ Topical capsaicin, considered first line in mild cases
  - neuropeptide from peppers (28–30)
  - disrupts cutaneous nociceptors providing analgesia (31)
  - side effects of topical use include burning and erythema at the site of administration (30)
  - High concentration capsaicin patches have better efficacy than topical cream (32)
- ○ Topical lidocaine, first line
  - Can be administered as gel, cream, spray, or plaster (33,34)
  - Blocks voltage-gated sodium channels
  - Uncertain efficacy with more high-quality studies needed to confirm efficacy
- Interventional therapies (16,17):
  - ○ Botulinum toxin type A injection
    - Inhibits acetylcholine release
    - Prevents pain by inhibiting release of substance P and calcitonin (35)
  - ○ Transcutaneous electrical nerve stimulation (TENS) (36)

- Low voltage delivered to skin for pain relief (37)
- Used as adjunct to pharmacologic management (38,39)
  ○ Sympathetic nerve blockade
- Unclear role in treating PHN, current data recommend against use (36,40)
- Combination of pharmacologic and interventional approaches often used (21)

## Conclusions

- PHN is a common, painful reaction following HZ infection
  ○ 1 million cases of HZ per year with 20% resulting in PHN
- Prevalent condition that significantly reduces the quality of life in affected individuals
- Increased nociception in dermatomal region following typical HZ rash
- Strongest risk factor is increasing age, and the FDA recommends all people age > 50 get vaccinated for prevention
- First-line treatments include topical capsaicin, lidocaine, and pharmacological management with TCAs and calcium channel $\alpha_2\delta$ ligands
  ○ Myriad other treatment options, many with conflicting evidence

## References

1. Johnson RW, Rice ASC. Clinical practice: Postherpetic neuralgia. *N Engl J Med*. 2014;**371**(16):1526–1533.

2. Sampathkumar P, Drage LA, Martin DP. Herpes zoster (Shingles) and postherpetic neuralgia. *Mayo Clin Proc*. 2009;**84**(3):274–280.

3. Insinga RP, Itzler RF, Pellissier JM, Saddier P, Nikas AA. The incidence of herpes zoster in a United States administrative database. *J Gen Intern Med*. 2005;**20**(8):748–753.

4. Massengill JS, Kittredge JL. Practical considerations in the pharmacological treatment of postherpetic neuralgia for the primary care provider. *J Pain Res*. 2014;**7**:125–132.

5. Johnson BH, Palmer L, Gatwood J et al. Annual incidence rates of herpes zoster among an immunocompetent population in the United States. *BMC Infect Dis*. 2015;**15**(1):1–5.

6. Forbes HJ, Thomas SL, Smeeth L et al. A systematic review and meta-analysis of risk factors for postherpetic neuralgia. *Pain*. 2016;**157**(1):30–54.

7. Head H, Campbell AW. The pathology of herpes zoster and its bearing on sensory localisation. *Brain*. 1900;**23**(3):353–362.

8. Hadley GR, Gayle JA, Ripoll J et al. Post-herpetic neuralgia: A review. *Curr Pain Headache Rep*. 2016;**20**(3):17. doi: 10.1007/s11916-016-0548-x.

9. Fields HL, Rowbotham M, Baron R. Postherpetic neuralgia: Irritable nociceptors and deafferentation. *Neurobiol Dis*. 1998;**5**(4):209–227.

10. Garry EM, Delaney A, Anderson HA et al. Varicella zoster virus induces neuropathic changes in rat dorsal root ganglia and behavioral reflex sensitisation that is attenuated by gabapentin or sodium channel blocking drugs. *Pain*. 2005;**118**(1–2):97–111.

11. Watson CPN, Deck JH, Morshead C, Van der Kooy D, Evans RJ. Post-herpetic neuralgia: Further post-mortem studies of cases with and without pain. *Pain*. 1991;**44**(2):105–117.

12. Woolf CJ, Max MB. Mechanism-based pain diagnosis: Issues for analgesic drug development. *Anesthesiology*. 2001;**95**(1):241–249.

13. Nalamachu S, Morley-Forster P. Diagnosing and managing postherpetic neuralgia. *Drugs Aging*. 2012;**29**(11):863–869.

14. Dworkin RH, Gnann JW, Oaklander AL et al. Diagnosis and assessment of pain associated with herpes zoster and postherpetic neuralgia. *J Pain*. 2008;**9** (Suppl 1):37–44.

15. Dooling KL, Guo A, Patel M et al. Recommendations of the advisory committee on immunization practices for use of herpes zoster vaccines. *Morb Mortal Wkly Rep*. 2018;**67**(3):103–108.

16. Finnerup NB, Attal N, Haroutounian S et al. Pharmacotherapy for neuropathic pain in adults: A systematic review and meta-analysis. *Lancet Neurol*. 2015;**14**(2):162–173.

17. Dworkin RH, O'Connor AB, Kent J et al. International association for the study of pain neuropathic pain special interest group. Interventional management of neuropathic pain: NeuPSIG recommendations. *Pain*. 2013;**154**(11):2249–2261.

18. Max MB. Treatment of post herpetic neuralgia: Antidepressants. *Ann Neurol*. 1994;**35**(Suppl 1):S50–S53.

19. Liang J, Liu X, Zheng J, Yu S. Effect of amitriptyline on tetrodotoxin-resistant $Na_v1.9$ currents in nociceptive trigeminal neurons. *Mol Pain*. 2013;**9**:31. doi: 10.1186/1744-8069-9-31.

20. Yalcin I, Choucair-Jaafar N, Benbouzid M et al. β2-adrenoceptors are critical for antidepressant treatment of neuropathic pain. *Ann Neurol*. 2009;**65** (2):218–225.

21. Dworkin RH, O'Connor AB, Audette J et al. Recommendations for the pharmacological management of neuropathic pain: An overview and literature update. *Mayo Clin Proc.* 2010;**85**(Suppl 3):S3–S14.

22. Attal N. Pharmacological treatments of neuropathic pain: The latest recommendations. *Rev Neurol (Paris).* 2019;**175**(1–2):46–50.

23. Bohnert AS, Ilgen MA, Trafton JA et al. Trends and regional variation in opioid overdose mortality among veterans health administration patients, fiscal year 2001 to 2009. *Clin J Pain.* 2014;**30**(7):605–612. doi: 10.1097/AJP.0000000000000011.

24. Johnson RW, Rice ASC. Postherpetic neuralgia. *N Engl J Med.* 2014;**371** (16):1526–1533.

25. Dworkin RH, O'Connor AB, Backonja M et al. Pharmacologic management of neuropathic pain: Evidence-based recommendations. *Pain.* 2007;**132** (3):237–251.

26. Finnerup NB, Otto M, McQuay HJ, Jensen TS, Sindrup SH. Algorithm for neuropathic pain treatment: An evidence based proposal. *Pain.* 2005;**118** (3):289–305.

27. McNicol ED, Midbari A, Eisenberg E. Opioids for neuropathic pain. *Cochrane Database Syst Rev.* 2013;(8):CD006146. doi: 10.1002/14651858 .CD006146.pub2.

28. Bernstein JE, Korman NJ, Bickers DR, Dahl MV, Millikan LE. Topical capsaicin treatment of chronic postherpetic neuralgia. *J Am Acad Dermatol.* 1989;**21**(2 Pt 1):265–270.

29. Backonja MM, Malan TP, Vanhove GF, Tobias JK. NGX-4010, a high-concentration capsaicin patch, for the treatment of postherpetic neuralgia: A randomized, double-blind, controlled study with an open-label extension. *Pain Med.* 2010;**11**(4):600–608.

30. Watson CP, Tyler KL, Bickers DR et al. A randomized vehicle-controlled trial of topical capsaicin in the treatment of postherpetic neuralgia. *Clin Ther.* 1993;**15**(3):510–526.

31. Anand P, Bley K. Topical capsaicin for pain management: Therapeutic potential and mechanisms of action of the new high-concentration capsaicin 8 patch. *Br J Anaesth.* 2011;**107**:490–502.

32. Derry S, Rice AS, Cole P, Tan T, Moore RA. Topical capsaicin (high concentration) for chronic neuropathic pain in adults. *Cochrane database Syst Rev.* 2017;**1**:CD007393.

33. de León-Casasola OA, Mayoral V. The topical 5% lidocaine medicated plaster in localized neuropathic pain: A reappraisal of the clinical evidence. *J Pain Res.* 2016;**9**:67–79.

34. Derry S, Wiffen PJ, Moore RA, Quinlan J. Topical lidocaine for neuropathic pain in adults. *Cochrane database Syst Rev.* 2014;**2014**(7):CD010958.

35. Cui M, Khanijou S, Rubino J, Aoki KR. Subcutaneous administration of botulinum toxin A reduces formalin-induced pain. *Pain.* 2004;**107**(1):125–133.

36. Lin C-S, Lin Y-C, Lao H-C, Chen C-C. Interventional treatments for postherpetic neuralgia: A systematic review. *Pain Physician.* 2019;**22**(3):209–228.

37. Sluka KA, Walsh D. Transcutaneous electrical nerve stimulation: Basic science mechanisms and clinical effectiveness. *J Pain.* 2003;4(3):109–121.

38. Barbarisi M, Pace MC, Passavanti MB et al. Pregabalin and transcutaneous electrical nerve stimulation for postherpetic neuralgia treatment. *Clin J Pain.* 2010;**26**(7):567–572.

39. Xû G, Xú G, Feng Y, Tang WZ, Lv ZW. Transcutaneous electrical nerve stimulation in combination with cobalamin injection for postherpetic neuralgia. *Am J Phys Med Rehabil.* 2014;**93**(4):287–298.

40. Wu CL, Marsh A, Dworkin RH. The role of sympathetic nerve blocks in herpes zoster and postherpetic neuralgia. *Pain.* 2000;**87**(2):121–129.

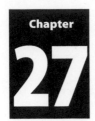

# Complex Regional Pain Syndrome (CRPS)

Alan D. Kaye and Nolan Weinstein

## CRPS

- Spontaneous regional pain
- Not confined to dermatomal distribution
- Develops after surgery, trauma, or minor event
- Pain greater than expected from inciting event
- May experience skin changes, autonomic dysfunction, motor and/or sensory changes (1)
- Negatively affects the quality of life (2)

## Epidemiology and Risk Factors

- Limited epidemiologic studies
  - Incidence found to be 0.55% in one study (3)
  - Found to be 0.07% in most recent study (4)
- Women affected 4× more frequently than men
- Upper extremities involved twice as much as lower
- Postmenopausal women most affected (3–7)
- Peak age of onset 45–55 in females (4)
- Other risk factors: depression, chronic headache, drug abuse (4)
- Protective factors: obesity, hypothyroidism, and diabetes associated with lower rates (4)
  - Lower baseline anxiety and reduced fear response also protective (8)
- Common inciting events: fracture, surgery, trauma, other minor event (9)

## Pathophysiology

- Unclear, controversial, and poorly understood (10)
- Multifactorial pathophysiology:
  - Inflammation following local trauma (11)

- Neurogenic inflammation out of proportion to injury (12,13)
- Peripheral nerve damage
○ Neurogenic inflammation results in overactivation of the sympathetic nervous system (14–16)
○ Central nervous system also implicated (11)
   - Motor dysfunction, impaired recognition, and neglect (17)
   - Abnormal response on fMRI (18)
○ Also described as an autoimmune disease (19)
   - Fracture results in B cell expression of IgM autoantibodies (20)
   - Led to the "IRAM" hypothesis (19):
     • Injury triggered
     • Regionally restricted
     • Autoantibody-mediated autoimmune disorder
     • Minimally destructive course

# Diagnosis

- Limited understanding of pathophysiology leads to difficult diagnosis
- Pain out of proportion following painful stimulus to a limb
- Divided into CRPS-1 and CRPS-2 (21,22)
   ○ CRPS-1: nociceptive pain
   ○ CRPS-2: neuropathic pain
- Diagnostic criteria as outlined by the International Association for the Study of Pain (IASP) in 1994 (21):
   ○ Inciting event
   ○ Continual allodynia, pain, or hyperalgesia
   ○ Edema, skin changes, abnormal motor activity
   ○ Absence of better explanation for symptoms
- Multiple other criteria have been developed since (23)
- These criteria were proven to have poor specificity and cause overdiagnosis (24)
- Newer diagnostic Budapest criteria (Table 27.1) have much better specificity than IASP criteria (0.79 vs. 0.41) (23)

**Table 27.1** The Budapest criteria, diagnostic criteria for CRPS as defined by an international consensus meeting held in Budapest (22,23)

| Budapest Criteria: Clinical Diagnostic Criteria for CRPS |
|---|
| Continuing pain, which is disproportionate to any inciting event |
| Must report at least one symptom in three of the four following categories:<br>– Sensory: Reports of hyperalgesia and/or allodynia<br>– Vasomotor: Reports of temperature asymmetry and/or skin color changes and/or skin color asymmetry<br>– Sudomotor/Edema: Reports of edema and/or sweating changes and/or sweating asymmetry<br>– Motor/Trophic: Reports of decreased range of motion and/or motor dysfunction (weakness, tremor, dystonia) and/or trophic changes (hair, nails, skin) |
| Must display at least one sign at time of evaluation in two or more of the following categories:<br>– Sensory: Evidence of hyperalgesia (to pinprick) and/or allodynia (to light touch and/or deep somatic pressure and/or joint movement)<br>– Vasomotor: Evidence of temperature asymmetry and/or skin color changes and/or asymmetry<br>– Sudomotor/Edema: Evidence of edema and/or sweating changes and/or sweating asymmetry<br>– Motor/Trophic: Evidence of decreased range of motion and/or motor dysfunction (weakness, tremor, dystonia) and/or trophic changes (hair, nails, skin) |
| There is no other diagnosis that better explains the signs and symptoms |
| – A sign is counted only if it is observed at the time of diagnosis<br>– Research criteria for CRPS are recommended that are more specific, but less sensitive than the clinical criteria; they require that four of the symptom categories and at least two sign categories be present |

# Treatment

- CRPS may spontaneously improve, but treatment should be aggressive
- Multimodal approach
- Various phenotypes in CRPS result in a variety of treatment options
- Difficult to observe clinical improvement from treatment
- Physical therapy and occupational therapy effective in reducing pain and increasing mobility (25–27)
  - 2016 Cochrane review concluded unclear evidence exhibiting benefits of PT/OT (28)

- Spinal cord stimulation (SCS) viable option after failing more conservative management
  - One study showed 95% response rate to SCS after 5 years (29)
  - Most effective within the first year of disease (30)
- Ketamine: commonly used but has only weak evidence supporting role in CRPS (31)
- Intrathecal baclofen
  - Upregulates GABAb receptors on afferent fibers, inhibiting neural transmission of nociceptive signals (32,33)
  - Shown to reduce pain in CRPS cohort, but has limited use due to significant side effect profile (34)
- Bisphosphonates
  - Have been shown to reduce pain in CRPS patients
  - Cochrane literature review showed low efficacy when compared to placebo (35,36)
- Immunoglobulin therapy
  - Proven to have no benefit (37–39)
- Vitamin C
  - High doses may confer protective benefit after surgery or trauma (40–44)
  - Reduces oxidative stress (45)
  - High-dose vitamin C reduces incidence of CRPS following distal radial fracture (43)
- Amputation
  - Controversial last resort in patients with CRPS
  - Does lead to improved overall quality of life and pain scores (46)
  - Insufficient evidence due to ethically ambiguous topic (22)

## Conclusions

- Challenging, poorly understood disease following local trauma or surgery
- Multifactorial pathophysiology involving pro-inflammatory state with autoimmune component
- Various diagnostic criteria available due to difficulty in diagnosis
- Devastating condition poorly affecting the quality of life
- Difficult to treat with numerous modalities available, most collecting low evidence in efficacy
- More research is needed to properly understand, diagnose, and treat CRPS

# References

1. Bruehl S. Complex regional pain syndrome. *BMJ*. 2016;**38**:82–86.

2. Van Velzen GAJ, Perez RSGM, Van Gestel MA et al. Health-related quality of life in 975 patients with complex regional pain syndrome type 1. *Pain*. 2014;**155**(3):629–634.

3. Sandroni P, Benrud-Larson LM, McClelland RL, Low PA. Complex regional pain syndrome type I: Incidence and prevalence in Olmsted county, a population-based study. *Pain*. 2003;**103**:199–207.

4. Elsharydah A, Loo NH, Minhajuddin A, Kandil ES. Complex regional pain syndrome type 1 predictors: Epidemiological perspective from a national database analysis. *J Clin Anesth*. 2017;**39**:34–37.

5. de Mos M, de Bruijn AGJ, Huygen FJPM et al. The incidence of complex regional pain syndrome: A population-based study. *Pain*. 2007;**129**(1–2):12–20.

6. Rewhorn MJ, Leung AH, Gillespie A, Moir JS, Miller R. Incidence of complex regional pain syndrome after foot and ankle surgery. *J Foot Ankle Surg*. 2014;**53**(3):256–258.

7. Jellad A, Salah S, Ben Salah Frih Z. Complex regional pain syndrome type I: Incidence and risk factors in patients with fracture of the distal radius. *Arch Phys Med Rehabil*. 2014;**95**(3):487–492.

8. Bean DJ, Johnson MH, Kydd RR. Relationships between psychological factors, pain, and disability in complex regional pain syndrome and low back pain. *Clin J Pain*. 2014;**30**(8):647–653.

9. Beerthuizen A, Stronks DL, Van'T Spijker A et al. Demographic and medical parameters in the development of complex regional pain syndrome type 1 (CRPS1): Prospective study on 596 patients with a fracture. *Pain*. 2012;**153**(6):1187–1192.

10. Birklein F, Schlereth T. Complex regional pain syndrome: Significant progress in understanding. *Pain*. 2015;**156**:S94–S103.

11. Marinus J, Moseley GL, Birklein F et al. Clinical features and pathophysiology of complex regional pain syndrome. *Lancet Neurol*. 2011;**10**(7):637–648.

12. Shi X, Wang L, Li X et al. Neuropeptides contribute to peripheral nociceptive sensitization by regulating interleukin-1β production in keratinocytes. *Anesth Analg*. 2011;**113**(1):175–183.

13. Sahbaie P, Shi X, Guo TZ et al. Role of substance P signaling in enhanced nociceptive sensitization and local cytokine production after incision. *Pain*. 2009;**145**(3):341–349.

14. Oaklander AL, Fields HL. Is reflex sympathetic dystrophy/complex regional pain syndrome type I a small-fiber neuropathy? *Ann Neurol*. 2009;**65**(6):629–638.

15. Albrecht PJ, Hines S, Eisenberg E et al. Pathologic alterations of cutaneous innervation and vasculature in affected limbs from patients with complex regional pain syndrome. *Pain*. 2006;**120**(3):244–266.

16. van der Laan L, ter Laak HJ, Gabreëls-Festen A, Gabreëls F, Goris RJ. Complex regional pain syndrome type I (RSD): Pathology of skeletal muscle and peripheral nerve. *Neurology*. 1998;**51**(1):20–25.

17. Reinersmann A, Maier C, Schwenkreis P, Lenz M. Complex regional pain syndrome: More than a peripheral disease. *Pain Manag*. 2013;**3**(6):495–502.

18. Hotta J, Saari J, Koskinen M et al. Abnormal brain responses to action observation in complex regional pain syndrome. *J Pain*. 2017;**18**(3):255–265.

19. Goebel A, Blaes F. Complex regional pain syndrome, prototype of a novel kind of autoimmune disease. *Autoimmun Rev*. 2013;**12**(6):682–686.

20. Guo T, Shi X, Li W et al. Passive transfer autoimmunity in a mouse model of complex regional pain syndrome. *Pain*. 2017;**158**(12):2410–2421. doi: 10.1097/j.pain.0000000000001046.

21. Merskey H, Bogduk N. *Classification of chronic pain: IASP pain terminology*. 1994. www.iasp-pain.org/publications/free-ebooks/classification-of-chronic-pain-second-edition-revised/.

22. Harden NR, Bruehl S, Perez RSGM, et al. Validation of proposed diagnostic criteria (the "Budapest Criteria") for Complex Regional Pain Syndrome. *Pain*. 2010;**150**(2):268–274. doi: 10.1016/j.pain.2010.04.030.

23. Harden RN, Bruehl S, Perez RSGM et al. Validation of proposed diagnostic criteria (the "Budapest Criteria") for complex regional pain syndrome. *Pain*. 2010;**150**(2):268–274.

24. Bruehl S, Harden RN, Galer BS et al. External validation of IASP diagnostic criteria for complex regional pain syndrome and proposed research diagnostic criteria. *Pain*. 1999;**81**(1–2):147–154.

25. Oerlemans HM, Oostendorp RAB, de Boo T et al. Adjuvant physical therapy versus occupational therapy in patients with reflex sympathetic dystrophy/complex regional pain syndrome type I. *Arch Phys Med Rehabil*. 2000;**81** (1):49–56

26. Rome L. The place of occupational therapy in rehabilitation strategies of complex regional pain syndrome: Comparative study of 60 cases. *Hand Surg Rehabil*. 2016;**35**(5):355–362.

27. Oerlemans HM, Oostendorp RA, de Boo T, Goris RJ. Pain and reduced mobility in complex regional pain syndrome I: Outcome of a prospective randomised controlled clinical trial of adjuvant physical therapy versus occupational therapy. *Pain*. 1999;**83**(1):77–83.

28. Smart KM, Wand BM, O'Connell NE. Physiotherapy for pain and disability in adults with complex regional pain syndrome (CRPS) types I and II.

*Cochrane Database Syst Rev.* 2016;**2**(2):CD010853. doi: 10.1002/14651858 .CD010853.pub2.

29. Kemler MA, Barendse GA, van Kleef M et al. Spinal cord stimulation in patients with chronic reflex sympathetic dystrophy. *N Engl J Med.* 2000;**343** (9):618–624.

30. Kumar K, Rizvi S, Bnurs SB. Spinal cord stimulation is effective in management of complex regional pain syndrome I: Fact or fiction. *Neurosurgery.* 2011;**69**(3):566–578.

31. Connolly SB, Prager JP, Harden RN. A systematic review of ketamine for complex regional pain syndrome. *Pain Med.* 2015;**16**(5):943–969.

32. Penn R, Kroin J. Intrathecal baclofen alleviates spinal cord spasticity. *Lancet.* 1984;**323**:1078. doi: 10.1016/s0140-6736(84)91487-9.

33. Melcangic M, Bowery NG. GABA and its receptors in the spinal cord. *Trends Pharmacol Sci.* 1996;**17**(12):457–462.

34. van Rijn MA, Munts AG, Marinus J et al. Intrathecal baclofen for dystonia of complex regional pain syndrome. *Pain.* 2009;**143**(1–2):41–47.

35. Ferraro MC, Cashin AG, Wand BM, et al. Interventions for treating pain and disability in adults with complex regional pain syndrome: An overview of systematic reviews (Review). *Cochrane Database Syst Rev.* 2013;**6**(6): CD009416. doi: 10.1002/14651858.CD009416.pub3.

36. Chevreau M, Romand X, Gaudin P, Juvin R, Baillet A. Bisphosphonates for treatment of complex regional pain syndrome type 1: A systematic literature review and meta-analysis of randomized controlled trials versus placebo. *Jt Bone Spine.* 2017;**84**(4):393–399.

37. O'Connell NE, Wand BM, McAuley J, Marston L, Moseley GL. Interventions for treating pain and disability in adults with complex regional pain syndrome: An overview of systematic reviews. In O'Connell NE, ed. *Cochrane batabase of systematic reviews.* John Wiley; 2013.

38. Goebel A, Bisla J, Carganillo R et al. Low-dose intravenous immunoglobulin treatment for long-standing complex regional pain syndrome: A randomized trial. *Ann Intern Med.* 2017;**167**(7):476–483.

39. Goebel A, Bisla J, Carganillo R et al. A randomised placebo-controlled Phase III multicentre trial: Low-dose intravenous immunoglobulin treatment for long-standing complex regional pain syndrome (LIPS trial). *NIHR Journals Library.* 2017. PMID: 29144634.

40. Jaiman A, Lokesh M, Neogi DS. Effect of vitamin C on prevention of complex regional pain syndrome type I in foot and ankle surgery. *Foot Ankle Surg.* 2011;**17**:207. doi: 10.1016/j.fas.2010.05.008.

41. Shibuya N, Humphers JM, Agarwal MR, Jupiter DC. Efficacy and safety of high-dose vitamin C on complex regional pain syndrome in extremity trauma

and surgery: Systematic review and meta-analysis. *J Foot Ankle Surg.* 2013;**52**(1):62–66.

42. Zollinger PE, Tuinebreijer WE, Breederveld RS, Kreis RW. Can vitamin C prevent complex regional pain syndrome in patients with wrist fractures? A randomized, controlled, multicenter dose-response study. *J Bone Joint Surg Am.* 2007;**89**(7):1424–1431.

43. Meena S, Sharma P, Gangary SK, Chowdhury B. Role of vitamin C in prevention of complex regional pain syndrome after distal radius fractures: A meta-analysis. *Eur J Orthop Surg Traumatol.* 2015;**25**(4):637–641.

44. Malay S, Chung KC. Testing the validity of preventing complex regional pain syndrome with vitamin C after distal radius fracture. *J Hand Surg Am.* 2014;**39**(11):2251–2257.

45. Kim JH, Kim YC, Nahm FS, Lee PB. The therapeutic effect of vitamin C in an animal model of complex regional pain syndrome produced by prolonged hindpaw ischemia-reperfusion in rats. *Int J Med Sci.* 2017;**14**(1):97–101.

46. Midbari A, Suzan E, Adler T et al. Amputation in patients with complex regional pain syndrome: A comparative study between amputees and non-amputees with intractable disease. *Bone Joint J.* 2016;**98**-B(4):548–554.

# Chapter 28

# Sickle Cell Disease

Vwaire Orhurhu and Nolan Weinstein

## Sickle Cell Acute Pain Crisis

- Umbrella term used to describe acute conditions resulting from sickle cell disease (1)
  - Most commonly used in reference to acute vaso-occlusive pain crisis
  - Can also result in:
    - Splenic sequestration crisis
    - Aplastic crisis
    - Hyperhemolytic crisis
    - Dactylitis
    - Acute chest syndrome
    - Priapism
- Results from autosomal recessive disorder sickle cell disease (SCD)
- Homologous Hemoglobin S (HbS), non-wild type allele
- Acute vaso-occlusive pain crisis results from (2):
  - HbS polymerization
  - Vaso-occlusion
  - Endothelial dysfunction
  - Impaired oxygen supply
  - Ischemic-reperfusion injury
  - Local inflammation
  - Most common chronic pain locations: back, abdomen, extremities (3)
- Acute pain crises often precipitated by infection, dehydration, acidosis, or stress (4)
- Acute pain crises are most common cause of hospitalization in SCD patients, resulting in $1.1 billion in annual healthcare costs (3)

# Epidemiology and Risk Factors

- SCD affects 1 in 2,500 children born in the United States each year (5)
- Approximately 100,000 adults affected in the United States (5)
- Annual global incidence of SCD is approximately 300,000 (6)
- Predominantly affects black Americans
- May be seen in patients as young as 6 months old, when HbS begins to replace HbF
  - Increases in intensity, duration, and frequency with increasing age (4)
- Acute pain crises have a 9% mortality rate in adults (2)

# Pathophysiology

- Single amino acid substitution of valine for glutamic acid in the beta-chain results in abnormal HbS
- Homozygous HbS alleles results in polymerization and then sickling of erythrocytes
- Erythrocytes become rigid and adhere to endothelium after release of adhesion molecules (1)
- Erythrocytes aggregate and cause small vessel occlusion and subsequent local ischemia
- Triggers a cycle of increased HbS formation as well as release of pro-inflammatory molecules and free radicals
  - Results in local reperfusion injuries
- Other pathophysiologic downstream effects:
  - Nitric oxide binding
  - Neutrophil adhesion and activation
  - Increased platelet activity
  - Hypercoagulation
- The above factors result in microvascular occlusion, injury, and then pain
- Some crises can be marked by an identifiable cause (dehydration, infection, stress, cold temperature); the majority are spontaneous

# Diagnosis

- Genetic screening for SCD is performed routinely in the United States

- Evaluated with thorough history and physical exam as well as lab testing:
  - CBC with differential, reticulocyte count, complete metabolic panel, liver function tests, type and screen
- Analysis for inciting cause often warranted such as infection or dehydration
- High suspicion for sickle cell pain crisis in SCD patients experiencing acute pain
  - Must rule out common alternative cause for pain at the site – for example, abdominal pain is a common location for sickle cell pain, though has a wide differential

## Treatment

- Analgesia is the main goal of therapy for patients experiencing vaso-occlusive pain crises (Tables 28.1 and 28.2)
- Numerous treatment modalities available
- Pharmacologic management typically involves escalation therapy from NSAIDS to opioids
  - One study showed in a cohort of 176 hospitalized patients for acute pain crises: 19% of patients received combination therapy of both opioids and NSAIDs, 48% received solely NSAID treatment, and 33% received opiate treatment (7)
  - Oxycodone and codeine are most commonly prescribed to SCD patients for use on "pain days" (8)
- Ketamine has been studied as a viable pain relief option
  - Appears to decrease pain scores in younger males but increase pain scores in older females (9)
- Other viable options include intranasal fentanyl, eptifibatide, and lidocaine patches, all outlined below
- Standard maintenance and prevention medication includes hydroxyurea by increasing HbF levels
  - Highly successful, decreasing all-cause mortality by 40% in one study (10)

## Conclusion

- "Sickle cell crisis" is a term used to capture myriad acute manifestations of sickle cell disease
- Underlying pathophysiology is due to polymerization of HbS, sickling of erythrocytes, and microvascular occlusion and injury

**Table 28.1** Adjunctive pharmaceutical analgesic treatments used in vaso-occlusive crisis

| Adjunctive Treatments | Efficacy | Adverse effects |
| --- | --- | --- |
| Ketamine (9,11,12) | – Decreased pain scores<br>– Decreased opioid-induced side effects<br>– Decreased opioid dosing requirements (90 mg less morphine equivalents per patient) | – Vivid dreams<br>– Light drowsiness |
| Ketamine/ Opioid Combination (13) | – Reduced pain scores in males and youth | – Increased pain scores in females and older patients |
| Intranasal fentanyl (14) | – Reduced time to initiation of analgesia<br>– Reduced length of stay | – None noted |
| Lidocaine 5% Patch (15) | – Decreased pain intensity in >50% | – 7.7% experienced lidocaine toxicity |
| Eptifibatide (16) | – Reduction in platelet aggregation, platelet release, platelet P-selectin<br>– Further studies needed to analyze pain reduction properties | – None noted |

- SCD and related pain are common in the United States, especially among Black Americans
- Routine newborn screening picks up the majority of cases and helps guide prevention and treatment of acute pain crises early on
- The mainstay of treating vaso-occlusive crises is analgesia and often achieved with NSAIDs, opioids, or combination therapy

# References

1. Borhade MB, Kondamudi NP. Sickle cell crisis. In *StatPearls*. 2022. pp. 365–379. Treasure Island (FL): StatPearls Publishing.

2. Sundd P, Gladwin MT, Novelli EM. Pathophysiology of sickle cell disease. *Annu Rev Pathol Mech Dis*. 2019;14(1):421058352. doi: 10.1146/annurev-pathmechdis-012418-012838.

**Table 28.2** Non-pharmaceutical management of pain

| Intervention | Treatment Protocol | Efficacy |
| --- | --- | --- |
| Hypnosis (17) | 30-minute hypnosis | – Moderate reduction in pain intensity<br>– May increase peripheral vasodilation |
| Virtual reality (18) | 15-minute VR session | – Reduced median pain intensity<br>– Decreased number of affected body areas<br>– Decreased qualitative measures of pain |
| Smartphone-guided cognitive behavioral therapy (19,20) | Personal cognitive behavioral therapy intervention delivered via web-based application | – >80% posttreatment retention<br>– Unclear pain reduction |

3. Dampier C, Palermo TM, Darbari DS et al. AAPT diagnostic criteria for chronic sickle cell disease pain. *J Pain*. 2017;**18**(5):490–498.

4. Brandow AM, DeBaun MR. Key components of pain management for children and adults with sickle cell disease. *Hematol Oncol Clin North Am*. 2018;**32**(3):535–550.

5. Strouse J. Sickle cell disease. *Handb Clin Neurol*. 2016;**138**:311–324.

6. Azar S, Wong TE. Sickle cell disease: A brief update. *Med Clin North Am*. 2017;**101**(2):375–393.

7. Cacciotti C, Vaiselbuh S, Romanos-Sirakis E. Pain management for sickle cell disease in the pediatric emergency department: Medications and hospitalization trends. *Clin Pediatr*. 2017;**56**:1109–1114.

8. Tran H, Gupta M, Gupta K. Targeting novel mechanisms of pain in sickle cell disease. *Blood*. 2017;**130**(22):2377–2385.

9. Nobrega R, Sheehy KA, Lippold C et al. Patient characteristics affect the response to ketamine and opioids during the treatment of vaso-occlusive episode-related pain in sickle cell disease. *Pediatr Res*. 2018;**83**(2):445–454.

10. Riley TR, Boss A, McClain D, Riley TT. Review of medication therapy for the prevention of sickle cell crisis. *Pharm Ther*. 2018;**43**(7):417–437.

11. Lubega FA, DeSilva MS, Munube D et al. Low dose ketamine versus morphine for acute severe vaso occlusive pain in children: A randomized controlled trial. *Scand J Pain.* 2018;**18**(1):19–27.

12. Palm N, Floroff C, Hassig TB, Boylan A, Kanter J. Low-dose ketamine infusion for adjunct management during vaso-occlusive episodes in adults with sickle cell disease: A case series. *J Pain Palliat Care Pharmacother.* 2018;**32**(1):20–26.

13. Young JR, Sawe HR, Mfinanga JA et al. Subdissociative intranasal ketamine plus standard pain therapy versus standard pain therapy in the treatment of paediatric sickle cell disease vaso-occlusive crises in resource-limited settings: Study protocol for a randomised controlled trial. *BMJ Open.* 2017;**7**(7): e017190.

14. Kelly GS, Stewart RW, Strouse JJ, Anders JF. Intranasal fentanyl improves time to analgesic delivery in sickle cell pain crises. *Am J Emerg Med.* 2018;**36** (7):1305–1307. doi: 10.1016/j.ajem.2017.11.015.

15. Rousseau V, Morelle M, Arriuberge C et al. Efficacy and tolerance of lidocaine 5% patches in neuropathic pain and pain related to vaso-occlusive sickle cell crises in children: A prospective multicenter clinical study. *Pain Pract.* 2018;**18**(6):788–797.

16. Brittain JE, Anea C, Desai P et al. Effect of eptifibatide on inflammation during acute pain episodes in sickle cell disease. *Am J of Hematol.* 2018;**93**: E99–E101.

17. Bhatt RR, Martin SR, Evans S et al. The effect of hypnosis on pain and peripheral blood flow in sickle-cell disease: A pilot study. *J Pain Res.* 2017;**10**:1635–1644.

18. Agrawal AK, Robertson S, Litwin L et al. Virtual reality as complementary pain therapy in hospitalized patients with sickle cell disease. *Pediatr Blood Cancer.* 2019;**66**(2):e27525. doi: 10.1002/pbc.27525.

19. Palermo TM, Zempsky WT, Dampier CD et al. iCanCope with sickle cell pain: Design of a randomized controlled trial of a smartphone and web-based pain self-management program for youth with sickle cell disease. *Contemp Clin Trials.* 2018;74:88–96.

20. Palermo TM, Dudeney J, Santanelli JP, Carletti A, Zempsky WT. Feasibility and acceptability of internet-delivered cognitive behavioral therapy for chronic pain in adolescents with sickle cell disease and their parents. *J Pediatr Hematol Oncol.* 2018;**40**(2):122–127.

# Breast Pain

Taylor Witten and Corey Moss

## Introduction and Epidemiology

- Breast cancer is the second most common cancer in males and females and the most common overall in the female population (2)
- Cosmetic breast surgery is commonly performed in the United States, with 520,000 procedures of the total 1.8 million cosmetic procedures in 2018 being related to the breast (1)
- The prevalence rates for persistent chronic pain following a cosmetic breast procedure are 25–60% (5)
  - The wide range here can be attributed to a number of factors, including individual patient threshold for pain, measures to assess pain, and if assessments were done prospectively or retrospectively (5)
- Postoperative chronic pain is defined as pain lasting 3 or more months and is different from the perioperative pain following a procedure (2)
  - This has been reported in several cosmetic breast procedures, including mastectomy with reconstruction, mammoplasty, and breast augmentation (1)
  - No evidence has been found to support the idea that the pain associated with each surgical procedure is dependent on how invasive the surgery is (2)
  - However, there have been studies that show there is a higher prevalence of chronic pain in procedures that include an axillary lymph node dissection likely because of the involvement of the intercostobrachial nerve (4)
  - Occasionally, the severity of breast pain can lead to a decline in physical activity and emotional well-being, resulting in a poor quality of life after breast surgery (3)

- In addition to lower quality of life in chronic pain patients after cosmetic surgery, another issue is overall dissatisfaction with the cosmetic results (2)
- Post-mastectomy pain syndrome is a specific etiology following cosmetic breast surgery
  - In Waltho and Rockwell's systematic review of this syndrome, the authors argue that, despite the nomenclature, the pain accompanied in this syndrome is not limited to mastectomy procedures (13,15)
    - Any surgery involving the breast parenchyma falls under this classification (13,15)
    - With this argument, one can apply their criteria of diagnosis to any cosmetic breast surgery (1,13)
  - Persistent pain following mastectomy was first reported in 1978 and has been named *post-mastectomy pain syndrome* (13)
  - This syndrome has a reported frequency of 4–100% and is defined as a chronic pain soon after mastectomy/lumpectomy affecting the anterior chest wall, axilla, or medial upper arm (13,14)

# Risk Factors

- The development of chronic pain in a patient can be multifactorial with patient demographics playing a large part (1)
- Patient risk factors associated with increased postoperative chronic pain:
  - Age <50 years old
    - This could be because younger patients have increased sensitivity to pain (3,10)
  - Larger breast size >500 ml (3)
    - This is not discussed enough in the literature but was demonstrated to be true in Monib's cohort (3)
  - BMI >25 (3,10)
  - Breast pain prior to the operation (6)
  - Non-white ethnicity (7)
  - Prior or concurrent radiotherapy/chemotherapy (7)
  - Psychological features of anxiety and depression (3)
- Each of the above risk factors must be carefully considered in patients who are being evaluated for the risk of postoperative chronic pain (1)

# Pathophysiology

- Where patients feel their chronic pain is dependent on the incision site for the procedure and the type of procedure performed (1)
- The most frequently damaged nerves during the cosmetic breast surgeries are the intercostal nerves followed by intercostobrachial and long thoracic nerve (1,8,12)
- The mechanism for nerve injury can vary from entrapment in scar tissue, direct mechanical injury, or compression via edema (11)
- Initial pain following a cosmetic procedure is defined as *acute pain*
- Nociceptors sense noxious stimuli via Aδ and C sensory nerves that trigger an inflammatory response driven by prostaglandins, histamine, bradykinin, and cytokines (9)
- This inflammatory response to noxious stimuli is termed primary hyperalgesia (1)
  - Aδ nerve fibers are lightly myelinated and fast conducting; these nerves are associated with sharp, localized pain (9)
  - C nerve fibers are unmyelinated and slow conducting; these nerves are associated with dull, diffuse pain (9)
- Persistent nociceptor stimulation in the periphery can lead to increased stimulation of the central nervous system, resulting in secondary hyperalgesia (1)
  - Secondary hyperalgesia is the transition from acute pain to chronic pain – the pain here is no longer due to noxious stimuli and is called allodynia (1)
  - The primary sensory neurons synapse with secondary afferent neurons in the dorsal horn of the spinal cord (9)
  - Repetitive depolarization in the dorsal horn stimulates the enhanced expression of genes that increase the excitability of nociceptive neurons via glutamate activation of NMDA, AMPA, and neurokinin1 receptors (1)
- The secondary afferent fibers ascend via the spinothalamic tract and transmit the signal of pain to the thalamus via third-order neurons; these third-order neurons then send the signal to the rest of the brain (9)

# Clinical Presentation and Diagnosis

- Initially, each patient following a cosmetic breast procedure experiences some level of acute pain
- The nerve injuries that are associated with chronic pain can be masked by this initial presentation (1)
- Workup for patients experiencing chronic breast pain includes a complete history and physical examination to exclude other causes of pain which include:
  - Fluid collections (11)
  - Infection (11)
  - Malignancy (11)
- A high index of suspicion is needed to identify nerve lesions; because of this, nerve injuries resulting in chronic pain are often misdiagnosed (11)
- Symptomology reported by patients includes sharp burning, itching, numbness, and pins and needles (1)
- The most common nerve deficit is hypoesthesia, with 8.72–9.56% of patients experiencing this symptom (12)
- The next most common nerve deficits following hypoesthesia were pain and hyperesthesia (12)
- Because of the many nerves that have the potential to be involved, it's important to look for specific features that could identify the nerve lesion
  - Examples include winged scapula for a long thoracic injury and medial arm pain with intercostobrachial injury (1,12)
- The criteria for the diagnosis of chronic pain syndrome following surgical breast procedures aren't well defined; however, Waltho and Rockwell's literature review states that the frequency should be pain present at least 4 days/week for greater than 12 hours/day (1,13)

# Treatment and Management

- Initial management includes a trial of medical management (NSAIDs, neuropathic pain medication) for at least 3 months (1,16)
  - The inhibition of COX 1 and 2 with NSAIDs aids in decreasing the inflammatory process and providing some pain relief (1)
  - Neuropathic pain medications include gabapentin and pregabalin to provide relief (1)

- o Opioids are effective but should be used with caution due to the risk of opioid dependence (18)
- Physical therapy and scar tissue massage can be included in the above conservative management (16,17)
- Many patients do not experience any relief from topical analgesics or other medical management as listed above (13,16)
- There are some studies that demonstrate a reduced incidence of chronic pain post-mastectomy and other breast procedures via either a paravertebral or pectoral nerve block perioperatively (19)
  - o There is evidence that pectoral blocks are more effective with fewer patients needing concurrent opioids for management (19)

# References

1. Urits I, Lavin C, Patel M et al. Chronic pain following cosmetic breast surgery: A comprehensive review. *Pain Ther.* 2020;9:71–82. https://doi.org/10.1007/s40122-020-00150-.

2. van Elk N, Steegers MA, van der Weij LP et al. Chronic pain in women after breast augmentation: Prevalence, predictive factors and quality of life. *Eur J Pain.* 2009;13(6):660–661.

3. Monib S, Abdelaziz MI. Epidemiology and predictive factors for persistent breast pain following breast-conserving surgery. *Cureus.* 2021;13(3):e14063. https://doi.org/10.7759/cureus.14063.

4. Wang L, Cohen JC, Devasenapathy N et al. Prevalence and intensity of persistent post-surgical pain following breast cancer surgery: A systematic review and meta-analysis of observational studies. *Br J Anaesth.* 2020;125(3):346–357. https://doi.org/10.1016/j.bja.2020.04.088.

5. Miaskowski C, Cooper B, Paul SM et al. Identification of patient subgroups and risk factors for persistent breast pain following breast cancer surgery. *J Pain.* 2012;13(12):1172–1187. https://doi.org/10.1016/j.jpain.2012.09.013.

6. Langford DJ, Schmidt B, Levine JD et al. Preoperative breast pain predicts persistent breast pain and disability after breast cancer surgery. *J Pain Symptom Manage.* 2015;49(6):981–994. https://doi.org/10.1016/j.jpainsymman.2014.11.292.

7. Fecho K, Miller NR, Merritt SA et al. Acute and persistent postoperative pain after breast surgery. *Pain Med.* 2009;10(4):708–715. https://doi.org/10.1111/j.1526-4637.2009.00611.x.

8. Ducic I, Seiboth LA, Iorio ML. Chronic postoperative breast pain: Danger zones for nerve injuries. *Plast Reconstr Surg.* 2011;127(1):41–46. https://doi.org/10.1097/PRS.0b013e3181f9587f.

9.  Fregoso G, Wang A, Tseng K, Wang J. Transition from acute to chronic pain: Evaluating risk for chronic postsurgical pain. *Pain Physician*. 2019;22 (5):479–488.

10. Kokosis G, Chopra K, Darrach H, Dellon AL, Williams EH. Re-visiting post-breast surgery pain syndrome: Risk factors, peripheral nerve associations and clinical implications. *Gland Surg*. 2019;8(4):407–415. https:// doi.org/10.21037/gs.2019.07.05.

11. Von Sperling ML, Høimyr H, Finnerup K, Jensen TS, Finnerup NB. Persistent pain and sensory changes following cosmetic breast augmentation. *Eur J Pain*. 2011;15(3):328–332.

12. Ducic I, Zakaria HM, Felder JM, Fantus S. Nerve injuries in aesthetic breast surgery: Systematic review and treatment options. *Aesthetic Surg J*. 2014;34 (6):841–856.

13. Waltho D, Rockwell G. Post-breast surgery pain syndrome: Establishing a consensus for the definition of post-mastectomy pain syndrome to provide a standardized clinical and research approach: A review of the literature and discussion. *Can J Surg*. 2016;59(5):342–350.

14. Classification of Chronic Pain. Descriptions of chronic pain syndromes and definitions of pain terms. Prepared by the International Association for the Study of Pain, Subcommittee on Taxonomy. *Pain Suppl*. 1986;3:S1–S226.

15. Couceiro TC, Valença MM, Raposo MC, Orange FA, Amorim MM. Prevalence of post-mastectomy pain syndrome and associated risk factors: A cross-sectional cohort study. *Pain Manag Nurs*. 2014;15(4):731–737. https:// doi.org/10.1016/j.pmn.2013.07.011.

16. Chopra K, Kokosis G, Slavin B, Williams E, Dellon AL. Painful complications after cosmetic surgery: Management of peripheral nerve injury. *Aesthet Surg J*. 2019;39(12):1427–1435. https://doi.org/10.1093/asj/sjy284.

17. Massingill J, Jorgensen C, Dolata J, Sehgal AR. Myofascial massage for chronic pain and decreased upper extremity mobility after breast cancer surgery. *Int J Ther Massage Bodyw Res Educ Pract*. 2018;11(3):4–9.

18. Dowell D, Haegerich TM, Chou R. CDC guideline for prescribing opioids for chronic pain – United States, 2016. *JAMA*. 2016;315(15):1624–1645.

19. Kulhari S, Bharti N, Bala I, Arora S, Singh G. Efficacy of pectoral nerve block versus thoracic paravertebral block for postoperative analgesia after radical mastectomy: A randomized controlled trial. *Br J Anaesth*. 2016;117 (3):382–386.

**Chapter 30**

# Post-thoracotomy Pain

Zahaan Eswani and Jamal Hasoon

## Post-thoracotomy Pain Syndrome (PTPS) or Chronic Post-thoracotomy Pain (CPTP)

- A musculoskeletal pain condition
- Definition of PTPS as per the International Association for the Study of Pain (IASP):
  - Pain that recurs or persists along a thoracotomy incision at least 2 months following the surgical procedure (1)
  - Chronic post-thoracotomy pain is defined as pain that recurs or persists along a thoracotomy scar >2 months after surgery (2)
  - The pain must also not be related to metastasis or other treatments (3)
- Acute pain following a thoracotomy is to be expected postoperatively. However, chronic pain after a thoracotomy can be debilitating and lead to long-term neuropathway along the incision site (1)
  - PTPS may cause significant perioperative and long-term morbidity and is noted for its intensity and duration (2)
- This chronic pain is a common complication post-thoracotomy (4)
- In terms of surgical procedures, thoracotomy has one of the greatest incidences of chronic postoperative pain and disability (2)
- If inadequately controlled in the immediate perioperative period, the pain from PTPS can prevent patients from taking adequate breaths, particularly large-volume breaths. This can lead to complications such as atelectasis and pneumonia (2)
- PTPS is often characterized as aching or tenderness, and it is localized to the area of incision in approximately 82% of cases (2)

# Epidemiology and Risk Factors

- The prevalence/incidence of PTPS varies greatly according to various sources:
  - The prevalence of PTPS ranges from 33% to 91% (4)
  - The incidence of chronic pain following thoracotomy is approximately 30–50% (2)
- PTPS can occur in 50% of postoperative patients with lung cancer; it is largely unrecognized (3)
- This wide variation is due to investigators not using a standardized set of criteria to classify patients as having post-thoracotomy pain. Some studies considered patients to have PTPS based on if they report whether pain was absent or present. Other studies required patients to have a certain level of pain intensity to be diagnosed with PTPS. Many studies involved questionnaires which can be impacted by recall bias (2)
- A representative study indicated APTPS incidence of 52% (32% mild, 16% moderate, 3% severe chronic postoperative pain) (2)

# Pathophysiology

- The exact pathologic mechanism for developing PTPS is unknown and is still being investigated (1,4)
- Believed to be a combination of somatic, visceral, and neuropathic pain components which are often complicated with central sensitization (1)
- Since nociceptive somatic afferent nerves arise from intercostal nerves, more pain may be caused via this pathway (1)
- Causes of PTPS from the procedure can include the following (3):
  - Trauma and compression of the intercostal nerves
    - Often caused by surgical compression due to instruments and ribs spreading
    - Common presentation is pain along the intercostal nerve pathway from spine to sternum and is typically characterized as a dull, prickly, cold, tingling, itchy sensation with no obvious external source
  - Fractured/compressed ribs (due to spreading)
    - Common presentation is severe pain radiating from the site of the removed/fractured/spread rib to the sternum

- ○ Inflammation of the chest muscles
  - ▪ Can be due to surgical and postsurgical causes
    - • Postsurgical causes include chest/draining tubes
  - ▪ Resulting inflammation can damage chest wall muscles, ribs, nerves, and the pulmonary lining of the lungs
  - ▪ The inflammation can incapacitate some patients. Therefore, it is important to be aware that even gentle stimulation can elicit intense/disabling pain during assessment
- ○ Atrophy of the chest muscles
  - ▪ Often due to ribs spreading
- ○ Scar tissue rubbing pleural cavity structures
  - ▪ Patient describes the pain as aching, tender, numb
  - ▪ Common presentation/major aggravating PTPS factors as reported by patients include physical exertion, weather changes, depression, lying on the operated side, sitting, walking, and working with the hand of the operated side
- As per the IASP, PTPS "is thought to be the result of injury to intercostal nerves, which transmit pain signals from the chest wall and costal plural" (2)
  - ○ Intercostal nerves may be injured during surgical resection, rib retraction, trocar placement, or suturing (2)
- PTPS may also be caused by nerve damage resulting from drainage mechanisms such as chest tubes and Jackson-Pratt tubing. Therefore, PTPS is also recognized as pain resulting from the installation of therapeutic chest drains and not from surgery alone (3)
- The surgical traumas (costochondral and costovertebral joint injuries, muscle and pleural damage, intercostal nerve injury) and pulmonary parenchymal damage and irritation (from chest tubes) contribute to a complex combination of myofascial and neuropathic pain (1), and the resulting inflammation, edema, fibrosis which lead to worsening nerve entrapment and irritation (1)
- Mediators (e.g., substance-p, glutamate, calcitonin gene-related peptide) are secreted and decrease the pain threshold via increasing nociceptor activity. This results in hypersensitization of the dorsal horn and upper cortex pain centers. Nociceptive stimuli reach the CNS and create functional changes and increase susceptibility to sensitization from future stimuli (1)

# Diagnosis

- Diagnostic criteria require a detailed medical history with temporal and clinical components (1)
- The pain must persist along a thoracotomy incision at least 2 months after surgery and not be related to metastasis or other treatments (1–3)
- Incisional side should be appropriately healed (3)
- Neuropathic and verbal pain descriptors include those mentioned as "common presentation" under pathophysiology
- Symptoms can be intermittent, continuous, or activity-based and are usually localized around the incision scar. Radiation to the back, shoulder, other chest wall locations is possible (1)
- The pain can also be described as:
  - Occasional or constant shooting or pinching sensations or a recurrent cramping, cutting, stabbing sensation (3)
  - Allodynia, aching, lancinating pain, and dysesthesias (1)
- Patients may state that anything touching the surgical scar area makes the pain worse (3)
- PTPS can be aggravated by comorbidities including anxiety, depression, fatigue, and dyspnea (3)
- Physical exam should include:
  - Palpation of the surgical area
    - Check for skin sensitivity. Can range from numbness/tingling to pain at the scar/along the intercostal nerve line
  - Movement of arm on the affected side
    - Move the arm of the affected side in both lateral and rotating motions, while checking for discomfort and pain
  - Flexion and extension of the arms and chest
- Chest CT and MRIs have been used to evaluate structural causes which can include local infection, porosity, tumor recurrence, or vertebral body collapse (1)
- Although not commonly tested, specific polymorphisms have been correlated with increased risk of chronic postsurgical pain (1)
- Clinical associations include (3):
  - Hypertension 66%
  - Coronary artery disease 26%

- ○ Obesity 26%
- ○ Diabetes mellitus 13%

# Treatment Modalities

## Development of New Surgical Techniques to Prevent the Development of PTPS (1)

1. The goal is to minimize nerve damage during the procedure (1)
2. This can be achieved by an integrated thoracotomy, retractor-free exposure, and neurovascular exclusion sutures which have been proven to be effective at reducing post-thoracotomy pain and analgesic use up to 6 months postoperatively (5)

## Anesthetic Techniques

1. One of the key predicting factors of the development of long-term PTPS is the development of severe postoperative pain. Therefore, many strategies have been developed to decrease the development of acute pain, including the following (1):

   a. Thoracic epidural analgesia
   b. IV/systemic opioid administration
   c. Neuromodulating medications
   d. Antidepressants
   e. Intercostal nerve blocks (continuous and single shot)
   f. Ultrasound-guided blocks

      i. Paravertebral, erector spinae, serratus anterior plane block

      ii. Ultrasound-guided blocks have increased in popularity due to ipsilateral blockade selectivity and decreased risk of sympathectomy

2. Ultrasound-guided serratus anterior plane blocks (SAPB) were noted to provide comparable analgesia to thoracic epidural analgesia (TEA) for acute post-thoracotomy pain (1,6)
3. An erector spinae plane block (ESPB) is an effective and safe alternative to TEA. It shows a superior analgesic profile compared to SAPB for patients undergoing posterolateral thoracotomy (1,7)
4. SAPB has been shown to be an effective alternative for post-thoracotomy analgesia. SAPB given postoperatively for a week may reduce the emergence of PTPS and reduce the need for pain therapy in patients (8)

# Pharmacologic Treatment

1. Calcium channel blockers
   a. Gabapentin and pregabalin are considered first-line agents for chronic neuropathic pain. It has been shown that perioperative administration decreases incidence of PTPS up to 3 months after surgery (1,9,10)
2. NMDA antagonists
   a. Ketamine and other NMDA antagonists can be used to treat PTPS. However, they have only proved beneficial in the immediate postoperative period and are not particularly effective for chronic pain after 2 months (1,11,12)

# Interventional Treatment

1. Thermal radiofrequency ablation of the intercostal nerves can be used for resistant PTPS after a successful diagnostic block (1,13,14)
2. Neuromodulation/nerve stimulation
   a. Peripheral nerve stimulation for post-thoracotomy pain has resulted in pain relief and reduced use of oral medications (1,15,16)
   b. Spinal cord stimulation for persistent PTPS is also a promising option (1,17,18)
   c. Dorsal root ganglion stimulation (DRG-S) for treatment of PTPS showed a decrease in pain scores, with relief maintained at 90 days and 12 months. Thoracic paravertebral blocks performed prior to DRG-S correlated with a positive outcome with treatment (1,19)

# Summary

- PTPS is a musculoskeletal pain condition defined by the IASP as pain that recurs or persists along a thoracotomy incision at least 2 months following the surgical procedure, and the pain must also not be related to metastasis or other treatments (1,3)
- The prevalence/incidence of PTPS varies greatly from 33% to 91%
- The exact pathologic mechanism for developing PTPS is unknown and is still being investigated but is believed to be a combination of somatic, visceral, and neuropathic pain components which are often complicated with central sensitization (1,4)
- Diagnostic criteria require a detailed medical history with temporal and clinical components

- Treatment includes the development of new surgical techniques to prevent the development of PTPS, anesthetic techniques (e.g., SAPB, TEA), pharmacological treatment (e.g., gabapentin and pregabalin, NMDA antagonists), and interventional treatment (e.g., thermal radiofrequency ablation, neuromodulation/nerve stimulation)

# References

1. Maloney J, Wie C, Pew S et al. Post-thoracotomy pain syndrome. *Curr Pain Headache Rep.* 2022;**26**(9):677–681. https://doi.org/10.1007/s11916-022-01069-z.

2. Khelemsky Y, Noto CJ. Preventing post-thoracotomy pain syndrome. *Mt Sinai J Med.* 2012;**79**(1):133–139. https://doi.org/10.1002/MSJ.21286.

3. Hopkins KG, Rosenzweig M. Post-thoracotomy pain syndrome: Assessment and intervention. *Clin J Oncol Nurs.* 2012;**16**(4):365–370. https://doi.org/10.1188/12.CJON.365-370.

4. Arends S, Böhmer AB, Poels M et al. Post-thoracotomy pain syndrome: Seldom severe, often neuropathic, treated unspecific, and insufficient. *Pain Rep.* 2020;**5**(2):e810. https://doi.org/10.1097/PR9.0000000000000810.

5. El-Hag-Aly MA, Hagag MG, Allam HK. If post-thoracotomy pain is the target, integrated thoracotomy is the choice. *Gen Thorac Cardiovasc Surg.* 2019;**67**(11):955–961. https://doi.org/10.1007/S11748-019-01126-2/TABLES/4.

6. Khalil AE, Abdallah NM, Bashandy GM, Kaddah TAH. Ultrasound-guided serratus anterior plane block versus thoracic epidural analgesia for thoracotomy pain. *J Cardiothorac Vasc Anesth.* 2017;**31**(1):152–158. https://doi.org/10.1053/J.JVCA.2016.08.023.

7. Elsabeeny WY, Ibrahim MA, Shehab NN, Mohamed A, Wadod MA. Serratus anterior plane block and erector spinae plane block versus thoracic epidural analgesia for perioperative thoracotomy pain control: A randomized controlled study. *J Cardiothorac Vasc Anesth.* 2021;**35**(10):2928–2936. https://doi.org/10.1053/J.JVCA.2020.12.047.

8. Reyad RM, Shaker EH, Ghobrial HZ et al. The impact of ultrasound-guided continuous serratus anterior plane block versus intravenous patient-controlled analgesia on the incidence and severity of post-thoracotomy pain syndrome: A randomized, controlled study. *Eur J Pain.* 2020;**24**(1):159–170. https://doi.org/10.1002/EJP.1473.

9. Gaber S, Saleh E, Elshaikh S et al. Role of perioperative pregabalin in the management of acute and chronic post-thoracotomy pain. *Open Access Maced J Med Sci.* 2019;**7**(12):1974–1978. https://doi.org/10.3889/OAMJMS.2019.556.

10. Fawzi HM, El-Tohamy SA. Effect of perioperative oral pregabalin on the incidence of post-thoracotomy pain syndrome. *Ain-Shams J Anaesthesiology.* 2014;**7**(2):143. https://doi.org/10.4103/1687-7934.133350.

11. Mendola C, Cammarota G, Netto R et al. S(+)-ketamine for control of perioperative pain and prevention of post thoracotomy pain syndrome: A randomized, double-blind study. *Minerva Anestesiol.* 2012;**78**(7):757–766. https://pubmed.ncbi.nlm.nih.gov/22441361/.

12. Israel JE, St Pierre S, Ellis E et al. Ketamine for the treatment of chronic pain: A comprehensive review. *Health Psychol Res.* 2021;**9**(1):1–12. https://doi.org /10.52965/001C.25535.

13. Abd-Elsayed A, Lee S, Jackson M. Radiofrequency ablation for treating resistant intercostal neuralgia. *Ochsner J.* 2018;**18**(1):91–93. https://doi.org/ 10.1043/TOJ-17-0043.

14. Engel AJ. Utility of intercostal nerve conventional thermal radiofrequency ablations in the injured worker after blunt trauma. *Pain Physician.* 2012;**15**: E711–E718. https://pubmed.ncbi.nlm.nih.gov/22996865/.

15. Theodosiadis P, Grosomanidis V, Samoladas E, Chalidis BE. Subcutaneous targeted neuromodulation technique for the treatment of intractable chronic postthoracotomy pain. *J Clin Anesth.* 2010;**22**(8):638–641. https://doi.org/10 .1016/J.JCLINANE.2009.10.018.

16. McJunkin TL, Berardoni N, Lynch PJ, Amrani J. An innovative case report detailing the successful treatment of post-thoracotomy syndrome with peripheral nerve field stimulation. *Neuromodulation Technol Neural Interface.* 2010;**13**(4):311–314. https://doi.org/10.1111/J.1525-1403 .2010.00277.X.

17. Graybill J, Conermann T, Kabazie AJ, Chandy S. Spinal cord stimulation for treatment of pain in a patient with post thoracotomy pain syndrome. *Pain Physician.* 2011;**14**(5):441–445. https://pubmed.ncbi.nlm.nih.gov/21927048/.

18. Wininger KL, Bester ML, Deshpande KK. Spinal cord stimulation to treat postthoracotomy neuralgia: Non-small-cell lung cancer: A case report. *Pain Manag Nurs.* 2012;**13**(1):52–59. https://doi.org/10.1016/J.PMN.2011.11.001.

19. lo Bianco G, Papa A, Gazzerro G et al. Dorsal root ganglion stimulation for chronic postoperative pain following thoracic surgery: A pilot study. *Neuromodulation.* 2021;**24**(4):774–778. https://doi.org/10.1111/NER.13265.

**Chapter 31**

# Multiple Sclerosis Pain

Salomon Poliwoda and Alan D. Kaye

- Pathophysiology
  - Multiple sclerosis (MS) is an autoimmune disorder of the central nervous system, causing inflammation with oligodendrocyte death and myelin sheath destruction (1)
- Clinical presentation and diagnosis
  - Classical symptoms of MS are fatigue, paresthesia, motor deficits, cognitive dysfunction, visual disturbances (due to optic neuritis), spasticity, depression, gait disturbance, and pain (2)
  - To make a formal diagnosis of MS, the 2017 McDonald criteria are used (1)
- Pain in MS
  - Pain in MS can present itself as headaches, extremity pain, back pain, neuropathic pain or, more specifically, trigeminal neuralgia (3)
  - Pain in MS can be severe and chronic enough to cause disability and decreased quality of life (4)
- Trigeminal neuralgia and MS
  - The prevalence of trigeminal neuralgia in the general population is less than 1%, whereas in patients with MS, the prevalence is up to 10% (5)
  - The first-line treatment for patients with trigeminal neuralgia without MS is carbamazepine. However, in patients with MS, there is no classical first-line pharmacological agent since the pathophysiology is different (6)
  - For this reason, patients with MS and trigeminal neuralgia may benefit early on with surgical management (6)

- One surgical option is a stereotactic radiosurgical procedure, which has shown to control symptoms in 88% of patients during a course of 14 months (7)
- Though surgical options are offered earlier in trigeminal neuralgia in patients with MS, these options are much more effective when this disease is not associated with MS (7)

- Headaches
  - Patients with MS are 50% more likely to suffer from headaches compared to people without MS (8)
  - There are two types of headaches that are common in MS depending on the type of disease presentation; in relapsing-remitting MS, there is a predominance of migraine without aura, and in progressive MS, there is a predominance of tension-type headaches (9)
  - There is no difference in treatment modalities for headaches in patients with MS vs. patients without MS (9)

- Neuropathic pain
  - The prevalence of neuropathic pain in MS can be as high as 86%, and it can manifest itself as back pain, headache, trigeminal neuralgia, or extremity pain (10)
  - When present, it is associated with MS that tends to be more severe, with a higher degree of disability (11)
  - Early treatment of these pains leads to better outcomes of MS itself (11)
  - Conventional methods to treat pain in these patients produce only a 50% reduction in symptomatology (12)
  - Some unconventional treatment modalities that have benefited patients are antidepressants, anticonvulsants, cannabinoids, low-dose naltrexone, and spinal stimulation (10)

- Advances in treatment options

  Medicinal cannabis

  - Cannabidiol (CBD) has been shown to be antioxidative, anti-inflammatory, antiemetic, antipsychotic, and neuro-protective (13)
  - Pain associated with spasticity is often present in MS, and cannabinoids have been shown to be beneficial with this type of symptomatology (14)

- Cannabinoids have been shown to be much more beneficial when used with combined pharmacological therapy as opposed to when it is used by itself (14)
- Cannabinoids may present with adverse effects such as headache, somnolence, nausea, dry cough, psychosis, decreased memory and cognition, cannabinoid hyperemesis syndrome, euphoria, and paranoia (15)

○ Physical therapy (PT) and exercise programs

- Both PT and exercise programs have been shown to reduce sensation of painful stimulation, as well as provide anti-inflammatory properties in patients with MS (16)
- Besides being beneficial with pain symptoms, both PT and exercise programs have been shown to reduce MS flare-ups and slow the progression of disease (16)
- One study showed that a 6-month yoga program on patients with MS provided significant improvement in the quality of life as well as with symptoms of fatigue, depression, and walking speed (17)
- Very few patients participate in these two treatment modalities due to lack of education (16)

○ Neuromodulation

- Neuromodulation consists of targeted electrical or chemical stimulation or inhibition; examples are intrathecal baclofen pumps, deep brain stimulation, spinal cord stimulation, and transcranial magnetic stimulation (18,19)
- Intrathecal baclofen pump with electrical stimulation has been beneficial for diffuse pain and spasticity (18)
- Deep brain stimulation has been shown to improve MS-related tremors as well as trigeminal neuralgia (18)
- Spinal cord stimulation helps to decrease overall pain sensation related to MS, and has also been shown to improve MS related bladder dysfunction (18)
- Transcranial magnetic stimulation has the potential for mitigation of symptoms as well as neurorehabilitation, but more studies are needed in this field (18)

# References

1. Ghasemi N, Razavi S, Nikzad E. Multiple sclerosis: Pathogenesis, symptoms, diagnoses and cell-based therapy. *Cell J*. 2017;**19**(1):1–10. https://doi.org/10.22074/cellj.2016.4867.

2. Monteleone F, Nicoletti CG, Stampanoni Bassi M et al. Nerve growth factor is elevated in the CSF of patients with multiple sclerosis and central neuropathic pain. *J Neuroimmunol*. 2018;**314**:89–93. https://doi.org/10.1016/j.jneuroim.2017.11.012.

3. Kalia LV, O'Connor PW. Severity of chronic pain and its relationship to quality of life in multiple sclerosis. *Mult Scler*. 2005;**11**(3):322–327. https://doi.org/10.1191/1352458505ms1168oa.

4. Young J, Amatya B, Galea MP, Khan F. Chronic pain in multiple sclerosis: A 10-year longitudinal study. *Scand J Pain*. 2017;**16**:198–203. https://doi.org/10.1016/j.sjpain.2017.04.070.

5. Fallata A, Salter A, Tyry T, Cutter GR, Marrie RA. Trigeminal neuralgia commonly precedes the diagnosis of multiple sclerosis. *Int J MS Care*. 2017;**19**(5):240–246. https://doi.org/10.7224/1537-2073.2016-065.

6. Zakrzewska JM, Wu J, Brathwaite TSL. A systematic review of the management of trigeminal neuralgia in patients with multiple sclerosis. *World Neurosurg*. 2018;**111**:291–306. https://doi.org/10.1016/j.wneu.2017.12.147.

7. Xu Z, Mathieu D, Heroux F et al. Stereotactic radiosurgery for trigeminal neuralgia in patients with multiple sclerosis: A multicenter study. *Neurosurgery*. 2019;**84**(2):499–505. https://doi.org/10.1093/neuros/nyy142.

8. La Mantia L, Prone V. Headache in multiple sclerosis and autoimmune disorders. *Neurol Sci*. 2015;**36**(Suppl 1):75–78. https://doi.org/10.1007/s10072-015-2146-9.

9. Husain F, Pardo G, Rabadi M. Headache and its management in patients with multiple sclerosis. *Curr Treat Options Neurol*. 2018;**20**(4):10. https://doi.org/10.1007/s11940-018-0495-4.

10. Murphy KL, Bethea JR, Fischer R. Neuropathic pain in multiple sclerosis: Current therapeutic intervention and future treatment perspectives. In: Zagon IS, McLaughlin PJ, eds, *Multiple Sclerosis: Perspectives in Treatment and Pathogenesis*. Brisbane: Codon Publications. 2017.

11. Solaro C, Cella M, Signori A et al. Identifying neuropathic pain in patients with multiple sclerosis: A cross-sectional multicenter study using highly specific criteria. *J Neurol*. 2018;**265**(4):828–835. https://doi.org/10.1007/s00415-018-8758-2.

12. Heitmann H, Biberacher V, Tiemann L et al. Prevalence of neuropathic pain in early multiple sclerosis. *Mult Scler*. 2016;**22**(9):1224–1230. https://doi.org/10.1177/1352458515613643.

13. Rice J, Cameron M. Cannabinoids for treatment of MS symptoms: State of the evidence. *Curr Neurol Neurosci Rep*. 2018;**18**(8):50. https://doi.org/10.1007/s11910-018-0859-x.

14. Landa L, Jurica J, Sliva J, Pechackova M, Demlova R. Medical cannabis in the treatment of cancer pain and spastic conditions and options of drug delivery in clinical practice. *Biomed Pap Med Fac Univ Palacky Olomouc Czech Repub*. 2018;**162**(1):18–25. https://doi.org/10.5507/bp.2018.007.

15. Jitpakdee T, Mandee S. Strategies for preventing side effects of systemic opioid in postoperative pediatric patients. *Paediatr Anaesth*. 2014;**24**(6):561–568. https://doi.org/10.1111/pan.12420.

16. Demaneuf T, Aitken Z, Karahalios A et al. Effectiveness of exercise interventions for pain reduction in people with multiple sclerosis: A systematic review and meta-analysis of randomized controlled trials. *Arch Phys Med Rehabil*. 2019;**100**(1):128–139. https://doi.org/10.1016/j.apmr.2018.08.178.

17. Kahraman T, Ozdogar AT, Yigit P et al. Feasibility of a 6-month yoga program to improve the physical and psychosocial status of persons with multiple sclerosis and their family members. *Explore (NY)*. 2018;**14**(1):36–43. https://doi.org/10.1016/j.explore.2017.07.006.

18. Abboud H, Hill E, Siddiqui J, Serra A, Walter B. Neuromodulation in multiple sclerosis. *Mult Scler*. 2017;**23**(13):1663–1676. https://doi.org/10.1177/1352458517736150.

19. Urits I, Adamian L, Fiocchi J et al. Advances in the understanding and management of chronic pain in multiple sclerosis: A comprehensive review. *Curr Pain Headache Rep*. 2019;**23**(8):59. https://doi.org/10.1007/s11916-019-0800-2.

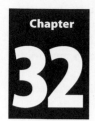

# Cerebral Palsy

Norris Talbot and Hisham Kassem

- Global mental and physical dysfunction or isolated disturbances in gait, cognition, growth, or sensation (1)
- Primarily noticed in developing children
  - Origins of genetic influence (2)
  - Trauma suffered during pregnancy or after within the first 2 years (2)
- Permanent disorders of the development of movement and posture, causing activity limitation, that are attributed to nonprogressive disturbances that occurred in the developing fetal or infant brain (3)
- Movement and coordination are large indicators
  - Poor motor functions overall
- Reduces quality of life from a motor perspective
  - Also reduces the quality of life for parental caretakers (4)

## Epidemiology and Risk Factors

- 2 to 3 out of 1,000 children in the United States (1,5)
- Estimated prevalence worldwide of 17 million (3)
- Significant proportion of children with CP live into adulthood
- One of the most prevalent physical disabilities in children
  - Primarily diagnosed after the age of 2 (6)
- Spasticity occurring in 80% of children with CP (7)
- 92% of cases traced to perinatal period (7)
- Risk factors:
  - Still developing a central cause for CP

- Chorioamnionitis, maternal urinary tract infection, neurotropic virus infection, and cytomegalovirus infection were associated with a higher risk for CP (8–13)
- Surviving twin after the co-twin's fetal death appears to have a higher risk for CP (8,14)
- Increased risk for CP after multiple gestation was seen in a large study from five populations (8,15)
- Intrauterine growth deviation (8,16,17)
- There does not appear to be a significant correlation from genetic studies thus far on CP (8)
- Trauma in perinatal asphyxiation (18)
- Other forms of trauma or cerebral malformation(1,8)

# Pathophysiology

- The main route comes from impaired and destructive developmental mechanisms (19)
- Environmental factors like ischemia and hypoxia
- Unilateral spastic CP related to infarct in middle cerebral artery, hemi-brain atrophy, brain malformations, and periventricular lesions (19)
- Intrapartum hypoxic-ischemic insult has caused a moderate to severe neonatal encephalopathy that subsequently results in cerebral palsy (20)
  - Metabolic acidosis in fetal umbilical cord arterial blood obtained at delivery (20)
  - Early onset of severe or moderate neonatal encephalopathy in infants born at 34 or more weeks' gestation (20)
  - Cerebral palsy of the spastic quadriplegic or dyskinetic type (20)
  - Exclusion of other identifiable etiologies, such as trauma, coagulation disorders, infectious conditions, or genetic disorders (20)
- Head injuries or trauma also can cause CP (7)
- Surefire method and determination is currently not available for 80% of cases (7)
  - Most pathophysiology is still being discovered

# Diagnosis

- Defining features:
  - Stiff muscles (spasticity) (7)
  - Uncontrollable movements (dyskinesia) (7)
  - Poor coordination (ataxia) (7)
  - Other/mixed
    - Spasticity is the most common symptom
- Can be diagnosed as early as 6 months of age (7)
- To help with diagnosis:
  - Recognition of a permanent, nonprogressive disorder of motor function in a child through a history and physical examination (7)

# Treatment: Interventional Approaches for Pain and Spasticity

- Botulinum Toxin Type A
  - Zinc-endopeptidase protein produced by bacteria of the clostridia species (21)
  - Toxin enters peripheral neuromuscular cholinergic nerve junctions via the vascular system
  - Interrupts cholinergic neurotransmitter release into the neuromuscular junction,
    - Causes flaccid paralysis of the muscle
  - Limited and varying evidence that supports the patient gait, range of motion, and satisfaction at follow-ups of 2–8 weeks and 12–16 weeks (21)
  - Adverse effects similar to placebo (21)
  - No serious differences between low and high doses (21)
  - Significantly decreases financial tolls on families and also contributes to a reduced risk of surgical interventions and shorter hospital stays (21)
  - Viable option for reducing spasticity in CP patients
    - Limitation: unknown on the length of effect and duration of the drug (21)
  - Otherwise, it has no significant differences in health problems compared to other solutions for CP spasticity and pain (21)
  - Reliable method to treat upper- and lower-extremity spasticity (22)

- ○ No high-quality evidence to support all its benefits
- Intrathecal baclofen
  - ○ Gamma-aminobutyric acid (GABA) agonist typically used orally to treat a wide array of musculoskeletal spasms in the general population (21)
  - ○ Has some basis in short-term benefits for CP, but the evidence is limited (21)
  - ○ Spinal injections and catheter-administered portions of ITB come with complications (21)
  - ○ Risk of assessment must be made over the price of the drug and the reassured quality of life
  - ○ Slow tapering of the drug must be used in cases of those at repeated high dose or else risk of stroke, hallucinations, fevers, altered mental statuses, and, in rare cases, of rhabdomyolysis and multiple organ system failure (23)
  - ○ Limited evidence to support ITB as a beneficial method
- Dorsal rhizotomy
  - ○ Irreversible spinal procedure performed by neurosurgery that permanently decreases muscle spasticity (21)
    - ▪ Utilized for children with gaits diagnosed as gross motor function classification type II or III (21)
      - • In more severe types IV and V, the procedure is performed to reduce spasticity and facilitate nursing care (21)
  - ○ Offers multiple benefits in terms of spasticity and quality of life
    - ▪ Hard to tell if it is better than other methods due to lack of control studies between methods SDR and ITB (21)
  - ○ Must be interpreted in the view of general surgical complications and the associated risks from surgery
- Dantrolene
  - ○ Muscle relaxant providing antispasmodic effects intracellularly to skeletal muscles (23)
  - ○ Primary use in malignant hyperthermia
    - ▪ Other uses now seen in muscle spasticity and traumatic brain injuries (23)
  - ○ Causes less sedation compared to other methods (23)

- ○ Has signs of hepatotoxicity
  - ▪ Liver function must be monitored (23)
- ○ Doses start at one a day, then increase to four, leading to difficulty for patients to adhere to this schedule (23)
- ○ Risks and concerns require more up-to-date studies and a larger quantity of studies
- Diazepam
  - ○ Benzodiazepine drug (23)
  - ○ Binds to BNZ1 and BNZ2 receptors and increases the affinity of GABA for GABA receptors
    - ▪ Increases summative inhibition of neuron firing (23)
  - ○ Taken IV, IM, orally, rectally, or parenterally (23)
  - ○ Used in skeletal muscle spasms, spasticity from upper motor neuron diseases, convulsive disorders, as well as its treatment of psychiatric conditions, like anxiety, as is a common use of benzodiazepines (23)
  - ○ Most useful for patients with the worst forms of CP symptoms
  - ○ Risk of abuse to liver and could cause immunodeficiency (23)
- Flexeril
  - ○ Centrally acting muscle relaxant (23)
  - ○ Functions over prolonged life – 18-hour half-life (23)
  - ○ Tapered cessation required in case of withdrawals
    - ▪ Dry mouth and drowsiness also experienced
  - ○ No clear use for centrally based muscle spasticity and would require more research to show more (23)
- Tizanidine
  - ○ Alpha-2 noradrenergic agonist (24)
  - ○ Works better than a placebo but equivalently to tizanidine, diazepam, and baclofen (23)
  - ○ Potential hepatotoxicity when used with fluoroquinolones (23)
  - ○ Also renal impairment likely due to renal excretion (23)
  - ○ Significant withdrawal problems (24)

## Summary

- CP is a neurological disorder that greatly affects movement and occurrence of muscle spasticity as well as other problems
- Significantly decreases the quality of life in patients

- Causes still not fully known, but prenatal complications as well as trauma during pregnancy can lead to higher risk
- Recommended for expecting mothers to not overexert themselves during pregnancy and keep consistent health checkups to prevent causative factors
- Current treatments to reduce spasticity and other symptoms involve: botulinum toxin type A, intrathecal baclofen, dorsal rhizotomy, dantrolene, diazepam, flexeril, and tizanidine
  - Each method presents some level of relief, but all come with their own existing risks and adverse effects
  - Patients must outweigh the risk over potential gain with the use of each treatment for pain and spasticity

# References

1. Krigger KW. Cerebral palsy: An overview. *Am Fam Physician*. 2006;**73**(1):91–100. www.aafp.org/pubs/afp/issues/2006/0101/p91.html.

2. Bonellie S, Currie D, Chalmers J. Comparison of risk factors for cerebral palsy in twins and singletons. *Dev Med Child Neurol*. 2022;**47**(9):587–591. https://doi.org/10.1111/J.1469-8749.2005.TB01208.X.

3. Graham HK, Rosenbaum P, Paneth N et al. Cerebral palsy. *Nat Rev Dis Primers*. 2016;**2**(1):1–25. https://doi.org/10.1038/nrdp.2015.82.

4. Guillamón N, Nieto R, Pousada M et al. Quality of life and mental health among parents of children with cerebral palsy: The influence of self-efficacy and coping strategies. *J Clin Nurs*. 2013;**22**(11–12):1579–1590. https://doi.org/10.1111/JOCN.12124.

5. Wimalasundera N, Stevenson VL. Cerebral palsy. *Pract Neurol*. 2016;**16**(3):184–194. https://doi.org/10.1136/PRACTNEUROL-2015-001184.

6. Byrne R, Noritz G, Maitre NL. Implementation of early diagnosis and intervention guidelines for cerebral palsy in a high-risk infant follow-up clinic. *Pediatr Neurol*. 2017;**76**:66–71. https://doi.org/10.1016/J.PEDIATRNEUROL.2017.08.002.

7. Vitrikas K, Dalton H, Breish D. Cerebral palsy: An overview. *Am Fam Physician*. 2020;**101**(4):213–220. https://doi.org/10.4274/hamidiyemedj.galenos.2021.72792.

8. Himmelmann K, Ahlin K, Jacobsson B, Cans C, Thorsen P. Risk factors for cerebral palsy in children born at term. *Acta Obstet Gynecol Scand*. 2011;**90**(10):1070–1081 https://doi.org/10.1111/j.1600-0412.2011.01217.x.

9. Bax M, Tydeman C, Flodmark O. Clinical and MRI correlates of cerebral palsy: The European cerebral palsy study. *JAMA*. 2006;**296**(13):1602–1608. https://doi.org/10.1001/JAMA.296.13.1602.

10. Pass RF, Fowler KB, Boppana SB, Britt WJ, Stagno S. Congenital cytomegalovirus infection following first trimester maternal infection: Symptoms at birth and outcome. *J Clin Virol*. 2006;**35**(2):216–220. https://doi.org/10.1016/J .JCV.2005.09.015.

11. Neufeld MD, Frigon C, Graham AS, Mueller BA. Maternal infection and risk of cerebral palsy in term and preterm infants. *J Perinatol*. 2005;**25**(2):108–113. https://doi.org/10.1038/SJ.JP.7211219.

12. Wu YW, Escobar GJ, Grether JK et al. Chorioamnionitis and cerebral palsy in term and near-term infants. *JAMA*. 2003;**290**(20):2677–2684. https://doi.org /10.1001/JAMA.290.20.2677.

13. Gibson CS, MacLennan AH, Goldwater PN et al. Neurotropic viruses and cerebral palsy: Population based case-control study. *BMJ*. 2006;**332** (7533):76–79. https://doi.org/10.1136/BMJ.38668.616806.3A.

14. Pharoah POD. Cerebral palsy in the surviving twin associated with infant death of the co-twin. *Arch Dis Child Fetal Neonatal Ed*. 2001;**84**(2):F111–F116. https://doi.org/10.1136/FN.84.2.F111.

15. Scher AI, Petterson B, Blair E et al. The risk of mortality or cerebral palsy in twins: A collaborative population-based study. *Pediatr Res*. 2002;**52** (5):671–681. https://doi.org/10.1203/00006450-200211000-00011.

16. Glinianaia SV, Jarvis S, Topp M et al. Intrauterine growth and cerebral palsy in twins: A European multicenter study. *Twin Res Hum Genet*. 2006;**9** (3):460–466. https://doi.org/10.1375/183242706777591209.

17. Jarvis S, Glinianaia SV, Torrioli MG et al. Cerebral palsy and intrauterine growth in single births: European collaborative study. *Lancet*. 2003;**362** (9390):1106–1111. https://doi.org/10.1016/S0140-6736(03)14466-2.

18. Reddihough DS, Collins KJ. The epidemiology and causes of cerebral palsy. *Aust J Physiother*. 2003;**49**(1):7–12. https://doi.org/10.1016/S0004-9514(14) 60183-5.

19. Upadhyay J, Tiwari N, Ansari MN. Cerebral palsy: Aetiology, pathophysiology and therapeutic interventions. *Clin Exp Pharmacol Physiol*. 2020;**47**(12):1891–1901. https://doi.org/10.1111/1440-1681.13379.

20. Hankins GDV, Speer M. Defining the pathogenesis and pathophysiology of neonatal encephalopathy and cerebral palsy. *Obstet Gynaecol*. 2003;**102** (3):628–636. https://doi.org/10.1016/S0029-7844(03)00574-X.

21. Jacquelin Peck B, Urits I, Kassem H et al. Interventional approaches to pain and spasticity related to cerebral palsy. *Psychopharmacol Bull*. 2020;**50**(4 Suppl 1):108–120.

22. Delgado MR, Hirtz FD, Aisen FM et al. Practice parameter: Pharmacologic treatment of spasticity in children and adolescents with cerebral palsy (an evidence-based review). *Neurology*. 2010;**74**(4):336–343.

23. Jacki Peck B, Urits I, Crane J et al. Oral muscle relaxants for the treatment of chronic pain associated with cerebral palsy. *Psychopharmacol Bull*. 2020;**50**(4 Suppl 1):142–162.

24. Sinatra R, Jahr J, Watkins-Pitchford J (Eds.). In *The essence of analgesia and analgesics*. Cambridge: Cambridge University Press. Published online January 1, 2022. pp. 375–378. https://doi.org/10.1017/CBO9780511841378 .094.

| Chapter 33 | # Myofascial Pain Syndrome
Cyrus Yazdi |

## Myofascial Pain Syndrome (MPS)

- A musculoskeletal pain condition
- Stems from localized trigger points
  - Taut regions comprising skeletal muscle and fascia (1)
- Neuropathic component with referred pain patterns
- Highly dependent on the patient's perception
- Often described as dull, aching, boring, and burning (2)
- Can be acute, although more commonly chronic
- Very detrimental to patient quality of life and costs on healthcare
  - Physical functioning, social functioning, emotional well-being, and energy, among others (9)

## Epidemiology and Risk Factors

- Affects up to 85% of the general population
  - Varying rates between males and females (3–5)
- Common risk factors for MPS
  - Overload on muscles
  - Ergonomic injuries
  - Psychological stress
  - Systemic disease
  - Underlying spine-related disorder (4)
- Clinical associations with MPS
  - Insomnia (6), vitamin D deficiency (7)
  - High rates of MPS found in Croatian war veterans with PTSD and depression (8)

# Pathophysiology

- Characterized by myofascial trigger points (MTrP)
  - Palpation can reproduce the patient's pain (10)
  - A snapping palpation or needle insertion can trigger a local twitch response (LTR), or rapid contractions of the muscle fibers around the frequently taut area
- Primary MTrP refers to the primary muscles affected
  - Can be felt as a taut band in superficial muscles
  - Taut band formation is hypothesized to be due to a deprivation of oxygen and nutrients from local constriction resulting from increased intracellular calcium release by trauma or excessive muscular stress (20,21)
- Secondary MTrP
  - Composed of synergistic and antagonistic muscles
- Satellite MTrP
  - Points between zones of primary and secondary MTrP
- Active MTrP
  - Spontaneously induces pain along with an associated pattern of referred pain
- Latent MTrP
  - Does not trigger a localized pain until it is palpated (10,11)
- The presence of MTrPs is supported by treatments, such as acupuncture and injections (e.g., saline, lidocaine), which target MTrPs (12)
- Mechanical and electrophysiological studies have further elucidated the mechanisms behind MTrP pain production (13)
  - The MTrP locus is composed of an active loci (motor) and a sensory locus (sensory)
  - Propagation of potentials along extrafusal fibers and the attenuation of pain through botulism treatment imply an endplate zone localization (14–17)
- Spontaneous electrical activity (SEA) stems from MTrPs, but not from non-MTrP sites (18)
  - EMG activity can be seen in electrodes inserted in taut bands that elicit LTRs (19)
  - Constant nociceptor stimulation from the primary muscle site contributes to localized and referred pain

- ○ MTrPs can be self-perpetuating due to central sensitization
  - Stemming from neuronal plasticity of the spinal cord's dorsal horn
  - May explain the referral patterns and satellite MTrPs (11)

## Diagnosis

- Diagnostic criteria require a detailed history and muscular palpation examination
- The presence of the treatable tender MTrPs and the referred pain pattern are pathognomonic for MPS (11)
- The taut MTrPs are more commonly found in the trunk, including the trapezius and neck, as opposed to the extremities
  - ○ Muscle weakness and decreased range of motion are commonly associated with these tight knots
- It is crucial to rule out other causes such as headaches, trauma, fibromyalgia, sedentary lifestyle, and other forms of neuropathic pain (22)
- Blood tests and imaging studies may not show apparent abnormalities
- Experimental data
  - ○ Transcranial magnetic stimulation (TMS) may demonstrate cortical disinhibition MPS (23)
    - Based on a hypothesis called central sensitization in which chronic pain can cause the CNS neurons to be hyperexcitable
    - The motor cortex's cortical alterations, especially intracortical facilitation (ICF) and intracortical inhibition (ICI), are involved in chronic pain and were investigated as diagnostic markers
  - ○ Magnetic resonance elastography (MRE) may objectively quantify physical properties of taut bands
    - Stiffness parameters on human patients correlated well with predictions by finite element simulation and gel replica experiments (24)
    - In contrast to the subjective touch of a health practitioner's fingers, MRE provides evidence as a proof of concept that MTrPs can be quantitatively characterized consistently
- MPS is prevalent among patients with other types of pain disorders (25)

- ○ Myofascial pelvic pain (MFPP) is characterized similarly to MPS, but with trigger points located in the pelvic floor musculature (26)
- Increased prevalence of MTrPs has been found in patients with migraines or tension type headaches (TTH) (27)
  - ○ Hypersensitivity of MTrPs related to central sensitization may be a contributing factor to lowered pressure pain thresholds, in the pericranial muscles of patients with TTH (28)
- Osteoarthritis (OA), the most common musculoskeletal pain disorder, has been hypothesized to be associated with MTrPs (29)
  - ○ Knee OA has been correlated to MTrPs in the lower extremity muscles (e.g., vastus lateralis, rectus femoris, gracilis) (30,31)
- MPS of the temporomandibular (TMJ) region is common, in patients with a history of TMJ trauma, and it can be mistakenly diagnosed as a TMJ disorder refractory to treatment (32)
- MPS is more prevalent in patients with spinal disorders, which include whiplash-associated disorder, lumbar disc herniation, idiopathic neck pain, and cervical radiculopathy (33)
- Fibromyalgia can be distinguished from MPS due to the presence of widespread pain and standardized bilateral, symmetric tender points (TP) (34)

## Non-pharmacologic Treatment Modalities

## Myofascial Release

- Myofascial release (MFR) may be beneficial in the treatment of MPR
- MFR can be performed in two different ways: direct or indirect
  - ○ Direct MFR involves slow, sustained pressure applied to areas of muscular tension (35,36)
    - ▪ Several kilograms of pressure may be applied directly into the affected area, with the goal of applying enough force to stretch the fascia
  - ○ Indirect MFR involves using the hands to hold the fascia in a gentle stretch, applying just a few grams of force along the direction of fascial restrictions, which allows the restricted fascia to unravel itself (37)
  - ○ Both techniques are thought to break fascial adhesions that have pathologically formed, reducing muscle stiffness (38)
  - ○ Advantages include simplicity of technique and a noninvasive nature

- Patients may administer therapy to themselves
- The data supporting the utility of MFR in clinical practice for MPS are underwhelming however
  - Only three out of eight studies demonstrated clinically significant at short-term follow-up (up to 2 months) (36)
  - MFR may increase joint ROM immediately post-intervention, but this effect seems to be short-lived, and may only last minutes (39)

## Dry Needling

- Dry needling (DN) is a minimally invasive procedure that involves the insertion of a thin filiform no-bore needle into myofascial trigger points without the addition of solutions or local pharmacological agents (40,41)
- The needle is inserted until it causes a local twitch response, and is then removed
- The effectiveness of DN may be explained by the gate control theory of pain
  - One type of sensory input, such as pain caused by trigger points, may be inhibited in the central nervous system by another type of input, in this case the needle (42–44)
  - In comparison of dry needling to other treatment modalities (e.g. sham dry needling, acupuncture), dry needling resulted in significant post-intervention reduction in pain intensity and functional improvement compared to alternate treatment (40)
  - Alternative treatments, such as lidocaine and corticosteroid injections, may provide superior efficacy (42)
  - DN may cause myofascial trigger points to transition from being active (spontaneously painful) to latent (painful only on palpation) (45)
    - If a patient achieves analgesia after the first treatment, they may be more likely to receive a sustained benefit and are thus better candidates for DN

## Acupuncture

- Acupuncture (AcP) dates back to ancient Chinese medicine
- Involves the insertion and subsequent manipulation of needles in specific points around the body (46)
- The needles are typically left inserted for a short period of time and may be gently shifted or twirled (47)

- Modern Western medicine suggests a mechanism of action similar to the gate control theory of DN (48,49)
  - Some have even argued that DN and AcP are similar (50)
  - DN targets myofascial trigger points, while the needling in acupuncture is directed at specific patterns or meridians along the human body
- AcP that targets trigger points in MPS may significantly decrease pain and reduce irritability after just one session (46)
  - There were no analgesic effects when considering the use of only traditional acupuncture points

## Transcutaneous Electrical Nerve Stimulation

- Transcutaneous electrical nerve stimulation (TENS) refers to the application of adhesive electrodes to the skin and subsequent electrical stimulation of painful areas (51)
  - Different combinations of intensity and frequency of electrical stimulation may be applied, but high frequency is usually paired with low intensity, and vice versa
- While there are no concrete guidelines describing what combination of these variables produces the greatest efficacy, it is believed that intensity is the most important factor, and that the treatment should produce a strong, but non-painful, sensation for maximum efficacy (52)
- The mechanism of action of TENS may be multifactorial, but it is believed that the muscle contractions induced by TENS may normalize the acetylcholine concentrations in the motor endplate, which may help relax taut bands of muscle (53)
- Research on the utility of TENS in MPS shows modest but favorable results, and, given its benign safety profile, may be a consideration in those who find it effective
  - Patients receiving TENS had significantly higher pain threshold and active ROM than those receiving sham treatment
  - TENS increased PPT and ROM in patients with trigger points in the trapezius, though effects were small and potentially clinically insignificant (53,54)

## Interferential Current Therapy

- Interferential current therapy (IFC) is the application of medium-frequency alternating currents

- ○ Purported to increase blood flow and reduce pain (55,56)
- Thought to be advantageous over TENS as it generates an amplitude modulated frequency (AMF), allowing it to penetrate more deeply than TENS
  - ○ Still TENS and IFC may have similar efficacy (57)
- A few small studies have shown that IFC may be beneficial in the treatment of MPS, but more research is needed to determine its efficacy (58)

## Biofeedback

- Biofeedback allows participants to receive real-time feedback on biological information like heart rate and muscle tone, which can then be interpreted by the participant and used to alter their behavior (59)
- Information is usually displayed to the patient by visual display, sound, or vibration
- Electromyogram biofeedback may provide information on the contraction of muscles to ensure activities like stretching and exercise are performed appropriately (60)
- Biofeedback requires active participation by the patient and is also targeted at improving coping skills and psychological response to pain (61)
- Its use in MPS specifically has only been scarcely studied, so little is known about its efficacy

# Pharmacologic Treatment Modalities

## Nonsteroidal Anti-inflammatory Drugs (NSAID)

- Nonsteroidal anti-inflammatory drugs (NSAIDs) are frequently used for pain relief; however, their use in chronic pain disorders is limited due to adverse effects
  - ○ These include, but are not limited to, dyspepsia, GI ulceration and bleeding, peripheral edema, and organ failure (62–64)
- NSAIDs help relieve pain via inhibition of cyclo-oxygenase (COX) enzyme and thus inhibition of prostaglandin synthesis which allows for reduced sensitization and excitation of peripheral nociceptors (65)
- There is limited literature on the efficacy of oral NSAIDs in the treatment of MPS

- There have been reports regarding the beneficial effects of topical administration (66)
  - Topical diclofenac sodium patch provided pain relief and improved function in patients with MPS of the upper trapezius when compared to control of menthol patch (66)

## Tri-Cyclic Antidepressants (TCA)

- Typical doses of amitriptyline range from 20 mg to 100 mg daily for the treatment of MPS (68)
- Tricyclics provide analgesia by inhibiting serotonin and norepinephrine reuptake along the descending spinal pain pathways. They also exert effects on sodium channels and histamine receptors (69,70)
- Studies investigating the efficacy of tricyclic antidepressants in myofascial pain syndrome have been positive (67,71–75)
- Amitriptyline and nortriptyline are both effective in reducing pain in patients with MPS
  - Nortriptyline may have increased efficacy, but further investigation is warranted (73)
- Amitriptyline has also been found effective in patients with chronic tension-type headaches and chronic pain associated with temporomandibular disorders (67,71)

## Muscle Relaxants

- Cyclobenzaprine provides analgesia by inhibiting reuptake of NE in locus coeruleus and inhibiting the descending serotonergic pathways in spinal cord (68)
- Clonazepam and other benzodiazepines act on chloride channels, enhancing GABA-A receptors, and resulting in inhibition at presynaptic and postsynaptic sites on the spinal cord (68,76,78–82)
- Muscle relaxants decrease skeletal muscle tone, thus alleviating the increased muscle activity seen in MPS (77)
  - Two reviews investigating use of cyclobenzaprine in treatment of MPS did not show benefit of cyclobenzaprine when compared to control
- Side effects may range from sedation, dizziness, and depression to anticholinergic effects and ataxia
  - Clonazepam is not recommended as long-term treatment option in chronic pain conditions due to potential for abuse and sedative effects but is a possibility for short-term relief (83)

- Both cyclobenzaprine and clonazepam have been shown to be effective in reducing pain intensity for temporomandibular disorders (79,80,82)
- Despite articles indicating benefits of muscle relaxants in MPS, there are other articles that have been unable to support any added benefit of muscle relaxants (84)

## Tizanidine

- Tizanidine is an alpha-2 adrenergic agonist that functions as a muscle relaxant by reducing release of excitatory neurotransmitters in the CNS (85)
  - There is evidence supporting the use of tizanidine in the treatment of several spasticity disorders, including myofascial pain syndrome (86–90)
    - 89% of patients with MPS were found to benefit with use of tizanidine
- Dosage usually begins at 2 mg orally and can be repeated every 6 to 8 hours. The dosage can be slowly increased by 2 to 4 mg per dose every 1 to 4 days (86)
- Although typically well tolerated, tizanidine can cause drowsiness, dizziness, hypotension, constipation, bradycardia, urinary frequency, dyskinesia, xerostomia, and blurred vision, among other adverse effects (68,86)
- In comparison of tizanidine to baclofen and diazepam for the treatment of spasticity, all three treatment options were equally effective (89)

## Interventional Treatment Modalities

### Local Injections

- Frequently utilized local injections involve use of a variety of drugs, including Botox, lidocaine, steroids, normal saline (91)
- Lidocaine functions as a nonspecific sodium channel blocker, stabilizing neuronal cell membranes and inhibiting nerve impulse initiation and conduction (68,69)
  - Possible side effects of lidocaine injections include anaphylaxis, CNS depression, seizures, arrhythmias (68)
  - Lidocaine injection therapy significantly reduced the degree and frequency of neck pain in patients after 6 months of treatment (92)

- 5% lidocaine patches provided pain relief when compared to placebo (93)
- In comparison of lidocaine injection to lidocaine patch, both were equally effective in relieving myofascial pain (94)
- In comparison of lidocaine injection with topical nimesulide (NSAID) gel for treatment of cervical myofascial trigger points, no difference in the efficacy between the two treatment groups was found (95)

- Botulinum toxin functions by preventing acetylcholine release at the neuromuscular junction and by preventing the release of pain neurotransmitters at primary sensory neurons in order to prevent muscle hyperactivity and spasm (76,96)

  - Possible adverse effects of Botox include excessive or adjacent unwanted muscle weakness, hypersensitivity reaction, anaphylaxis, autonomic dysreflexia, respiratory compromise, urinary retention, myasthenia gravis, and facial paralysis (1,68)
  - Data are conflicting for use of botulinum toxin in the management of temporomandibular dysfunction (97–99)
  - Significant benefit in the use of botulinum toxin myofascial pain syndromes has been demonstrated (99–102)

    - Botox combined with myofascial release physical therapy was effective in managing myofascial pelvic pain (102)
    - Botox was significantly more effective compared to placebo in the treatment of MPS (100)

## Conclusions

- Myofascial pain syndrome is characterized by localized, taut regions comprising skeletal muscle and fascia, termed trigger points and is an increasingly prevalent complaint (1)
- Pharmacologic interventions with evidence to support their use in MPS include muscle relaxants such as benzodiazepines, tizanidine, and cyclobenzaprine, TCAs, topical agents such as diclofenac gel and lidocaine patches, as well as injection therapy of botulinum toxin or lidocaine
- Other modalities with evidence to support their use include acupuncture, dry needling, and, to a certain extent, TENS therapy

# References

1. Wheeler AH, Carolina N. Myofascial pain disorders: Theory to therapy. *Drugs*. 2004;**64**(1):45–62.

2. Harden RN, Bruehl SP, Gass S, Niemiec C, Barbick B. Signs and symptoms of the myofascial pain syndrome: A national survey of pain management providers. *Clin J Pain*. 2000;**16**(1):64–72.

3. Fleckenstein J, Zaps D, Rüger LJ et al. Discrepancy between prevalence and perceived effectiveness of treatment methods in myofascial pain syndrome: Results of a cross-sectional, nationwide survey. *BMC Musculoskelet Disord*. 2010;**11**:32. doi: 10.1186/1471-2474-11-32.

4. Gerwin RD. Classification, epidemiology, and natural history of myofascial pain syndrome. *Curr Pain Headache Rep*. 2001;**5**(5):412–420.

5. Vázquez-Delgado E, Cascos-Romero J, Gay-Escoda C. Myofascial pain syndrome associated with trigger points: A literature review. (I): Epidemiology, clinical treatment and etiopathogeny. *Med Oral Patol Oral Cir Bucal*. 2009;**14**(10):e494–e498.

6. Lin WC, Shen CC, Tsai SJ, Yang AC. Increased risk of myofascial pain syndrome among patients with insomnia. *Pain Med (United States)*. 2017;**18**(8):1557–1565.

7. Bartley J, Reid D, Morton RP. Prevalence of vitamin D deficiency among patients attending a general otolaryngology clinic in South Auckland. *Ann Otol Rhinol Laryngol*. 2009;**118**(5):326–328.

8. Vidaković B, Uljanić I, Perić B, Grgurević J, Sonicki Z. Myofascial pain of the head and neck among Croatian war veterans treated for depression and posttraumatic stress disorder. *Psychiatr Danub*. 2016;**28**(1):73–76.

9. Brodsky M, Spritzer K, Hays RD, Hui KK. Change in health-related quality-of-life at group and individual levels over time in patients treated for chronic myofascial neck pain. *J Evidence-Based Complement Altern Med*. 2017;**22**(3):365–368.

10. Celik D, Mutlu EK. Clinical implication of latent myofascial trigger point topical collection on myofascial pain. *Curr Pain Headache Rep*. 2013;**17**(8):353. doi: 10.1007/s11916-013-0353-8. PMID: 23801006.

11. Money S. Pathophysiology of trigger points in myofascial pain syndrome. *J Pain Palliat Care Pharmacother*. 2017;**31**(2):158–159.

12. Baldry P. Management of myofascial trigger point pain. *Acupunct Med*. 2002;**20**(1):2–10.

13. Hong CZ, Simons DG. Pathophysiologic and electrophysiologic mechanisms of myofascial trigger points. *Arch Phys Med Rehabil*. 1998;**79**(7):863–872.

14. Simons DG. Clinical and etiological update of myofascial pain from trigger points. *J Musculoskelet Pain.* 1996;4(1–2):93–122.

15. Juan FJ. Use of botulinum toxin-A for musculoskeletal pain in patients with whiplash associated disorders [ISRCTN68653575]. *BMC Musculoskelet Disord.* 2004;5(1):5. doi: 10.1186/1471-2474-5-5. PMID: 15018625; PMCID: PMC356919.

16. Acquadro MA, Borodic GE. Treatment of myofascial pain with botulinum A toxin. *Anesthesiology.* 1994;80(3):705–706.

17. Zhou JY, Wang D. An update on botulinum toxin A injections of trigger points for myofascial pain. *Curr Pain Headache Rep.* 2014;18(1):386. doi: 10.1007/s11916-013-0386-z. PMID: 24338700.

18. Ge H-Y, Fernández-de-Las-Peñas C, Yue S-W. Myofascial trigger points: Spontaneous electrical activity and its consequences for pain induction and propagation. *Chin Med.* 2011;6:13. doi: 10.1186/1749-8546-6-13. PMID: 21439050; PMCID: PMC3070691.

19. Simons DG, Dexter JR. Comparison of local twitch responses elicited by palpitation and needling of myofascial trigger points. *J Musculoskelet Pain.* 1995;3(1):49–61.

20. Bengtsson A, Henriksson KG, Larsson J. Reduced high-energy phosphate levels in the painful muscles of patients with primary fibromyalgia. *Arthritis Rheum.* 1986;29(7):817–821.

21. Jafri MS. Mechanisms of myofascial pain. *Int Sch Res Not.* 2014;2014:523924. oi: 10.1155/2014/523924. PMID: 25574501; PMCID: PMC4285362.

22. Graff-Radford SB. Myofascial pain: Diagnosis and management. *Curr Pain Headache Rep.* 2004;8(6):463–467.

23. Thibaut A, Zeng D, Caumo W, Liu J, Fregni F. Corticospinal excitability as a biomarker of myofascial pain syndrome. *PAIN Rep.* 2017;2(3):e594. doi: 10.1097/PR9.0000000000000594. PMID: 29392210; PMCID: PMC5741300.

24. Chen Q, Basford J, An K-N. Ability of magnetic resonance elastography to assess taut bands. *Clin Biomech (Bristol, Avon).* 2008;23(5):623–629.

25. Fricton J. Myofascial pain. *Oral Maxillofac Surg Clin North Am.* 2016;28(3):289–311.

26. Bonder JH, Chi M, Rispoli L. Myofascial pelvic pain and related disorders. *Phys Med Rehabil Clin North Am.* 2017;28(3):501–515.

27. Do TP, Heldarskard GF, Kolding LT, Hvedstrup J, Schytz HW. Myofascial trigger points in migraine and tension-type headache. *J Headache Pain.* 2018;19(1):84. doi: 10.1186/s10194-018-0913-8. PMID: 30203398; PMCID: PMC6134706.

28. Palacios-Ceña M, Wang K, Castaldo M et al. Trigger points are associated with widespread pressure pain sensitivity in people with tension-type headache. *Cephalalgia*. 2018;**38**(2):237–245.

29. Cambron J. A new era for the Journal of Bodywork and Movement Therapies. *J Bodyw Mov Ther*. 2019;**23**(1):1–2.

30. Bajaj P, Bajaj P, Graven-Nielsen T, Arendt-Nielsen L. Trigger points in patients with lower limb osteoarthritis. *J Musculoskelet Pain*. 2001;**9** (3):17–33.

31. Henry R, Cahill CM, Wood G et al. Myofascial pain in patients waitlisted for total knee arthroplasty. *Pain Res Manag*. 2012; **17**(5):321–327.

32. Peral-Cagigal B, Pérez-Villar Á, Redondo-González L-M et al. Temporal headache and jaw claudication may be the key for the diagnosis of giant cell arteritis. *Med Oral Patol Oral Cir Bucal*. 2018;**23**(3):e290–e294.

33. Chiarotto A, Clijsen R, Fernandez-De-Las-Penas C, Barbero M. Prevalence of myofascial trigger points in spinal disorders: A systematic review and meta-analysis. Presented as an abstract and poster to the World Confederation of Physical Therapy Congress, May 1–4, 2015, Singapore. *Arch Phys Med Rehabil*. 2016;**97**(2):316–337.

34. Bourgaize S, Newton G, Kumbhare D, Srbely J. A comparison of the clinical manifestation and pathophysiology of myofascial pain syndrome and fibromyalgia: Implications for differential diagnosis and management. *J Can Chiropr Assoc*. 2018;**62**(1):26–41.

35. Ajimsha MS, Al-mudahka NR. Effectiveness of myofascial release: Systematic review of randomized controlled trials. *J Bodyw Mov Ther*. 2015;**19**(1):102–112.

36. Laimi K, Mäkilä A, Bärlund E et al. Effectiveness of myofascial release in treatment of chronic musculoskeletal pain: A systematic review. *Clin Rehabil*. 2018;**32**(4):440–450.

37. Ajimsha MS, Daniel B, Chithra S. Effectiveness of myofascial release in the management of chronic low back pain in nursing professionals. *J Bodyw Mov Ther*. 2014;**18**(2):273–281.

38. Kalichman L, Ben David C. Effect of self-myofascial release on myofascial pain, muscle flexibility, and strength: A narrative review. *J Bodyw Mov Ther*. 2017;**21**(2):446–451.

39. Beardsley C, Škarabot J. Effects of self-myofascial release: A systematic review. *J Bodyw Mov Ther*. 2015;**19**(4):747–758.

40. Liu L, Huang QM, Liu QG et al. Evidence for dry needling in the management of myofascial trigger points associated with low back pain: A systematic review and meta-analysis. *Arch Phys Med Rehabil*. 2018;**99** (1):144–152.

41. Espejo-Antúnez L, Tejeda JFH, Albornoz-Cabello M et al. Dry needling in the management of myofascial trigger points: A systematic review of randomized controlled trials. *Complement Ther Med.* 2017;**33**:46–57.

42. Rodríguez-Mansilla J, Gonzalez-Sanchez B. Effectiveness of dry needling on reducing pain intensity in patients with myofascial pain syndrome: A meta-analysis. *J Tradit Chinese Med.* 2016;**36**(1):1–13. doi: 10.1016/s0254-6272(16)30001-2. PMID: 26946612.

43. Furlan AD, van Tulder M, Cherkin D et al. Acupuncture and dry-needling for low back pain: An updated systematic review within the framework of the cochrane collaboration. *Spine.* 2005;**30**(8):944–963. doi: 10.1097/01.brs.0000158941.21571.01. PMID: 15834340.

44. Abbaszadeh-Amirdehi M, Nakhostin Ansari N, Naghdi S, Olyaei G. Neurophysiological and clinical effects of dry needling in patients with upper trapezius myofascial trigger points. *J Bodyw Mov Ther.* 2017;**21**(1):48–52.

45. Gerber LH, Sikdar S, Aredo JV et al. Beneficial effects of dry needling for treatment of chronic myofascial pain persist for 6 weeks after treatment completion. *PM&R.* 2017;**9**(2):105–112.

46. Wang R, Li X, Zhou S et al. Manual acupuncture for myofascial pain syndrome: A systematic review and meta-analysis. *Acupunct Med.* 2017;**35**(4):241–250.

47. Mayo Clinic. *Acupuncture.* 2019. pp. 2–5.

48. Chou LW, Hsieh YL, Chen HS et al. Remote therapeutic effectiveness of acupuncture in treating myofascial trigger point of the upper trapezius muscle. *Am J Phys Med Rehabil.* 2011;**90**(12):1036–1049.

49. Hsieh Y, Hong C, Liu S, Chou L. Acupuncture at distant myofascial trigger spots enhances endogenous opioids in rabbits: A possible mechanism for managing myofascial pain. *Acupunct Med.* 2016;**34**(4):302–309.

50. Fan A, He H. Dry needling is acupuncture. *Acupunct Med.* 2016;**34**(3):241. doi: 10.1136/acupmed-2015-011010. Epub 2015 Dec 15. PMID: 26672062.

51. Gibson W, Bm W, Meads C, Mj C, Ne OC. Transcutaneous electrical nerve stimulation (TENS) for chronic pain: An overview of cochrane reviews (Review). *Cochrane Database Syst Rev.* 2019;**2**(2):CD011890. doi: 10.1002/14651858.CD011890.pub2.

52. Sluka KA, Bjordal JM, Marchand S, Rakel BA. What makes transcutaneous electrical nerve stimulation work? Making sense of the mixed results in the clinical literature. *Phys Ther.* 2013;**93**(10):1397–1402.

53. Rodríguez-Fernández ÁL, Garrido-Santofimi V, Güeita-Rodríguez J, Fernández-de-las-Peñas C. Effects of burst-type transcutaneous electrical nerve stimulation on cervical range of motion and latent myofascial trigger point pain sensitivity. *Arch Phys Med Rehabil.* 2011;**92**(9):1353–1358.

54. Gemmell H, Hilland A. Immediate effect of electric point stimulation (TENS) in treating latent upper trapezius trigger points: A double blind randomised. *J Bodyw Mov Ther*. 2011;**15**(3):348–354.

55. Fuentes JP, Olivo SA, Magee DJ, Gross DP. Effectiveness of interferential current therapy in the management of musculoskeletal pain: A systematic review and meta-analysis. *Phys Ther*. 2010;**90**(9):1219–1238.

56. Albornoz-Cabello M, Maya-Martín J, Domínguez-Maldonado G, Espejo-Antúnez L, Heredia-rizo AM. Effect of interferential current therapy on pain perception and disability level in subjects with chronic low back pain: A randomized controlled trial. 2017;**31**(2):242–249. doi: 10.1177/0269215516639653. Epub 2016 Jul 10. PMID: 26975312.

57. Cadena de Almeida C, Maldaner de Silva VZ, Cipriano Junior G, Eloin Liebano R, Joao Luiz QD. Transcutaneous electrical nerve stimulation and interferential current demonstrate similar effects in relieving acute and chronic pain: A systematic review with meta-analysis. *Brazilian J Phys Ther*. 2018;**22**(5):347–354.

58. Dissanayaka T, Pallegama R, Suraweera H, Johnson MI, Kariyawasam AP. Comparison of the effectiveness of transcutaneous electrical nerve stimulation and interferential therapy on the upper trapezius in myofascial pain syndrome. *Am J Phys Med Rehabil*. 2016;**95**(9):663–672.

59. Giggins OM, Persson UM, Caulfield B. Biofeedback in rehabilitation. *J Neuroeng Rehabil*. 2013;**10**(1):60. doi. 10.1186/1743-0003-10-60. PMID: 23777436; PMCID: PMC3687555.

60. Srinivasan AK, Kaye JD, Moldwin R. Myofascial dysfunction associated with chronic pelvic floor pain: Management strategies. *Curr Pain Headache Rep*. 2007;**11**(5):359–364. doi: 10.1007/s11916-007-0218-0. PMID: 17894926.

61. Nestoriuc Y, Martin A, Rief W, Andrasik F. Biofeedback treatment for headache disorders: A comprehensive efficacy review. *Appl Psychophysiol Biofeedback*. 2008;**33**(3):125–140.

62. Whelton A. Renal and related cardiovascular effects of conventional and COX-2-specific NSAIDs and non-NSAID analgesics. *Am J Ther*. 2000;**7**(2):63–74.

63. Laine L. Gastrointestinal effects of NSAIDs and coxibs. *J Pain Symptom Manage*. 2003;**25**(2):32–40.

64. Rainsford K. Profile and mechanisms of gastrointestinal and other side effects of nonsteroidal anti-inflammatory drugs (NSAIDs). *Am J Med*. 1999;**107**(6):27–35.

65. Cashman JN. The mechanisms of action of NSAIDs in analgesia. *Drugs*. 1996;**52**(Suppl 5):13–23.

66. Hsieh L-F, Hong C-Z, Chern S-H, Chen C-C. Efficacy and side effects of diclofenac patch in treatment of patients with myofascial pain syndrome of the upper trapezius. *J Pain Symptom Manage.* 2010;**39**(1):116–125.

67. Plesh O, Curtis D, Levine J, McCall WD. Amitriptyline treatment of chronic pain in patients with temporomandibular disorders. *J Oral Rehabil.* 2000;**27**(10):834–841.

68. Huang-Lionnet JH, Hameed H, Cohen SP. Pharmacologic management of myofascial pain. In *Essentials of pain medicine.* 4th ed. 2018. pp. 475–484. doi: 10.1016/B978-0-323-40196-8.00053-X.

69. Gallagher RM. Management of neuropathic pain: Translating mechanistic advances and evidence-based research into clinical practice. *Clin J Pain.* 2006;**22**(Suppl 1):S2–S8.

70. Obata H. Analgesic mechanisms of antidepressants for neuropathic pain. *Int J Mol Sci.* 2017;**18**(11): 2483. doi: 10.3390/ijms18112483.

71. Bendtsen L, Jensen R. Amitriptyline reduces myofascial tenderness in patients with chronic tension-type headache. *Cephalalgia.* 2000;**20**(6):603–610.

72. Haviv Y, Rettman A, Aframian D, Sharav Y, Benoliel R. Myofascial pain: An open study on the pharmacotherapeutic response to stepped treatment with tricyclic antidepressants and gabapentin. *J Oral Facial Pain Headache.* 2015;**29**(2):144–151.

73. Haviv Y, Zini A, Sharav Y, Almoznino G, Benoliel R. Nortriptyline compared to amitriptyline for the treatment of persistent masticatory myofascial pain. *J Oral Facial Pain Headache.* 2018;**33**(1):7–13. doi: 10.11607/ofph.1886.

74. Czarnetzki C, Elia N, Lysakowski C et al. Dexamethasone and risk of nausea and vomiting and postoperative bleeding after tonsillectomy in children. *JAMA.* 2008;**300**(22):2621–2630. doi: 10.1001/jama.2008.794. PMID: 19066382.

75. Annaswamy TM, De Luigi AJ, O'Neill BJ, Keole N, Berbrayer D. Emerging concepts in the treatment of myofascial pain: A review of medications, modalities, and needle-based interventions. *PM&R.* 2011;**3**(10):940–961.

76. Heir GM. The efficacy of pharmacologic treatment of temporomandibular disorders. *Oral Maxillofac Surg Clin North Am.* 2018;**30**(3):279–285.

77. McNeill C. Management of temporomandibular disorders: concepts and controversies. *J Prosthet Dent.* 1997;**77**(5):510–522. doi: 10.1016/s0022-3913(97)70145-8. PMID: 9151272.

78. Loveless MS, Fry AL. Pharmacologic therapies in musculoskeletal conditions. *Med Clin North Am.* 2016;**100**(4):869–890.

79. Häggman-Henrikson B, Alstergren P, Davidson T et al. Pharmacological treatment of oro-facial pain: Health technology assessment including a systematic review with network meta-analysis. *J Oral Rehabil.* 2017;**44** (10):800–826.

80. Herman CR, Schiffman EL, Look JO, Rindal DB. The effectiveness of adding pharmacologic treatment with clonazepam or cyclobenzaprine to patient education and self-care for the treatment of jaw pain upon awakening: A randomized clinical trial. *J Orofac Pain.* 2002;**16**(1):64–70.

81. Fishbain DA, Cutler RB, Rosomoff HL, Rosomoff RS. Clonazepam open clinical treatment trial for myofascial syndrome associated chronic pain. *Pain Med.* 2000;**1**(4):332–339.

82. Harkins S, Linford J, Cohen J, Kramer T, Cueva L. Administration of clonazepam in the treatment of TMD and associated myofascial pain: A double-blind pilot study. *J Craniomandib Disord.* 1991;**5**(3):179–186.

83. Hersh EV, Balasubramaniam R, Pinto A. Pharmacologic management of temporomandibular disorders. *Oral Maxillofac Surg Clin North Am.* 2008;**20** (2):197–210.

84. Leite FM, Atallah ÁN, El Dib R et al. Cyclobenzaprine for the treatment of myofascial pain in adults. *Cochrane Database Syst Rev.* 2009;(3):CD006830. doi: 10.1002/14651858.CD006830.

85. Beebe FA, Barkin RL, Barkin S. A clinical and pharmacologic review of skeletal muscle relaxants for musculoskeletal conditions. *Am J Ther.* 2005;**12** (2):151–171.

86. Ghanavatian S, Derian A. *Tizanidine.* StatPearls; 2018.

87. Shakespeare D, Boggild M, Young CA. Anti-spasticity agents for multiple sclerosis. *Cochrane Database Syst Rev.* 2003;(4):CD001332. doi: 10.1002/14651858.CD006830.

88. Malanga GA, Gwynn MW, Smith R, Miller D. Tizanidine is effective in the treatment of myofascial pain syndrome. *Pain Physician.* 2002;**5**(4):422–432.

89. Groves L, Shellenberger MK, Davis CS. Tizanidine treatment of spasticity: A meta-analysis of controlled, double-blind, comparative studies with baclofen and diazepam. *Adv Ther.* 1998;**15**(4):241–251.

90. Malanga G, Reiter RD, Garay E. Update on tizanidine for muscle spasticity and emerging indications. *Expert Opin Pharmacother.* 2008;**9** (12):2209–2215.

91. Jaiswal M, Sanyal RP, Goswami S. Revalidation of trigger point injection in myofascial pain syndrome, assessed by pain disability score. *Int J Sci Study.* 2017;**172**.

92. Xie P, Qin B, Yang F et al. Lidocaine injection in the intramuscular innervation zone can effectively treat chronic neck pain caused by MTrPs in the trapezius muscle. *Pain Physician*. 2015;**18**(5):E815–E826.

93. Firmani M, Miralles R, Casassus R. Effect of lidocaine patches on upper trapezius EMG activity and pain intensity in patients with myofascial trigger points: A randomized clinical study. *Acta Odontol Scand*. 2015;**73**(3):210–218.

94. Affaitati G, Fabrizio A, Savini A et al. A randomized, controlled study comparing a lidocaine patch, a placebo patch, and anesthetic injection for treatment of trigger points in patients with myofascial pain syndrome: Evaluation of pain and somatic pain thresholds. *Clin Ther*. 2009;**31**(4):705–720.

95. Affaitati G, Costantini R, Tana C et al. Effects of topical vs. injection treatment of cervical myofascial trigger points on headache symptoms in migraine patients: A retrospective analysis. *J Headache Pain*. 2018;**19**(1):104. doi: 10.1186/s10194-018-0934-3.

96. Borg-Stein J, Simons DG. Myofascial pain. *Arch Phys Med Rehabil*. 2002;**83**:S40–S47.

97. Awan KH, Patil S, Alamir AWH et al. Botulinum toxin in the management of myofascial pain associated with temporomandibular dysfunction. *J Oral Pathol Med*. 2019;**48**(3):192–200. doi: 10.1111/jop.12822.

98. Machado E, Machado P, Wandscher VF et al. A systematic review of different substance injection and dry needling for treatment of temporomandibular myofascial pain. *Int J Oral Maxillofac Surg*. 2018;**47**(11):1420–1432.

99. Baker JS, Nolan PJ. Effectiveness of botulinum toxin type A for the treatment of chronic masticatory myofascial pain: A case series. *J Am Dent Assoc*. 2017;**148**(1):33–39.

100. Khalifeh M, Mehta K, Varguise N, Suarez-Durall P, Enciso R. Botulinum toxin type A for the treatment of head and neck chronic myofascial pain syndrome. *J Am Dent Assoc*. 2016;**147**(12):959–973.

101. Kwanchuay P, Petchnumsin T, Yiemsiri P et al. Efficacy and safety of single botulinum toxin type A (Botox®) injection for relief of upper trapezius myofascial trigger point: A randomized, double-blind, placebo-controlled study. *J Med Assoc Thai*. 2015;**98**(12):1231–1236.

102. Halder GE, Scott L, Wyman A et al. Botox combined with myofascial release physical therapy as a treatment for myofascial pelvic pain. *Investig Clin Urol*. 2017;**58**(2):134–139. doi: 10.4111/icu.2017.58.2.134.

# Post-stroke Pain

Alan D. Kaye, Norris Talbot, and Vijay Kurup

## Dejerine Roussy Syndrome

- Central post-stroke pain (CPSP) (1)
- A type of hemidystonia typically in regions affected by stroke (1)
- Pain and sensory abnormalities to the specific parts of the body that correspond to the effected brain area (2)
- Diverse range of sensory symptoms (3)
- Associated with mild motor symptoms with relative sparing of joint position and vibration sensations (3)
- Splits into three components:
  - Spontaneous, constant pain described as burning, aching, pricking, freezing, and squeezing (1)
  - Spontaneous, intermittent component present in 15% of cases and lasting for a few seconds to minutes, intense in severity, and described as shooting and lancinating (1)
  - 66% of patients have hyperalgesia, hyperesthesia, and/or allodynia (1)

## Epidemiology and Risk Factors

- The incidence report of post-stroke pain can be underdiagnosed and mistreated frequently (4)
- The prevalence is between 8% and 46% (1,3)
  - Wide variation in prevalence rates is attributed to heterogeneity of lesions in the patient populations surveyed, study designs, onset of strokes (3)
- Some studies have shown higher prevalence in patients with lateral medullary syndrome (Wallenberg syndrome) (1)
  - Wallenberg syndrome – clinical presentation of the infarct in the territory of posterior inferior cerebellar artery (5)

- The exact diagnosis of Dejerine Roussy syndrome can be confounded due to the similar nature of shoulder pain, painful shoulder spasticity, primary headaches like a tension-type headache, or various musculoskeletal pains particularly affecting knees and hips (1)
- Can occur within 3 to 6 months of a stroke (6)
  ○ Possible to occur within 1 month (7)
- Risk Factors:
  ○ Age is currently undetermined to be a factor (1)
  ○ Sex of patient saw predominance in females in some results (8)
  ○ Dejerine Roussy presumably happens after a cerebrovascular accident (2)
    ▪ As a result, any increased risk of stroke should increase the risk of Dejerine Roussy syndrome

## Pathophysiology

- Thought to result from a lesion in any part of the central nervous system (9)
- Any lesion on the spinothalamic tract, anywhere throughout its course in the central nervous system (CNS), can cause central post-stroke pain (10)
- CPSP can commonly occur secondary to damage that is limited to the spinothalamic tract and thalamocingulate pathway (9)
- Pain manifests contralateral to the lesion and most commonly involving the upper extremities (9)
- Central imbalance (abnormal nociception and thermal sensation) might occur due to abnormal integration between normally functioning dorsal-medial lemniscus pathway and the damaged spinothalamic tract within the multisynaptic paleo-spinothalamic pathway (1,11)
- Central disinhibition etiological theory – stroke affecting the lateral thalamus causes central disinhibition by the deafferentation of the thalamic nucleus, which causes the activation of cortical areas resulting in pain (1)
  ○ The slow return of neuronal fibers can help explain the onset of pain
- Central sensitization is the increased synaptic efficacy of the central afferent neurons leading to spontaneous pain or nociception on suboptimal stimulus (1)

○ Through other evidence, some suggestions about the damage of central neurons from *N*-methyl-*D*-aspartate-receptor activation in central sensitization

## Diagnosis

- Pain symptoms of CPSP are often characterized as burning, freezing, squeezing, heavy pressure, electric, stabbing, and lacerating (12–14)

  ○ The symptoms can vary, so it is important to constantly listen to the patient and interpret the symptoms accordingly

- Infarcted area of the brain can be visualized by CT or MRI (2)
- History of stroke and onset of pain after the stroke, peripheral pain corresponding to a central lesion, confirmation of that lesion with imaging, and the taking away other nociceptive/neuropathic causes of pain (2)

  ○ Lack of inflammation and local tissue damage are signs
  ○ Allodynia or dysesthesia to touch or cold

- Difficult to pin down symptoms due to the wide variation
- More confusion in that CPSP (Dejerine Roussy) is not distinctly a lesion of the spinothalamic tract (1)

  ○ While similar, a spinothalamic legion is considered pseudo-thalamic pain and treatment varies significantly (1)

- Differential diagnosis includes multiple sclerosis (MS), syringomyelia, conversion disorder, and cervical disk herniation (15)

  ○ Effects secondary to lesions in MS will not be as likely to manifest in CPSP and have different timeline
  ○ Syringomyelia can be visible on imaging of the spinal cord
  ○ Cervical disk herniation is hard to differentiate due to similar peripheral symptoms

## Treatment and Management

- Minimally invasive therapeutic options

  ○ Requires increased medicative doses only providing a 30–40% reduction in pain (16)
  ○ Antidepressants and anticonvulsants affect the hypersensitivity of nerves but do not selectively act on damaged nerves, can result in adverse effects (16)
  ○ These factors of adverse effects and problems pharmacologically have led to newer treatments for pain management (17)

- Botulin toxin injection
  - Therapeutic modality for spasticity including stroke, multiple sclerosis, cerebral palsy, and spinal cord injury (18)
  - One study showed significantly lower pain scores from a week 1 follow-up to a week 4 follow-up (16)
  - BTX as a whole in many of the studies was shown to reduce pain over different periods of time (16)
- Deep brain stimulation
  - Old technique from the 1950s with low understanding of its mechanisms (19)
  - DBS targets have included the ventral posterior medial/ventral posterior lateral thalamic nuclei, left centromedian thalamic nuclei, posterior limb of the internal capsule, the periaqueductal/periventricular gray matter, and the anterior cingulate cortex (16)
    - Bilateral DBS favored over unilateral (16)
    - Improved quality of life and pain in eleven patients who underwent bilateral DBS of the anterior cingulate cortex (16)
  - DBS targets a network allowing for a multifaceted approach to pain management (16)
- Transcranial stimulation
  - Stimulation through surgically implanted epidural electrodes in DBS can contribute to analgesic effects in CPSP patients (20)
    - Problems with invasive surgery and long-term electrode use
- Transcranial magnetic stimulation
  - Noninvasive, use of magnetic fields can allow modulation of nerve cell activity in focal brain areas (20)
  - A high-frequency TMS showed that it can modulate cortical neuronal excitability and reduce neuropathic pain, especially in CPSP (20)
  - Multiple TMS sessions could be a tool to manage neuropathic pain (16)
  - Treatment effects thought to be similar to motor cortex stimulation (MCS) (20)
    - MCS the only surgical procedure approved by the FDA for treatment of CPSP (16)

- May exhibit an analgesic effect by facilitating blood flow to the affected area (16)

  - No persistent evidence for analgesic effects 3 months after therapy (16)

- Transcranial direct current stimulation

  - Similar to TMS in that it's a safe, viable method of noninvasive brain stimulation (16)
  - Stimulation of motor cortex of the affected hemisphere and stimulation of hemisphere contralateral to the pain site (21)
  - tDCS with virtual reality helped improve gait, pain management, and vegetative reactions in children with cerebral palsy and post-stroke pain (16)
  - Anodal stimulation of tDCS helped improve variability of sensory differentiation in CPSP (16)
  - The possible mechanisms of tDCS therapy including inhibition of ascending pain transmission by thalamic nuclei, upregulation of motor cortex activation, or manipulation of corticothalamic fibers (22)
  - Predicting electrical current in the brain after infarction and cerebral spinal fluid influx can affect different therapies

    - Noted that TMS and tDCS both have low focality which may cause these techniques to be less sensitive to mislocalization than epidural brain stimulation (EBS) (16)
      - Could explain why TMS and tDCS output more consistent therapeutic effects in patients with CPSP

- Neuromodulation

  - Helpful for treatment of neuropathic pain, peripheral neuropathy, and complex regional pain stimulation; however, it is not a definitive recommendation for CPSP (23)
  - Spinal cord stimulator therapy was utilized and had positive effects on six of eight tested patients (23)
  - Current studies to test the effects of pharmacological drugs on the efficiency of the spinal cord stimulator therapy (16)

    - For example, those with ketamine-sensitive pain experienced greater pain reductions from SCS (16)

- Advances in Therapy

  - Motor cortex stimulation has proven to be somewhat effective for CPSP and even other neuropathic pains such as atypical facial pain, phantom limb pain, and complex region pain syndrome (16)

- Increased effects for those with treatment-resistant spontaneous burning superficial pain (16)

○ Mirror therapy

- In one case of a 50-year-old woman, it created a reduction in pain by following up a year later (16)

○ Diffusion tensor tractography

- Visualization of the spinothalamic tract (16)
- Diagnosis of CPSP becomes more straightforward
  - Comparisons can be made directly against prior imaging studies to compare the size and integrity of the spinothalamic tract (16)

○ Use of caloric vestibular stimulation to reduce pain and somatoparaphrenia (24)

- Injection of cold water into the ear canal of the patient (16)
- Recent case study associated it with significant improvements in motor skills, pain, and somatic delusions in impaired patients (16)
  - The injection induced horizontal nystagmus and vertigo in healthy patients (16)

○ Stellate ganglion block

- Selective sympathetic block (16)
- Case study of a woman with refractory, lancinating, severe pain on the right side of her face and hand status post right basal ganglia/left thalamic stoke (25)
  - Refused DBS due to invasive nature and switched to stellate ganglion block (25)
  - Patient endorsed 3-day pain-free period followed by an interval of decreasing pain (25)
  - Two more injections led to half a year of pain-free period (25)
- Stellate ganglion looks like a promising option for short-term relief, but more evidence is required to prove it (16)

# Conclusions

- CPSP, Dejerine Roussy syndrome, is a specific injury resulting from usually ischemic stroke
- Diagnosing and discovering direct mechanisms are still works in process
- The syndrome is also hard to differentiate among other similar ones due to the varying symptomatic responses in individuals
- Many different therapy processes and management systems are being studied to find an efficient and safe way to reduce the pain in individuals with CPSP
- Seen in the treatments and management section, some techniques are invasive while others are not
  - Transcranial stimulation is invasive
    - Leads to many other complications that come with surgical procedures
  - Other methods are not as invasive and have some existing evidence of reducing pain
- Many of the treatments and management of CPSP still need more evidence to fully figure out their mechanisms of action and the consistent effects of the treatments
- The different methods appear to have promising results and future research can help to uncover that potential

# References

1. Jahngir MU, Qureshi AI. Dejerine Roussy syndrome. *StatPearls*. Published online July 4, 2022. www.ncbi.nlm.nih.gov/books/NBK519047/.

2. Klit H, Finnerup NB, Jensen TS. Central post-stroke pain: Clinical characteristics, pathophysiology, and management. *Lancet Neurol*. 2009;8(9):857–868. https://doi.org/10.1016/S1474-4422(09)70176-0.

3. Kumar B, Kalita J, Kumar G, Misra UK. Central poststroke pain: A review of pathophysiology and treatment. *Anesth Analg*. 2009;108(5):1645–1657. https://doi.org/10.1213/ANE.0B013E31819D644C.

4. Delpont B, Blanc C, Osseby GV et al. Pain after stroke: A review. *Rev Neurol (Paris)*. 2018;174(10):671–674. https://doi.org/10.1016/J.NEUROL.2017.11.011.

5. Gasca-González OO, Pérez-Cruz JC, Baldoncini M, Macías-Duvignau MA, Delgado-Reyes L. Neuroanatomical basis of Wallenberg syndrome. *Cir Cir*. 2020;88(3):376–382. https://doi.org/10.24875/CIRU.19000801.

6. Canavero S, Bonicalzi V. Central pain of brain origin. *Central Pain Syndrome*. Published online December 24, 2007:9–112. https://doi.org/10.1017/CBO9780511585692.003.

7. Leijon G, Boivie J, Johansson I. Central post-stroke pain: Neurological symptoms and pain characteristics. *Pain*. 1989;**36**(1):13–25. https://doi.org/10.1016/0304-3959(89)90107-3.

8. Hansen AP, Marcussen NS, Klit H et al. Pain following stroke: A prospective study. *Eur J Pain*. 2012;**16**(8):1128–1136. https://doi.org/10.1002/J.1532-2149.2012.00123.X.

9. Akyuz G, Kuru P. Systematic review of central post stroke pain. *Am J Phys Med Rehabil*. 2016;**95**(8):618–627. https://doi.org/10.1097/PHM.0000000000000542.

10 Zheng Y, Xu L, Dong N, Li F. NLRP3 inflammasome: The rising star in cardiovascular diseases. *Front Cardiovasc Med*. 2022;**9**:927061. doi: 10.3389/fcvm.2022.927061. PMID: 36204568; PMCID: PMC9530053.

11. Whiting BB, Whiting AC, Whiting DM. Thalamic deep brain stimulation. *Prog Neurol Surg*. 2018;**33**:198–206. https://doi.org/10.1159/000481104.

12. Kumar A, Bhoi SK, Kalita J, Misra UK. Central poststroke pain can occur with normal sensation. *Clin J Pain*. 2016;**32**(11):955–960. https://doi.org/10.1097/AJP.0000000000000344.

13. Şahin-Onat Ş, Ünsal-Delialioğlu S, Kulaklı F, Özel S. The effects of central post-stroke pain on quality of life and depression in patients with stroke. *J Phys Ther Sci*. 2016;**28**(1):96–101. https://doi.org/10.1589/JPTS.28.96.

14. Paolucci S, Iosa M, Toni D et al. Prevalence and time course of post-stroke pain: A multicenter prospective hospital-based study. *Pain Med (United States)*. 2016;**17**(5):924–930. https://doi.org/10.1093/PM/PNV019.

15. Lim TH, Choi SI, Yoo JI et al. Thalamic pain misdiagnosed as cervical disc herniation. *Korean J Pain*. 2016;**29**(2):119–122. https://doi.org/10.3344/KJP.2016.29.2.119.

16. Urits I, Gress K, Charipova K et al. Diagnosis, treatment, and management of Dejerine-Roussy syndrome: A comprehensive review. *Curr Pain Headache Rep*. 2020;**24**(9):48. https://doi.org/10.1007/S11916-020-00887-3.

17. Chen CC, Chuang YF, Huang ACW, Chen CK, Chang YJ. The antalgic effects of non-invasive physical modalities on central post-stroke pain: A systematic review. *J Phys Ther Sci*. 2016;**28**(4):1368–1373. https://doi.org/10.1589/JPTS.28.1368.

18. Park JH, Park HJ. Botulinum toxin for the treatment of neuropathic pain. *Toxins (Basel)*. 2017;**9**(9):260. https://doi.org/10.3390/TOXINS9090260.

19. Ward M, Mammis A. Deep brain stimulation for the treatment of Dejerine-Roussy syndrome. *Stereotact Funct Neurosurg*. 2017;**95**(5):298–306. https://doi.org/10.1159/000479526.

20. Jin Y, Xing G, Li G et al. High frequency repetitive transcranial magnetic stimulation therapy for chronic neuropathic pain: A meta-analysis. *Pain Physician*. 2015;**18**(6):E1029–E1046. https://doi.org/10.36076/ppj.2015/18/e1029.

21. Morishita T, Hyakutake K, Saita K et al. Pain reduction associated with improved functional interhemispheric balance following transcranial direct current stimulation for post-stroke central pain: A case study. *J Neurol Sci*. 2015;**358**(1–2):484–485. https://doi.org/10.1016/J.JNS.2015.08.1551.

22. Bae SH, Kim GD, Kim KY. Analgesic effect of transcranial direct current stimulation on central post-stroke pain. *Tohoku J Exp Med*. 2014;**234**(3):189–195. https://doi.org/10.1620/TJEM.234.189.

23. Yamamoto T, Watanabe M, Obuchi T et al. Importance of pharmacological evaluation in the treatment of poststroke pain by spinal cord stimulation. *Neuromodulation*. 2016;**19**(7):744–751. https://doi.org/10.1111/NER.12408.

24. Spitoni GF, Pireddu G, Galati G et al. Caloric vestibular stimulation reduces pain and somatoparaphrenia in a severe chronic central post-stroke pain patient: A case study. *PLoS One*. 2016;**11**(3):e0151213. https://doi.org/10.1371/JOURNAL.PONE.0151213.

25. Liao C, Yang M, Liu P, Zhong W, Zhang W. Thalamic pain alleviated by stellate ganglion block: A case report. *Medicine*. 2017;**96**(5):e6058. https://doi.org/10.1097/MD.0000000000006058.

# Chronic Abdominal Pain

Alan D. Kaye and Zahaan Eswani

- Pain is defined by the International Association for the Study of Pain (IASP) as "an unpleasant sensory and emotional experience associated with, or resembling that associated with, actual or potential tissue damage" (1)
- CAP is a constant or recurrent pain that lasts for more than 3 months (1,2)
- Abdominal pain is a common symptom of the gastrointestinal (GI) system and can be associated with various diseases of the abdomen or extra-abdominal diseases. The pain may occur at various locations with varying intensities and propagation and is often associated with other symptoms (2)

## Epidemiology and Risk Factors

- Abdominal pain is the most common GI symptom, and it is a leading cause for inpatient and outpatient visits (1)
- International prevalence is between 22% and 25%, with more women reporting abdominal pain than men (24% versus 17%) (1)
- Abdominal pain has been found to be the second most common pain after back pain. Nineteen percent of the Middle Eastern population suffers from chronic pain (3)
- The prevalence of chronic abdominal pain in low- and middle-income countries is estimated to be 17% of the general elderly population (4,5)
- Chronic pain is specifically associated with females, advanced age, multiple pain sites, mood, psychosomatic disorders, predictive of healthcare costs (4,5)
- Almost 1/3 of cases of CAP occur in people under 20 years old with a steady decrease in prevalence toward old age (1)
- Irritable bowel syndrome (IBS) 1–4% global prevalence
- Functional dyspepsia (FD) 2–7% global prevalence

- Functional constipation 7–11% global prevalence
- Unspecified bowl disorder 0–11% global prevalence
- Chronic abdominal wall pain (CAWP) is commonly overlooked and is responsible for 2–3% of cases of CAP. The prevalence of CAWP can rise to 30% in cases with no identifiable organic cause and is four times more common in women aged 30–50
- The most common cause of CAWP is abdominal cutaneous nerve entrapment syndrome which accounts for 10–30% of cases of CAP (1,6)

## Pathophysiology

- Many diseases such as the following can cause CAP (1,2)
  - Gastroesophageal reflux disease (GERD)
  - Chronic gastritis
  - Gastric and duodenal ulcers
  - Crohn's disease
  - Centrally mediated abdominal pain syndrome (CAPS)
  - Chronic pancreatitis (CP)
  - Functional gastrointestinal disorders (FGIDs) (1)
    - Irritable bowel syndrome (IBS) 1–4% global prevalence
    - Functional Dyspepsia (FD) 2–7% global prevalence
    - Functional constipation 7–11% global prevalence
    - Unspecified bowl disorder 0–11% global prevalence
- CAP can arise from GI disease and extraintestinal conditions which involve the genitourinary tract, domino wall, thorax, and spine and which often result in significant declines in function and quality of life (1)
- As per the IASP, CAP can be classified into abdominal wall pain, abdominal pain of visceral origin, abdominal pain syndromes of generalized diseases, and FGIDs (1,7)
- CAP is divided into visceral, somatosensory, and functional pain. Visceral pain is that of the deep, internal abdominal structures, somatic pain is that of nociceptors in superficial tissue (e.g., skin) or the musculoskeletal system, and functional pain relates primarily to visceral or central hypersensitivity (1,8)
- CAP in geriatric patients is typically due to peptic ulcer disease, biliary colic, diverticular disease, chronic mesenteric ischemia, and colon cancer (1)

- Visceral pain is transmitted to the brain via vagal, thoracolumbar, and lumbosacral afferent nerves (9,10)
- Non-referred visceral pain is characterized as diffuse, dull, and midline, or epigastric due to the afferent nervous system to this region being supplied by bilateral splanchnic nerves (9,11)
- Referred pain is characterized as aching or near the body's surface and is accompanied by skin hyperalgesia and increased abdominal wall muscle tone. Referred pain presents in a dermatomal distribution which correlates with the site of the spinal cord level of the affected visceral organ (9)

## Diagnosis

- Diagnostic criteria require a detailed medical history
- Upper abdominal pain tends to arise from biliary, pancreatic, gastric, and duodenal pathology. Mid-abdominal pain can be caused by the small bowel. Lower abdominal pain arises from the colon, bladder, or reproductive organs (1)
- Physical exam of the abdomen includes (1)
  - Inspection
    - Note any surgical scars
  - Auscultation
    - Note any bruits which can indicate chronic mesenteric ischemia
  - Palpation
    - Light/deep palpation can help to localize pain to a specific abdominal quadrant, for masses, ascites, hernias, and organomegaly
  - Rectal examination
    - Note any active bleeding, mass, signs of constipation, pelvic floor dysfunction, high anal resting tone
- CBC with differential, CMP, lipase, urinalysis should be performed (9)
- Abdominal imaging such as ultrasound, CT, MRI are usually ordered as part of the initial workup (9)

# Treatment Modalities

## Anesthetic Techniques

The celiac plexus is the largest autonomic plexus, and it is located in the retroperitoneum at the roots of the celiac trunk and superior mesenteric artery (SMA). It is made up of paired celiac ganglia and superior mesenteric and aorticorenal ganglia which are presynaptic fibers of the sympathetic splanchnic nerves (T5 to T12) (12)

1. Celiac plexus neurolysis

   a. Neurolytic agents like ethanol and phenol are used to destroy the nerves of the celiac plexus permanently. This is often reserved for malignant disease such as pancreatic cancer (13)
   b. Most performed by injection of 50–100% ethanol or (less likely) 3–20% phenol (12)
   c. Ethanol causes irreversible damage and concentrations over 50%. Since Espinal may cause temporary severe pain, it is recommended to add a long-acting anesthetic like bupivacaine. The most utilized mixture contains 95–100% ethanol, bupivacaine, and iodinated contrast in a 6:3:1 ratio (12,14,15)

2. Celiac plexus blocking agents

   a. Local anesthetics (e.g., bupivacaine, lidocaine) are often used with steroids and ethanol to counteract pain (13)

## Pharmacologic Treatment (9)

1. Antispasmodic drugs
2. Antidepressants and psychological treatment
3. Drugs acting on opioid receptors
4. 5-HT3 receptor antagonists
5. Bile acid sequestrants
6. Antibiotics
7. Intestinal secretagogues
8. Gamma-aminobutyric acid analogs

## Interventional Treatment

1. Spinal cord stimulation

   a. Appears to be a useful therapeutic option for patients with severe visceral pain (16)

## Lifestyle Modifications

1. Exercise
   a. Shown to improve overall GI symptoms and anxiety (9,10)
   b. Yoga has been shown to be beneficial in reducing symptom severity and IBS (9,17)
   c. Exercise for 20–60 minutes resulted in significant improvement in IBS symptoms and psychological symptoms over a 12-week period. This was confirmed with a median follow-up of 5.2 years. Evidence suggests that reduced physical activity may be related to levels of pain intensity in children with chronic pain (9,18)

2. Dietary modifications
   a. Can help in patients with IBS
   b. Thought to be due to altered gut microbiota, sensitivity to gastrocolic reflux, insoluble fiber exacerbating symptoms, and antigens in food altering intestinal epithelial barrier (9,10,19)

## Conclusions

- CAP is a constant or recurrent pain that lasts for more than 3 months (1,2)
- Abdominal pain is the most common GI symptom, and it is a leading cause for inpatient and outpatient visits. International prevalence is between 22% and 25%, with more women reporting abdominal pain than men (24% versus 17%) (1)
- Many diseases processes can cause CAP (1,2)
- Treatments include: celiac plexus neurolysis, celiac plexus blocking agent, various pharmacologic treatment, spinal cord stimulation, and lifestyle modifications (9)

## References

1. Sabo CM, Grad S, Dumitrascu DL. Chronic abdominal pain in general practice. *Dig Dis.* 2021;**39**(6):606–614. https://doi.org/10.1159/000515433.

2. Lukic S, Mijac D, Filipovic B et al. Chronic abdominal pain: Gastroenterologist approach. *Dig Dis.* 2022;**40**(2):181–186. https://doi.org/10.1159/000516977.

3. El-Metwally A, Shaikh Q, Aldiab A et al. The prevalence of chronic pain and its associated factors among Saudi Al-Kharj population; a cross sectional study. *BMC Musculoskelet Disord.* 2019;**20**(1):177. https://doi.org/10.1186/S12891-019-2555-7.

4.  Jackson T, Thomas S, Stabile V et al. Chronic pain without clear etiology in low- and middle-income countries: A narrative review. *Anesth Analg.* 2016;**122**(6):2028–2039. https://doi.org/10.1213/ANE.0000000000001287.

5.  Jackson T, Thomas S, Stabile V et al. A systematic review and meta-analysis of the global burden of chronic pain without clear etiology in low- and middle-income countries: Trends in heterogeneous data and a proposal for new assessment methods. *Anesth Analg.* 2016;**123**(3):739–748. https://doi.org /10.1213/ANE.0000000000001389.

6.  Koop H, Koprdova S, Schürmann C. Chronic Abdominal Wall Pain: A Poorly Recognized Clinical Problem. *Dtsch Arztebl Int.* 2016;**113**:51–57. www .aerzteblatt.de/int/archive/article/173620/Chronic-abdominal-wall-pain-a-p oorly-recognized-clinical-problem.

7.  Aziz Q, Giamberardino MA, Barke A et al. The IASP classification of chronic pain for ICD-11: Chronic secondary visceral pain. *Pain.* 2019;**160**(1):69–76. https://doi.org/10.1097/J.PAIN.0000000000001362.

8.  Wilson PR. Chronic abdominal pain: An evidence-based, comprehensive guide to clinical management. *Pain Med.* 2015;**16**(12):2412–2413. https://doi .org/10.1111/PME.12849.

9.  Stemboroski L, Schey R. Treating chronic abdominal pain in patients with chronic abdominal pain and/or irritable bowel syndrome. *Gastroenterol Clin North Am.* 2020;**49**(3):607–621. https://doi.org/10.1016/J.GTC.2020.05.001.

10.  Camilleri M. Management options for irritable bowel syndrome. *Mayo Clin Proc.* 2018;**93**(12):1858–1872. https://doi.org/10.1016/J.MAYOCP.2018.04.032.

11.  Pichetshote N, Pimentel M. An approach to the patient with chronic undiagnosed abdominal pain. *Am J Gastroenterol.* 2019;**114**(5):726–732. htt ps://doi.org/10.14309/AJG.0000000000000130.

12.  Cornman-Homonoff J, Holzwanger DJ, Lee KS, Madoff DC, Li D. Celiac plexus block and neurolysis in the management of chronic upper abdominal pain. *Semin Intervent Radiol.* 2017;**34**(4):376–386. https://doi.org/10.1055/S-0037-1608861.

13.  Urits I, Jones MR, Orhurhu V et al. A comprehensive review of the celiac plexus block for the management of chronic abdominal pain. *Curr Pain Headache Rep.* 2020;**24**(9):42. https://doi.org/10.1007/S11916-020-00878-4.

14.  Bahn BM, Erdek MA. Celiac plexus block and neurolysis for pancreatic cancer. *Curr Pain Headache Rep.* 2013;**17**(2):310. https://doi.org/10.1007/S1 1916-012-0310-Y.

15.  Dolly A, Singh S, Prakash R et al. Comparative evaluation of different volumes of 70% alcohol in celiac plexus block for upper abdominal malignsancies. *South Asian J Cancer.* 2016;**5**(4):204–209. https://doi.org/10 .4103/2278-330X.195346.

16. Kapural L, Nagem H, Tlucek H, Sessler DI. Spinal cord stimulation for chronic visceral abdominal pain. *Pain Med.* 2010;**11**(3):347–355. https://doi.org/10.1111/J.1526-4637.2009.00785.X.

17. Johannesson E, Simrén M, Strid H, Bajor A, Sadik R. Physical activity improves symptoms in irritable bowel syndrome: A randomized controlled trial. *Am J Gastroenterol.* 2011;**106**(5):915–922. https://doi.org/10.1038/AJG.2010.480.

18. Kichline T, Cushing CC, Ortega A, Friesen C, Schurman JV. Associations between physical activity and chronic pain severity in youth with chronic abdominal pain. *Clin J Pain.* 2019;**35**(7):618–624. https://doi.org/10.1097/AJP.0000000000000716.

19. Drossman DA. Functional gastrointestinal disorders: History, pathophysiology, clinical features and Rome IV. *Gastroenterology.* 2016;**150**(6):1262–1279. https://doi.org/10.1053/J.GASTRO.2016.02.032.

**Chapter 36**

# Chronic Pelvic Pain

Taylor Witten, Nazir Noor, and Corey Moss

## Introduction and Epidemiology

- Urologic chronic pelvic pain syndrome is defined as pain found in the pelvic area that lasts greater than 3 months in the absence of other causes that limits functioning (1)
  - Chronic pelvic pain and its associated factors can have a severe impact on a patient's quality of life (1,4)
  - Patients diagnosed with chronic pelvic pain syndrome typically also have a significant financial burden with estimated annual medical care costs amounting to $3,017 per Medicare patient and $6,534 per non-Medicare patient (4)
- This syndrome encompasses three chronic pelvic disorders:
  1. Interstitial cystitis also known as bladder pain syndrome prevalent in both men and women (1,2)
  2. Provoked vestibulodynia in women (1,2)
  3. Chronic prostatitis in men (1,2)
  - Chronic pelvic pain syndrome is one of the many diseases shared by urologic and gynecologic professions (1,3)
- Prostatitis specifically is classified by the National Institutes of Health (NIH) into four categories:
  - I and II are acute and chronic bacterial prostatitis and account for 5–10% of all cases (12)
    - These classes are clearly associated with bacterial infection
  - III is the most common and encompasses chronic pelvic pain syndrome (12)
  - IV is asymptomatic inflammatory prostatitis diagnosed incidentally when evaluating for infertility (12)
- Chronic pelvic pain syndrome accounts for approximately 2 million medical visits a year (4)

- This syndrome is more common in women overall (3)
- The chronic prostatitis in men that leads to pelvic pain syndrome is the third most common genitourinary diagnosis in men behind benign prostatic hyperplasia and prostate cancer (4)

- The MAPP Research network has shown that patients who report pain below the pelvis often have more severe symptoms and more flares than those who just report pain at the pelvic region (2)
- Common symptoms of pelvic pain syndrome are urogenital pain, urinary tract symptoms, sexual dysfunction, and psychosocial factors (4,7)
- More specifically:
  - The symptoms reported with bladder pain syndrome is characterized by urinary frequency, urgency, and pelvic pain (2)
  - Provoked vestibulodynia symptoms are difficulty with sexual intercourse and soreness located in the vestibule (1)
  - Chronic prostatitis is often characterized by pain in the perineum, penis, testicles, and suprapubic region (2)
- The urogenital pain is often the first symptom patients notice (4)
- Sexual dysfunction can be seen in a variety of forms, including erectile dysfunction, ejaculatory dysfunction, and decreased libido (5)
- Patients with the symptoms above often experience anxiety and depression and will even show worse mental health scores than other patient cohorts (4,6)

## Pathophysiology

- Studies have shown a variety of etiologies, including infectious, neurologic, physiologic, immunologic, and endocrinologic (4)
- Infectious:
  - The diagnosis of chronic pelvic pain syndrome is dependent on ruling out any cause of infection
  - Despite this, there are some studies that suggest infection could be a potential cause, but the data are limited and there are several studies that contradict this finding (8,9)
  - Though infection is not proven as a direct etiology, there are studies that demonstrate men have a higher likelihood of being diagnosed with chronic pelvic pain syndrome if they have had a prior infection like prostatitis or urethritis (10)

- Immunologic:
  - A dysregulated immune response has been demonstrated to be a potential cause for chronic pelvic pain syndrome prompted by various catalysts such as infection, trauma, or voiding dysfunction (4)
  - There is an imbalance of cytokines with an increase in pro-inflammatory IFN-α, IL-6, and IL-8 and a decrease in anti-inflammatory IL-10 (12)
  - Studies have shown an autoimmune response involving self-reactive T cells to prostate-specific antigen and other seminal proteins (11)

- Neurologic:
  - Irritation and inflammation of the pelvis results in the release of nerve growth factor (NGF)
    - NGF is a neuropeptide released from mast cells that can hypersensitize peripheral nerve fiber endings (12,13)
    - The amount of nerve growth factor present can also be correlated to the pain severity felt by a patient and can even play a role in central nervous system sensitization (13,14)
  - Inflammation of the pelvic region can result in microstructural changes and reorganization of the brain and spinal cord (12,15)

- Pelvic floor dysfunction:
  - Weakness, tenderness, or cramps in the pelvic floor muscles (16)
  - It is unknown whether this is truly a cause of chronic pelvic pain or occurs as a result of the pain (17)

- Endocrinologic:
  - There is evidence that local inflammation can lead to decreased steroid hormone production (12)
  - In a rat model with prostatitis, inflammation was demonstrated to inhibit 5α reductase activity and lower levels of dihydrotestosterone, effectively increasing testosterone levels (18,19)
    - This is significant because the study found that the increased levels of testosterone were able to block estradiol and its ability to produce pro-inflammatory markers (19)

# Clinical Presentation and Diagnosis

- Because the etiology of chronic pelvic pain syndrome is complex and can present in a variety of ways, the presentation and diagnosis are equally complex (4)
- This is often a diagnosis of exclusion ruling out other causes of pain including malignancy, injury, and infectious causes (4)
- A physical exam should include an abdominal exam, digital rectal exam, and pelvic floor evaluation (4)
- There is a wide range of signs/symptoms reported by patients with chronic pelvic pain syndrome, including:
  - Pain of the perineum, suprapubic region, testicles/penis, lower back, abdomen, groin, and rectum (4,7)
  - Muscle tenderness in abdominal and pelvic regions (7)
  - Functional bowel symptoms (IBS) (7)
  - Urinary symptoms such as weak stream, straining, urgency, nocturia (4,7)
  - Decreased libido and ejaculatory dysfunction (7)
  - Anxiety, depression, and decreased quality of life causing limitations to a patient's activity (7)
- In 1999, the National Institutes of Health developed a Chronic Prostatitis Symptom Index as a way to evaluate a male patient's pain severity, urinary symptoms, and quality of life (20)
- A new approach to classifying chronic pelvic pain syndromes is the UPOINT system which stratifies patients into symptom-led phenotypes (21)
  - This system has seven domains, including urinary symptoms, psychosocial dysfunction, organ-specific findings, infection, muscle tenderness, sexual dysfunction, and neurologic symptoms (21)
- Provoked vestibulodynia is a subgroup of the chronic pelvic pain syndrome characterized by vulvar discomfort, dyspareunia, and vestibular tenderness (16)
  - Often diagnosed by a history and Q-tip test (16)
- Painful bladder syndrome/interstitial cystitis presents with the frequent need to urinate, urgency, interrupted sleep, anxiety, and even difficulty with intercourse (1)
  - The diagnosis of this often begins with manual examination of the pelvis to identify any rigidity or sensitivity followed by urinalysis and cultures (1,7)

- An infectious etiology can be ruled out with urinalysis and cultures of the urine, semen, and cervical discharge (7)
  - This should include sexually transmitted infections (7)
- Pelvic floor dysfunction can be excluded via pelvic floor ultrasound (17)

## Treatment and Management

- Identifying patients' symptom pattern is important because this will guide treatment (7)
- Similar to other chronic pain syndromes in which the etiology is multifactorial and unknown, treatment can be varied (1)
- Patients should be referred to a pain specialist when initial treatments fail (7)
- Though not proven as an etiology, if an infectious process is suspected as the source of chronic pelvic pain syndrome, studies have shown that antibiotic treatment is relatively ineffective but can still be used as first-line therapy (1,7)
  - Look at alternative treatments such as anti-inflammatory medications as a possibility when antimicrobials fail (1)
- Endocrinologic etiologies can be treated with finasteride, a 5α reductase inhibitor, in order to increase the levels of testosterone in the body and decrease inflammation (12,23)
- Studies have proven that alpha-adrenergic antagonists such as tamsulosin and terazosin can reduce symptoms such as pain and urinary symptoms (22)
  - These should be considered as an initial treatment option for patients with voiding lower urinary tract symptoms (22)
  - If no relief following 4–6 weeks, another treatment option should be considered (7)
- Pain management includes anti-inflammatory, antidepressants, neuromodulators, and immunologic agents
  - These should be considered due to the potential for a dysregulated immune response as a cause (24)
  - NSAIDs such as celecoxib should be offered for short-term treatment only due to adverse effects
    - These have shown a significant improvement in pelvic pain, but this is largely limited because of the duration of therapy (24)

- ○ The use of opioids is typically avoided because of the risk of use dependence
- ○ GABA analogs, tricyclic antidepressants, or selective serotonin-noradrenaline reuptake inhibitors can be considered for neuropathic pain (1,7,25)
- Pelvic floor physical therapy and myofascial trigger point release should be considered especially in patients who haven't responded to pharmacotherapy (26)
  - ○ This includes a series of stretches and exercises designed to strengthen the pelvic floor muscles (27)
  - ○ It addition to pain management, it has also shown improvement in sexual dysfunction (27)
- Surgery is a last resort when traditional treatment fails (1)

# References

1. Grinberg K, Sela Y, Nissanholtz-Gannot R. New insights about chronic pelvic pain syndrome (CPPS). *Int J Environ Res Public Health*. 2020;**17**(9):3005. https://doi.org/10.3390/ijerph17093005.

2. Clemens JQ, Mullins C, Ackerman AL et al. Urologic chronic pelvic pain syndrome: Insights from the MAPP research network. *Nat Rev Urol*. 2019;**16**(3):187–200. https://doi.org/10.1038/s41585-018-0135-5.

3. Ahangari A. Prevalence of chronic pelvic pain among women: An updated review. *Pain Physician*. 2014;**17**:141–147.

4. Pena VN, Engel N, Gabrielson AT, Rabinowitz MJ, Herati AS. Diagnostic and management strategies for patients with chronic prostatitis and chronic pelvic pain syndrome. *Drugs Aging*. 2021;**38**(10):845–886. https://doi.org/10.1007/s40266-021-00890-2.

5. Lee SWH, Liong ML, Yuen KH et al. Adverse impact of sexual dysfunction in chronic prostatitis/chronic pelvic pain syndrome. *Urology*. 2008;**71**(1):79–84.

6. Collins MM, Pontari MA, O'Leary MP et al. Quality of life is impaired in men with chronic prostatitis: The chronic prostatitis collaborative research network. *J Gen Intern Med*. 2001;**16**(10):656–662.

7. Rees J, Abrahams M, Doble A, Cooper A, Prostatitis Expert Reference Group (PERG). Diagnosis and treatment of chronic bacterial prostatitis and chronic prostatitis/chronic pelvic pain syndrome: A consensus guideline. *BJU Int*. 2015;**116**(4):509–525. https://doi.org/10.1111/bju.13101.

8. Hou DS, Long WM, Shen J et al. Characterisation of the bacterial community in expressed prostatic secretions from patients with chronic prostatitis/chronic pelvic pain syndrome and infertile men: A preliminary investigation. *Asian J Androl*. 2012;**14**(4):566–573. https://doi.org/10.1038/aja.2012.30.

9.  Weidner W, Schiefer HG, Krauss H et al. Chronic prostatitis: A thorough search for etiologically involved microorganisms in 1,461 patients. *Infection.* 1991;**19**(Suppl 3):S119–S125. https://doi.org/10.1007/BF01643680.

10. Pontari MA, McNaughton-Collins M, O'Leary MP et al. A case-control study of risk factors in men with chronic pelvic pain syndrome. *BJU Int.* 2005;**96** (4):559–565.

11. Alexander RB, Brady F, Ponniah S. Autoimmune prostatitis: Evidence of T cell reactivity with normal prostatic proteins. *Urology.* 1997;**50**(6):893–899. https://doi.org/10.1016/S0090-4295(97)00456-1.

12. Pontari MA, Ruggieri MR. Mechanisms in prostatitis/chronic pelvic pain syndrome. *J Urol.* 2004;**172**(3):839–845. https://doi.org/10.1097/01. ju.0000136002.76898.04.

13. Ishigooka M, Zermann D, Doggweiler R, Schmidt RA. Similarity of distributions of spinal c-fos and plasma extravasation after acute chemical irritation of the bladder and the prostate. *J Urol.* 2000;**164**(5):1751–1756.

14. Miller LJ, Fischer KA, Goralnick SJ et al. Nerve growth factor and chronic prostatitis/chronic pelvic pain syndrome. *Urology.* 2002;**59**(4):603–608.

15. Woodworth D, Mayer E, Leu K et al. Unique microstructural changes in the brain associated with urological chronic pelvic pain syndrome (UCPPS) revealed by diffusion tensor MRI, super-resolution track density imaging, and statistical parameter mapping: A MAPP network neuroimaging study. *PLoS One.* 2015,**10**(10). e0140250.

16. Næss I, Bø K. Pelvic floor muscle function in women with provoked vestibulodynia and asymptomatic controls. *Int Urogynecol J.* 2015;**26** (10):1467–1473. https://doi.org/10.1007/s00192-015-2660-6.

17. Davis SN, Morin M, Binik YM, Khalife S, Carrier S. Use of pelvic floor ultrasound to assess pelvic floor muscle function in urological chronic pelvic pain syndrome in men. *J Sex Med.* 2011;**8**(11):3173–3180.

18. Diserio GP, Carrizo AE, Pacheco-Rupil B, Nowotny E. Effect of male accessory glands autoaggression on androgenic cytosolic and nuclear receptors of rat prostate. *Cell Mol Biol.* 1992;**38**:201–207.

19. Naslund MJ, Strandberg JD, Coffey DS. The role of androgens and estrogens in the pathogenesis of experimental nonbacterial prostatitis. *J Urol.* 1988;**140** (5):1049–1053.

20. Litwin MS, McNaughton-Collins M, Fowler FJ et al. The National Institutes of Health chronic prostatitis symptom index: Development and validation of a new outcome measure. *J Urol.* 1999;**162**(2):369–375.

21. Shoskes DA, Nickel JC, Rackley RR, Pontari MA. Clinical phenotyping in chronic prostatitis/chronic pelvic pain syndrome and interstitial cystitis: A management strategy for urologic chronic pelvic pain syndromes. *Prostate Cancer Prostatic Dis.* 2009;**12**(2):177–183.

22. Evliyaoğlu Y, Burgut R. Lower urinary tract symptoms, pain and quality of life assessment in chronic non-bacterial prostatitis patients treated with alpha-blocking agent doxazosin; versus placebo. *Int Urol Nephrol.* 2002;**34**(3):351–356. https://doi.org/10.1023/a:1024487604631.

23. Leskinen M, Lukkarinen O, Marttila T. Effects of finasteride in patients with inflammatory chronic pelvic pain syndrome: A double-blind, placebo-controlled, pilot study. *Urology.* 1999;**53**(3):502–505. https://doi.org/10.1016/s0090-4295(98)00540-8.

24. Zhao WP, Zhang ZG, Li XD et al. Celecoxib reduces symptoms in men with difficult chronic pelvic pain syndrome (Category IIIA). *Braz J Med Biol Res.* 2009;**42**(10):963–967. https://doi.org/10.1590/s0100-879x2009005000021.

25. Pontari MA, Krieger JN, Litwin MS et al. Pregabalin for the treatment of men with chronic prostatitis/chronic pelvic pain syndrome: A randomized controlled trial. *Arch Intern Med.* 2010;**170**(17):1586–1593. https://doi.org/10.1001/archinternmed.2010.319.

26. Anderson RU, Wise D, Sawyer T, Chan C. Integration of myofascial trigger point release and paradoxical relaxation training treatment of chronic pelvic pain in men. *J Urol.* 2005;**174**(1):155–160.

27. Anderson RU, Wise D, Sawyer T, Chan CA. Sexual dysfunction in men with chronic prostatitis/chronic pelvic pain syndrome: Improvement after trigger point release and paradoxical relaxation training. *J Urol.* 2006;**176**(4 Pt 1):1534–1539. https://doi.org/10.1016/j.juro.2006.06.010.

# Chapter 37

# Postsurgical Nerve Entrapment
Zohal Sarwary

- Nerve entrapment is defined as pressure neuropathy from chronic nerve compression
- Frequently underdiagnosed and undertreated (1)
- Contributes to increased morbidity, financial burden, functional impairment, loss of work, and increases medical dependence (2,3)

## Epidemiology

- Cutaneous nerve entrapment is not an uncommon occurrence after surgery (up to 30% of patients) (1)
- Most significantly associated with hernia repair and procedures utilizing a Pfannenstiel incision (4)
- Most frequently involved nerves include: iliohypogastric, ilioinguinal, and genitofemoral nerves (1)
- Laparoscopic procedures are associated with significantly higher rates of postoperative pain than open procedures (4)
- Prevalent in adult as well as pediatric populations, predominantly female teenagers with pain most frequently presenting in the right lower quadrant (5)

## Pathophysiology

- Incision of nerve during surgery causes formation of a neuroma, incorporation of the nerve during closing, or constriction from adhesions
- Lengthening incision increases risk of developing nerve entrapment (6)

## Presentation

- Pain is commonly postural, continuous with intermittent exacerbations, local or diffuse with possible radiation

- Present with worsening pain described as sharp pain exacerbation in the setting of more mild chronic pain (7)
- Pain on palpation suggests the presence of a neuroma instead of nerve entrapment alone (8)
- Worsens in days prior to menses in females secondary to inflammation
- Symptoms may present soon after surgery or several years later

## Diagnosis

- Careful history and physical exam narrows down differential diagnosis
  - Positive Carnett sign on abdominal palpation indicates ACNES (anterior cutaneous nerve entrapment syndrome) (9)
  - "Arch and twist" maneuver (standing, hyperextending, and rotating trunk) reproduces pain (4)
  - Dermatomal pattern of sensory disturbances
- Diagnosis of exclusion
- Confirmed by temporary relief of pain after nerve block (8)
  - Threshold of at least 50% pain relief
  - Electrical stimulation may be efficacious in helping support diagnosis (10)

## Treatment

- Pharmacotherapy:
  - First line: NSAIDs and transdermal local anesthetics (10)
  - Second line: Oral and transdermal narcotics, antiepileptics (gabapentin/pregabalin), antidepressants (amitriptyline), and anxiolytics (9,10)
  - Pharmacotherapy generally ineffective
- Psychical therapy
- Majority of cases require further intervention for complete pain relief
  - Injections: local anesthetics, corticosteroids, alcohol, or phenol (11)
    - Efficacious
    - Less invasive
    - Must avoid major landmarks during administration, ultrasound guidance useful in finding trigger points (5,12,13)

- Most utilized block for ACNES:
  - Trigger point injections
  - TAP block
  - Rectus sheath block
- Botulinum toxin injection and neuromodulation (9)
○ Neuroablative therapy
○ Cryoanalgesic ablation
○ Surgery

- Isolate, transect, and implant ends to surrounding muscles to prevent neuroma formation (14,15)
- Ligate nerves with fine-braided polyester suture and apply alcohol or 12% phenol
- End-to-end nerve anastomosis, epineural ligation and flap (16,17)
- Neurectomy has a risk of worsening chronic neuropathic pain (10)
- Endoscopic retroperitoneal neurectomy (ERN) shown to be as effective as traditional open neurectomy (13)

## Conclusions

- There are simple and accurate methods to identify nerve entrapment; however, it is still underdiagnosed and undertreated
- Giving postsurgical nerve entrapment more attention will decrease morbidity, improve outcomes, and decrease healthcare worker costs
- Providers should be highly suspicious of postsurgical nerve entrapment, particularly when patients present with over 1 to 2 months of unresolved pain (1)
- Nonoperative management includes pharmacotherapy, psychical therapy, and injections
- Injections and blocks should be performed under ultrasound guidance
- Neuroablative therapy and cryoanalgesic ablation are still being explored and need to be further studied
- Refractory neuropathic pain unresolved with pharmacotherapy and nonoperative procedures should undergo neurectomy

## References

1. Charipova K, Gress K, Berger AA et al. A comprehensive review and update of post-surgical cutaneous nerve entrapment. *Curr Pain Headache Rep*. 2021;

25(2):11. Published online 1916. https://doi.org/10.1007/s11916-020-00924-1/Published.

2. Bay-Nielsen M, Perkins FM, Kehlet H. Pain and functional impairment 1 year after inguinal herniorrhaphy: A nationwide questionnaire study. *Ann Surg.* 2001;**233**(1):1–7. https://doi.org/10.1097/00000658-200101000-00001.

3. Poobalan AS, Bruce J, King PM et al. Chronic pain and quality of life following open inguinal hernia repair. *Br J Surg.* 2002;**88**(8):1122–1126. https://doi.org/10.1046/J.0007-1323.2001.01828.X.

4. Madura JA, Madura JA, Copper CM, Worth RM. Inguinal neurectomy for inguinal nerve entrapment: An experience with 100 patients. *Am J Surg.* 2005;**189**(3):283–287. https://doi.org/10.1016/j.amjsurg.2004.11.015.

5. Kifer T, Mišak Z, Jadrešin O, Hojsak I. Anterior cutaneous nerve entrapment syndrome in children: A prospective observational study. *Clin J Pain.* 2018;**34**(7):670–673. https://doi.org/10.1097/AJP.0000000000000573.

6. Luijendijk RW, Jeekel J, Storm RK et al. The low transverse Pfannenstiel incision and the prevalence of incisional hernia and nerve entrapment. *Ann Surg.* 1997;**225**(4):365–369. doi: 10.1097/00000658-199704000-00004.

7. Melville K, Schultz EA, Dougherty JM. Ilionguinal-iliohypogastric nerve entrapment. *Ann Emerg Med.* 1990;**19**(8):925–929. https://doi.org/10.1016/S0196-0644(05)81572-0.

8. Liszka T, Dellon A, Manson P. Iliohypogastric nerve entrapment following abdominoplasty. *Plast Reconstr Surg.* 1994;**93**(1):181–184. https://doi.org/10.1097/00006534-199401000-00030.

9. Chrona E, Kostopanagiotou G, Damigos D, Batistaki C. Anterior cutaneous nerve entrapment syndrome: Management challenges. *J Pain Res.* Published online 2017;**10**;145–156. https://doi.org/10.2147/JPR.S99337.

10. Fanelli RD, DiSiena MR, Lui FY, Gersin KS. Cryoanalgesic ablation for the treatment of chronic postherniorrhaphy neuropathic pain. *Surg Endosc.* 2003;**17**(2):196–200. https://doi.org/10.1007/S00464-002-8840-8.

11. Xu Z, Tu L, Zheng Y et al. Fine architecture of the fascial planes around the lateral femoral cutaneous nerve at its pelvic exit: An epoxy sheet plastination and confocal microscopy study. *Lab Invest J Neurosurg.* 2019;**131**:1860–1868. https://doi.org/10.3171/2018.7.JNS181596.

12. Kifer T, Mišak Z, Jadrešin O, Hojsak I. Anterior cutaneous nerve entrapment syndrome in children: A prospective observational study. *Clin J Pain.* 2018;**34**(7):670–673. https://doi.org/10.1097/AJP.0000000000000573.

13. Giger U, Wente MN, Büchler MW et al. Endoscopic retroperitoneal neurectomy for chronic pain after groin surgery. *Br J Surg.* 2009;**96**(9):1076–1081. https://doi.org/10.1002/BJS.6623.

14. Lee CH, Dellon AL. Surgical management of groin pain of neural origin. *J Am Coll Surg.* 2000;**191**(2):137–142. https://doi.org/10.1016/S1072-7515(00)00319-7.

15. Starling JR, Harms BA. Diagnosis and treatment of genitofemoral and ilioinguinal neuralgia. *World J Surg.* 1989;**13**(5):586–591. https://doi.org/10.1007/BF01658875.

16. Aszmann OC, Korak KJ, Rab M et al. Neuroma prevention by end-to-side neurorraphy: An experimental study in rats. *J Hand Surg.* 2003;**28**(6):1022–1028. https://doi.org/10.1016/S0363-5023(03)00379-4.

17. Yüksel F, Kişlaoğlu E, Durak N, Uçar C, Karacaoğlu E. Prevention of painful neuromas by epineural ligatures, flaps and grafts. *Br J Plast Surg.* 1997;**50**;182–185.

# Cancer Pain

Pranav Bhargava and Alan D. Kaye

## Introduction/Overview

- Pain is quite common in patients with cancer, especially those with metastatic disease (1)
- Oncologic pain implications
  - Decreased quality of life
  - Can be an indicator of the progression of a tumor
  - Psychosocial effects such as anxiety and depression (2)
- Cancer pain divided into an acute and chronic form (1)
- Advances have been made in both oncology and pain management. The application of pain management into clinical oncology is still a work in progress (3)
- Pain management that is sufficient and consistent is difficult in cancer patients (4,5)
- Inadequate pain management most prevalent in:
  - Children (6)
  - Underserved communities (7)
  - Geriatric patients (8)
  - Outpatients with metastatic progression of disease (9)
- Most common reasons for undertreatment of cancer (10,11)
  - Fear of overprescribing
  - Lack of knowledge as to what entails adequate treatment
  - Patient apprehension to taking opioids

## Epidemiology and Risk Factors

- Prevalence of cancer may be increasing due to advances in screening and treatment (12–14)
- Little is known about the prevalence of pain
  - Prevalence varies depending on the cancer type and stage

- One meta-analysis calculations of prevalence rates of cancer pain in certain subgroups include (15):
  - Patients after curative treatment → 33%
  - Patients undergoing treatment → 59%
  - Patients with advanced disease → 64%
  - Patients at all disease stages → 53%
- Highest prevalence of cancer pain in those with head and neck cancers → 70% (15)

## Pathophysiology

- Cancer pain is dependent on tumor type and location (16)
- Mechanisms of pain (17)
  - Secondary to tumor
  - Secondary to treatment
- Tumor as the cause of pain
  - Tumor itself can secrete mediators that lead to angiogenesis and peripheral sensitization (16)
  - Primary and secondary tumors often deposit in the bone and can cause pain by (18):
    - Structural disruption of the bone
      - Resulting disruption of periosteum, marrow, and cortex → Pain
    - Direct tumor infiltration in metastatic disease (19)
    - Inflammatory mediator release
    - Alteration of osteoclast activity
  - Treatment-related pain causes (20)
    - Secondary to surgery
      - Persistent postsurgical pain (PPSP) can occur. This is defined by lasting pain 2 months following a procedure. It is often reported in cancer patients (21)
        - PPSP is thought to be caused by pathologic neural plasticity and limited to the dermatome/territory that the surgery was completed in (17,22,23)
        - PPSP most prevalent in patients who underwent thoracotomy, breast surgery, and limb amputation (17)

- Secondary to chemotherapy
  - Chemotherapy can cause chemotherapy-induced peripheral neuropathy (CIPN) by affecting long sensory nerves. It may be associated with the infusion of platinum compounds, vinca alkaloids, and taxanes (17,24)
- Secondary to radiotherapy
  - Pain can be caused by the damage to nonmalignant tissue (25)
    - Early-onset pain occurs in tissues with high cell turnover such as mucosa
    - Late-onset pain often occurs in nerves and muscle tissue
- More targeted approaches may be needed to reduce stress on nonmalignant tissue. May be important in reduction of treatment-associated pain

# Diagnosis

## Presentation

- History and physical exam are essential to properly diagnose cancer pain (26)
  - Description of the pain must include the following:
    - Location
    - Intensity
    - Character
    - Radiation
    - Duration
    - Timing
    - Inciting/alleviating factors
  - Cancer patients may have pain at various anatomic regions (26)
    - Additionally, each anatomic region must be assessed including the viscera, bone, and nervous tissue (26)
- Cancer pain is often difficult to classify as acute and chronic. (26) Pain often described as continuous ("background pain") or intermittent (27)
  - Can also be "breakthrough pain," which is an increase in pain intensity from the "background pain" (28)
  - 50% of patients with cancer experience "breakthrough pain" (28)

- Some cancer pain can be classified into specific pain syndromes based on groups of signs and symptoms. Classifying patients into pain syndromes can help in the selection of treatment
  - For example, the International Association for the Study of Pain (IASP) Task Force has a published syndromic classification of pain caused by solid tumors (29). Other pain syndromes have been described in those with hematologic malignancies (30,31)
- Classification systems do exist, although there is not a universally accepted system that properly identifies pain in cancer patients (32–34)
  - Edmonton Classification System for Cancer Pain is one such system that uses five domains to identify/diagnose pain accurately. This is not widely used in clinical medicine (35)
    - Domains include:
      - Mechanism of pain
      - Incidental pain
      - Psychologic distress
      - Addictive behavior
      - Cognitive function

## Evaluation

- Cancer pain requires an accurate evaluation for better long-term management. Likert-type systems to describe pain intensity do not consider the complex biopsychosocial nature of cancer pain (36,37)
- Some assessments go further than superficial descriptors (i.e., severity). These include the Brief Pain Inventory (BPI) and the McGill Pain Questionnaire (MPQ) (38,39)
  - MPQ looks at pain intensity, visual analog scale (VAS) assessment, and pain descriptors. (40) MPQ-SF is a shortened version of MPQ and is better in detection of neuropathic pain.
  - BPI looks at both severity of pain and patients' experience of the pain (41)
- Using various assessment tools can determine treatment (42)

## Differential Diagnosis

- Not all pain is due to malignancy (43)
  - 17% may be secondary to anticancer treatment
  - 10% may be due to factors other than their cancer

## Prognosis

- The Cancer Pain Prognostic Scale (CPPS) can aid in predicting if a patient will achieve pain relief from treatment in cancer patients with moderate to severe pain. A score from 0 to 17 is reported. Higher scores indicate a greater likelihood to achieve pain relief (44)
  - CPPS uses formula that incorporates:
    - Pain severity
    - Emotional well-being
    - Daily opioid requirement

## Treatment Modalities

- Both pharmacologic and non-pharmacologic treatments in conjunction should be included in the standard of care for cancer pain (45)

## Non-pharmacologic Interventions

- Interventional procedures
  - Used in cases when analgesia could not be achieved despite high doses of pharmacologic treatment (46)
  - Procedures include neuroablative procedures, soft tissue injections, and neuraxial analgesia (47,48)
- Physical therapy
- Occupational therapy
- Behavioral medicine treatments
  - Takes into account psychological and social factors such as anxiety, catastrophizing, and somatization (49)
  - Treatments include cognitive-behavioral therapy (CBT), stress management, and relaxation imagery (49)
- Alternative methods including acupuncture and massage may have some benefit (50)

## WHO Pain Ladder

- The pain ladder is a stepwise approach to provide appropriate analgesia for cancer pain (51)
  - According to the ladder, non-opioid medications are first line. After this, weak opioids can be considered followed by consideration for strong opioids (51)

- ○ Morphine has now been replaced with semi-synthetic opioids such as oxycodone and hydrocodone as the gold standard for treatment of cancer pain (52)
- Outside of opioids, osteogenic pain from bony metastasis can get relief from nonsteroidal anti-inflammatory drugs, and neuropathic pains can be treated with anticonvulsants and antidepressants (45)
- "Breakthrough" pain can be treated with rapid-acting opioids (53,54)

## Patient Education

- Education is essential to ensure proper efficacy of treatment. Poor compliance and inadequate management of pain can be overcome with proper education (49,55)

## Conclusions

- Cancer pain affects a large portion of those with cancerous disease processes. Metastatic disease tends to be associated with more pain
- Pain can come from the cancer itself or from the treatment
- More work is needed to standardize the evaluation and treatment of cancer pain. Further work is needed to take into account each individual's unique circumstances

## References

1. Cherny NI. The management of cancer pain. *CA Cancer J Clin.* 2000;**50** (2):20–70.

2. Li X-M, Xiao W-H, Yang P, Zhao H-X. Psychological distress and cancer pain: Results from a controlled cross-sectional survey in China. *Sci Rep.* 2017;7(1):39397. https://doi.org/10.1038/srep39397.

3. Breivik H, Cherny N, Collett B et al. Cancer-related pain: A pan-European survey of prevalence, treatment, and patient attitudes. *Ann Oncol Off J Eur Soc Med Oncol.* 2009;**20**(8):1420–1433.

4. World Health Organization. *Cancer pain relief: With a guide to opioid availability.* 2nd ed. World Health Organization; 1996. p. ita reproduced in Quaderni di Sanità Pubblica, Anno 21, febbraio 1998.

5. World Health Organization. *Cancer pain relief.* World Health Organization; 1986. p. 74.

6. Wolfe J, Grier HE, Klar N et al. Symptoms and suffering at the end of life in children with cancer. *N Engl J Med.* 2000;**342**(5):326–333. https://doi.org/10.1056/NEJM200002033420506.

7. Cleeland CS, Gonin R, Baez L, Loehrer P, Pandya KJ. Pain and treatment of pain in minority patients with cancer. The Eastern Cooperative Oncology Group Minority Outpatient Pain Study. *Ann Intern Med*. 1997;**127**(9):813–816.

8. Bernabei R, Gambassi G, Lapane K et al. Management of pain in elderly patients with cancer. SAGE Study Group. Systematic Assessment of Geriatric Drug Use via Epidemiology. *JAMA*. 1998;**279**(23):1877–1882.

9. Cleeland CS, Gonin R, Hatfield AK et al. Pain and its treatment in outpatients with metastatic cancer. *N Engl J Med*. 1994;**330**(9):592–596. https://doi.org/10.1056/NEJM199403033300902.

10. Klepstad P, Kaasa S, Cherny N, Hanks G, de Conno F. Pain and pain treatments in European palliative care units: A cross sectional survey from the European Association for Palliative Care Research Network. *Palliat Med*. 2005;**19**(6):477–484.

11. Weiss SC, Emanuel LL, Fairclough DL, Emanuel EJ. Understanding the experience of pain in terminally ill patients. *Lancet (London, England)*. 2001;**357**(9265):1311–1315.

12. Stewart BW, Wild CP. *World cancer report 2014*. World Health Organization; 2014.

13. Glaser AW, Fraser LK, Corner J et al. Patient-reported outcomes of cancer survivors in England 1–5 years after diagnosis: A cross-sectional survey. *BMJ Open*. 2013;**3**(4):e002317. doi: 10.1136/bmjopen-2012-002317. PMID: 23578682; PMCID: PMC3641492.

14. Elliott J, Fallows A, Staetsky L et al. The health and well-being of cancer survivors in the UK: Findings from a population-based survey. *Br J Cancer*. 2011;**105**(Suppl 1):S11–S20.

15. van den Beuken-van Everdingen MHJ, de Rijke JM, Kessels AG et al. Prevalence of pain in patients with cancer: A systematic review of the past 40 years. *Ann Oncol Off J Eur Soc Med Oncol*. 2007;**18**(9):1437–1449.

16. Le Bitoux M-A, Stamenkovic I. Tumor-host interactions: The role of inflammation. *Histochem Cell Biol*. 2008;**130**(6):1079–1090.

17. Magee D, Bachtold S, Brown M, Farquhar-Smith P. Cancer pain: Where are we now? *Pain Manag*. 2019;**9**(1):63–79.

18. Blair JM, Zhou H, Seibel MJ, Dunstan CR. Mechanisms of disease: Roles of OPG, RANKL and RANK in the pathophysiology of skeletal metastasis. *Nat Clin Pract Oncol*. 2006;**3**(1):41–49.

19. Reis-Pina P, Lawlor PG, Barbosa A. Cancer-related pain management and the optimal use of opioids. *Acta Med Port*. 2015;**28**(3):376–381.

20. Jost LM. ESMO minimum clinical recommendations for the management of cancer pain. *Ann Oncol Off J Eur Soc Med Oncol*. 2005;**16**(Suppl 1):i83–i85.

21. Hucker T, Winter N, Chou J. Challenges and advances in pain management for the cancer patient. *Curr Anesthesiol Rep.* 2015;**5**. doi: 10.1007/s40140-015-0120-y.

22. Humble SR, Dalton AJ, Li L. A systematic review of therapeutic interventions to reduce acute and chronic post-surgical pain after amputation, thoracotomy or mastectomy. *Eur J Pain.* 2015;**19**(4):451–465.

23. Andreae MH, Andreae DA. Regional anaesthesia to prevent chronic pain after surgery: A cochrane systematic review and meta-analysis. *Br J Anaesth.* 2013;**111**(5):711–720.

24. Seretny M, Currie GL, Sena ES et al. Incidence, prevalence, and predictors of chemotherapy-induced peripheral neuropathy: A systematic review and meta-analysis. *Pain.* 2014;**155**(12):2461–2470.

25. Marín A, Martín M, Liñán O et al. Bystander effects and radiotherapy. *Rep Pract Oncol Radiother J Gt Cancer Cent Pozn Polish Soc Radiat Oncol.* 2015;**20**(1):12–21.

26. Caraceni A, Shkodra M. Cancer pain assessment and classification. *Cancers (Basel).* 2019;**11**(4):510. doi: 10.3390/cancers11040510. PMID: 30974857.

27. Portenoy RK, Hagen NA. Breakthrough pain: Definition, prevalence and characteristics. *Pain.* 1990;**41**(3):273–281.

28. Deandrea S, Corli O, Consonni D et al. Prevalence of breakthrough cancer pain: A systematic review and a pooled analysis of published literature. *J Pain Symptom Manage.* 2014;**47**(1):57–76.

29. Portenoy RK, Ahmed E. Cancer pain syndromes. *Hematol Oncol Clin North Am.* 2018;**32**(3):371–386.

30. Niscola P, Tendas A, Scaramucci L et al. Pain in malignant hematology. *Expert Rev Hematol.* 2011;**4**(1):81–93.

31. Niscola P, Cartoni C, Romani C et al. Epidemiology, features and outcome of pain in patients with advanced hematological malignancies followed in a home care program: An Italian survey. *Ann Hematol.* 2007;**86**(9):671–676.

32. Fainsinger RL, Nekolaichuk C, Lawlor P et al. An international multicentre validation study of a pain classification system for cancer patients. *Eur J Cancer.* 2010;**46**(16):2896–2904.

33. Knudsen AK, Brunelli C, Klepstad P et al. Which domains should be included in a cancer pain classification system? Analyses of longitudinal data. *Pain.* 2012;**153**(3):696–703.

34. Knudsen AK, Brunelli C, Kaasa S et al. Which variables are associated with pain intensity and treatment response in advanced cancer patients? Implications for a future classification system for cancer pain. *Eur J Pain.* 2011;**15**(3):320–327.

35. Fainsinger RL, Nekolaichuk CL. A "TNM" classification system for cancer pain: The edmonton classification system for cancer pain (ECS-CP). *Support Care Cancer Off J Multinatl Assoc Support Care Cancer.* 2008;**16**(6):547–555.

36. Capelli G, De Vincenzo RI, Addamo A et al. Which dimensions of health-related quality of life are altered in patients attending the different gynecologic oncology health care settings? *Cancer.* 2002;**95**(12):2500–2507.

37. Korfage IJ, Essink-Bot M-L, Mols F et al. Health-related quality of life in cervical cancer survivors: A population-based survey. *Int J Radiat Oncol Biol Phys.* 2009;**73**(5):1501–1509.

38. Kumar SP. Utilization of brief pain inventory as an assessment tool for pain in patients with cancer: A focused review. *Indian J Palliat Care.* 2011;**17**(2):108–115.

39. Ngamkham S, Vincent C, Finnegan L et al. The McGill Pain Questionnaire as a multidimensional measure in people with cancer: An integrative review. *Pain Manag Nurs Off J Am Soc Pain Manag Nurses.* 2012;**13**(1):27–51.

40. Dworkin RH, Turk DC, Revicki DA et al. Development and initial validation of an expanded and revised version of the short-form McGill Pain Questionnaire (SF-MPQ-2). *Pain.* 2009;**144**(1–2):35–42.

41. Cleeland CS, Ryan KM. Pain assessment: Global use of the brief pain inventory. *Ann Acad Med Singapore.* 1994;**23**(2):129–138.

42. de Wit R, van Dam F, Abu-Saad HH et al. Empirical comparison of commonly used measures to evaluate pain treatment in cancer patients with chronic pain. *J Clin Oncol Off J Am Soc Clin Oncol.* 1999;**17**(4):1280. doi: 10.1200/JCO.1999.17.4.1280. PMID: 10561190.

43. Grond S, Zech D, Diefenbach C, Radbruch L, Lehmann KA. Assessment of cancer pain: A prospective evaluation in 2266 cancer patients referred to a pain service. *Pain.* 1996;**64**(1):107–114.

44. Hwang SS, Chang VT, Fairclough DL, Kasimis B. Development of a cancer pain prognostic scale. *J Pain Symptom Manage.* 2002;**24**(4):366–378.

45. Portenoy RK. Treatment of cancer pain. *Lancet (London, England).* 2011;**377**(9784):2236–2247.

46. Miguel R. Interventional treatment of cancer pain: The fourth step in the World Health Organization analgesic ladder? *Cancer Control.* 2000;**7**(2):149–156.

47. Vayne-Bossert P, Afsharimani B, Good P, Gray P, Hardy J. Interventional options for the management of refractory cancer pain: What is the evidence? *Support Care Cancer Off J Multinatl Assoc Support Care Cancer.* 2016;**24**(3):1429–1438.

48. Urits I, Jones MR, Orhurhu V et al. A comprehensive review of the celiac plexus block for the management of chronic abdominal pain. *Curr Pain Headache Rep.* 2020;**24**(8):42.

49. Liu WC, Zheng ZX, Tan KH, Meredith GJ. Multidimensional treatment of cancer pain. *Curr Oncol Rep.* 2017;**19**(2):10.

50. Hu C, Zhang H, Wu W et al. Acupuncture for pain management in cancer: A systematic review and meta-analysis. *Evid Based Complement Alternat Med.* 2016;**2016**:1720239.

51. Anekar AA, Cascella M. *WHO analgesic ladder.* World Health Organization; 2021.

52. Caraceni A, Hanks G, Kaasa S et al. Use of opioid analgesics in the treatment of cancer pain: Evidence-based recommendations from the EAPC. *Lancet Oncol.* 2012;**13**(2):e58–e68.

53. Caraceni A, Davies A, Poulain P et al. Guidelines for the management of breakthrough pain in patients with cancer. *J Natl Compr Canc Netw.* 2013;**11**(Suppl 1):S29–S36.

54. Fallon M, Giusti R, Aielli F et al. Management of cancer pain in adult patients: ESMO clinical practice guidelines. *Ann Oncol Off J Eur Soc Med Oncol.* 2018;**29**(Suppl 4):iv166–iv191.

55. Gunnarsdottir S, Donovan HS, Serlin RC, Voge C, Ward S. Patient-related barriers to pain management: The barriers questionnaire II (BQ-II). *Pain.* 2002;**99**(3):385–396.

**Chapter**

# 39

# Neuromodulation

Nazir Noor and Jamal Hasoon

- Spinal cord stimulation (SCS) and peripheral nerve stimulation (PNS) are treatment modalities that take advantage of gate theory of nociception first described by Ronald Melzack and Patrick Wall in 1965 (1–3)
- Types of neuromodulation: (1,2)
  - ○ SCS
  - ○ Dorsal root ganglion stimulation (DRG)
  - ○ PNS
- Important modality in the wake of increased use of opioids in chronic pain patients and increased rates of opioid use disorder and dependence (2)
- Some indications of neuromodulation, such as SCS, include failed back surgery syndrome (FBSS), complex regional pain syndrome (CRPS), neuropathic and ischemic pain, including refractory angina pectoris (RAP) (2,4)
- Psychologic screening necessary in determining patient selection for SCS treatment (5)
- Trial period of SCS essential for predicting outcomes and further identifying which patients should undergo permanent SCS implantation (5)
- Conventional SCS works by delivering electrical impulses at specific frequencies to dorsal columns of spinal cord, with the objective of producing paresthesia overlapping with existing distribution of pain, thus distorting perception of delivered pain (5)
  - ○ Success dependent upon pain surgeon's ability to provide coverage over patients' distribution of pain and patients' willingness to tolerate possible induced sensations of paresthesia (5)

- Lead type, anesthesia, waveform programming are considerations for optimal patient-specific management of chronic pain with SCS (5)
- Long-term cost-effectiveness for treatment of chronic pain compared to alternative treatment modalities (5)

## Indications

- FDA approval exists for several SCS systems for chronic intractable pain of trunk, upper and lower extremities (unilateral or bilateral), FBSS, low back and leg, CRPS type I and II, neuropathic pain (5)
- Evidence for retractable angina pectoris (RAP) is developing, as well (5)
- FBSS – condition where patients experience recurring low back pain following prior spinal surgery (5)
  - 10–30% of patients experience postoperative low back pain (6)
  - SCS has been demonstrated to successfully treat this pain with low morbidity rates compared with reoperation (6)
  - SCS shown to be more effective than conservative medical management at improving pain relief, quality of life, and functional capacity (7)
  - Success of SCS may also be mode dependent, as burst stimulation and high-frequency (10 kHz) therapies have shown more significant pain relief when compared to tonic stimulation (8–10)
- CRPS – form of chronic pain, usually affecting single limb, typically arising after sustaining injury or having surgery; Budapest criteria is used to help diagnosis CRPS (e.g., hyperesthesia, allodynia, temperature asymmetry, skin color changes, edema, decreased range-of-motion, trophic changes) (5,11)
  - Level I evidence studies comparing SCS with physical therapy to physical therapy alone demonstrated significant pain relief of >3 points on visual analog scale (VAS) and improvement of the quality of life at 6-month and 2-year follow-up (12,13)
- RAP – anginal pain commonly caused by coronary artery disease (CAD) unresponsive to antianginal medications; symptoms include episodes of heavy, pressure-like chest pain (5)
  - Initial concerns for SCS masking myocardial ischemia; however, early studies demonstrated antianginal effects without increased risk of ischemia

- ○ Small RCT ($n = 17$) demonstrated improved cardiac treadmill stress testing and reduced nitrate intake among SCS patients; results were replicated by future RCTs and case series (14–16)
- ○ Mannheimer et al. conducted larger-scale RCT ($n = 100$) comparing SCS with coronary artery bypass surgery (CABG); CABG patients performed significantly better on exercise tolerance testing, but both SCS and CABG groups experienced adequate symptom relief without significant difference between the two cohorts (17)
- ○ Mixed evidence exists for use of SCS in peripheral vascular ischemia, critical limb ischemia, and wound healing (18,19)

## Patient Selection

- Patients selected for SCS must have tried other treatment modalities, such as medication, steroid injections, and/or PT (5,20)
- Once selected for SCS, psychiatric comorbidities must be assessed, MRI eligibility for spine imaging (or CT if MRI contraindicated), preoperative surgical risk, and expected response to a trial of SCS (5,20)
- Contraindications (5,20)
  - ○ Bleeding diathesis
  - ○ Sepsis
  - ○ Cognitive impairments
  - ○ Unresolved or poorly managed psychological disorders (e.g., major depressive disorder, anxiety, personality disorder, substance use, posttraumatic stress disorder)
  - ○ Tobacco use is a relative contraindication, as it has been associated with early SCS failure
- Realistic outcomes should be explained to patients, such as unlikelihood of 100% relief (~50% reduction is more likely) (5,20)

## Trialing

- Unlike other spine surgeries, SCS allows for opportunity of a trial period prior to permanent implantation requiring no incision which allows clinician and patient to gauge potential benefits of a permanent implantation (5,21)
- Trial periods are typically 5–7 days with close follow-up and involvement of the device representatives, as attempts are made to provide the optimal mode settings to provide the best pain relief (5,21)

- At the end of the trial, clinician and patient must consider if pain relief, quality of life, and/or functionality improved by at least 50% and/or if permanent implantation is worthwhile (5,21)
  - Common instruments to assess these findings include: (5,21)
    - VAS for pain reduction
    - McGill Pain Questionnaire
    - Oswestry Disability Index
- The trial determines optimal lead placement (5,21)
  - If "sweet spot" of lead is at tip of lead, the permanent implant leads should be placed higher, so the "sweet spot" is in the middle
  - Lead location for back and leg coverage varies among devices and waveforms
  - For high-frequency (10 kHz) lead placement should always be at T9–10 levels
  - For arm and neck pain, cervical leads placed either with a retrograde paddle from occiput to C3 or one/two leads depending on symptoms in a "blooming flower" configuration up to C1–2 levels
  - For RAP, lead placement typical at T4–6 levels

## Technical Considerations

- After successful SCS trial, several decisions must be made: (5)
  1. Should patient undergo percutaneous or paddle implantation?
  2. Are there any technical nuances that must be considered?
  3. Should the procedure be performed asleep or awake?
  4. What waveform should be used?
- Lead type: percutaneous versus paddle leads
  - Percutaneous leads
    - Less invasive procedure (22)
    - Less likely to result in postoperative complications (2.2% compared to 3.4% in patients with paddle leads) (22)
    - Better for patients with multiple comorbidities (23)
  - Paddle leads
    - Requires more invasive surgery via hemilaminotomy (23)
    - May have higher satisfaction and pain relief (23)

- Similar rates of lead migration for both percutaneous and paddle leads, but less extreme for paddle leads (24)
- Contacts of paddle leads all face epidural space, allowing for more effective energy delivery (25)

- Some reports have suggested placement of permanent implant while patient is asleep has similar or superior outcomes compared with awake placement (26–30)
- Goal of SCS is to reduce pain by 50% via multimodal approach, with SCS being one of the many modes of analgesia (31)
  - Medications may be used concurrently with SCS to optimize pain relief (32,33)
  - Baclofen with SCS has been shown to produce greater pain relief than SCS alone (32,33)
  - Patients on opioids at time of implantation who continue opioid use at similar doses post-SCS implantation tend to have poorer long-term outcomes (34)
- Habituation, meaning patients become accustomed to the effects of stimulation, is a feared complication of SCS (32,33)
  - This is minimized by varying the signal and its focal point, thus creating alternating waveforms (32,33)

# References

1. Moayedi M, Davis KD. Theories of pain: From specificity to gate control. *J Neurophysiol.* 2013;**109**(1):5–12. https://pubmed.ncbi.nlm.nih.gov/23034364/.

2. Viswanath O, Urits I, Bouley E et al. Evolving spinal cord stimulation technologies and clinical implications in chronic pain management. *Curr Pain Headache Rep.* 2019;**23**(6):39. https://doi.org/10.1007/s11916-019-0778-9.

3. Urits I, Schwartz R, Smoots D et al. Peripheral neuromodulation for the management of headache. *Anesthesiol Pain Med.* 2020;**10**(6):1–10. https://pubmed.ncbi.nlm.nih.gov/34150578/.

4. Börjesson M, Andréll P, Mannheimer C. Spinal cord stimulation for long-term treatment of severe angina pectoris: What does the evidence say? *Future Cardiol.* 2011;7(6):825–833. https://pubmed.ncbi.nlm.nih.gov/22050067/.

5. Rock AK, Truong H, Park YL, Pilitsis J. Spinal cord stimulation. *Neurosurg Clin North Am.* 2019;**30**(2):169–194.

6. North RB, Kidd DH, Farrokhi F, Piantadosi SA. Spinal cord stimulation versus repeated lumbosacral spine surgery for chronic pain: A randomized, controlled trial. *Neurosurgery.* 2005;**56**(1):98–106. https://pubmed.ncbi.nlm.nih.gov/15617591/.

7.  Kumar K, Taylor RS, Jacques L et al. The effects of spinal cord stimulation in neuropathic pain are sustained: A 24-month follow-up of the prospective randomized controlled multicenter trial of the effectiveness of spinal cord stimulation. *Neurosurgery*. 2008;**63**(4):762–768. https://pubmed .ncbi.nlm.nih.gov/18981888/.

8.  Deer T, Slavin KV, Amirdelfan K et al. Success using neuromodulation with BURST (SUNBURST) study: Results from a prospective, randomized controlled trial using a novel burst waveform. *Neuromodulation Technol Neural Interface*. 2018;**21**(1):56–66.

9.  Kapural L, Yu C, Doust MW et al. Novel 10-kHz high-frequency therapy (HF10 therapy) is superior to traditional low-frequency spinal cord stimulation for the treatment of chronic back and leg pain: The SENZA-RCT randomized controlled trial. *Anesthesiology*. 2015;**123** (4):851–860. https://pubmed.ncbi.nlm.nih.gov/26218762/.

10. Kapural L, Yu C, Doust MW et al. Comparison of 10-kHz high-frequency and traditional low-frequency spinal cord stimulation for the treatment of chronic back and leg pain: 24-month results from a multicenter, randomized, controlled pivotal trial. *Neurosurgery*. 2016;**79**(5):667–676.

11. Harden RN, Bruehl S, Perez RSGM et al. Validation of proposed diagnostic criteria (the "Budapest Criteria") for complex regional pain syndrome. *Pain*. 2010;**150**(2):268–274. doi: 10.1016/j.pain.2010.04.030.

12. Barolat G, Schwartzman R, Woo R. Epidural spinal cord stimulation in the management of reflex sympathetic dystrophy. *Stereotact Funct Neurosurg*. 1989;**53**(1):29–39. https://pubmed.ncbi.nlm.nih.gov/2740656/.

13. Kemler MA, Barendse GAM, van Kleef M et al. Spinal cord stimulation in patients with chronic reflex sympathetic dystrophy. *N Engl J Med*. 2000;**343** (9):618–624. https://pubmed.ncbi.nlm.nih.gov/10965008/.

14. Mannheimer C, Eliasson T, Andersson B et al. Effects of spinal cord stimulation in angina pectoris induced by pacing and possible mechanisms of action. *BMJ*. 1993;**307**(6902):477–480. https://pubmed.ncbi.nlm.nih.gov/840 0930/.

15. Eliasson T, Jern S, Augustinsson LE, Mannheimer C. Safety aspects of spinal cord stimulation in severe angina pectoris. *Coron Artery Dis*. 1994;**5** (10):845–850. https://pubmed.ncbi.nlm.nih.gov/7866604/.

16. Hautvast RWM, Dejongste MJL, Staal MJ, Van Gilst WH, Lie KI. Spinal cord stimulation in chronic intractable angina pectoris: A randomized, controlled efficacy study. *Am Heart J*. 1998;**136**(6):1114–1120. https://pubmed .ncbi.nlm.nih.gov/9842028/.

17. Mannheimer C, Eliasson T, Augustinsson LE et al. Electrical stimulation versus coronary artery bypass surgery in severe angina pectoris: The ESBY

study. *Circulation*. 1998;**97**(12):1157–1163. https://pubmed.ncbi.nlm.nih.gov /9537342/.

18. Augustinsson L-E. Epidural spinal electrical stimulation in peripheral vascular disease. *Pacing Clin Electrophysiol*. 1987;**10**(1 Pt 2):205–206. https:// pubmed.ncbi.nlm.nih.gov/2436178/.

19. Robaina FJ, Dominguez M, Diaz M, Rodriguez JL, De Vera JA. Spinal cord stimulation for relief of chronic pain in vasospastic disorders of the upper limbs. *Neurosurgery*. 1989;**24**(1):63–67. https://pubmed.ncbi.nlm.nih.gov/27 84547/.

20. De La Cruz P, Fama C, Roth S et al. Predictors of spinal cord stimulation success. *Neuromodulation*. 2015;**18**(7):599–602. https://pubmed .ncbi.nlm.nih.gov/26119040/.

21. Haider S, Owusu-Sarpong S, Peris Celda M et al. A single center prospective observational study of outcomes with tonic cervical spinal cord stimulation. *Neuromodulation*. 2017;**20**(3):263–268. https://pubmed.ncbi.nlm.nih.gov/27 491956/.

22. Babu R, Hazzard MA, Huang KT et al. Outcomes of percutaneous and paddle lead implantation for spinal cord stimulation: A comparative analysis of complications, reoperation rates, and health-care costs. *Neuromodulation*. 2013;**16**(5):418–427. https://pubmed.ncbi.nlm.nih.gov/23647789/.

23. North RB, Kidd DH, Petrucci L, Dorsi MJ. Spinal cord stimulation electrode design: A prospective, randomized, controlled trial comparing percutaneous with laminectomy electrodes: Part II-clinical outcomes. *Neurosurgery*. 2005;**57**(5):990–995. https://pubmed.ncbi.nlm.nih.gov/16284568/.

24. Veizi E, Hayek SM, North J et al. Spinal cord stimulation (SCS) with anatomically guided (3D) neural targeting shows superior chronic axial low back pain relief compared to traditional SCS-LUMINA study. *Pain Med*. 2017;**18**(8):1534–1548. https://pubmed.ncbi.nlm.nih.gov/28108641/.

25. North RB, Kidd DH, Olin JC, Sieracki JM. Spinal cord stimulation electrode design: Prospective, randomized, controlled trial comparing percutaneous and laminectomy electrodes-part I: Technical outcomes. *Neurosurgery*. 2002;**51**(2):381–389. https://pubmed.ncbi.nlm.nih.gov/12182776/.

26. Roth SG, Lange S, Haller J et al. A prospective study of the intra- and postoperative efficacy of intraoperative neuromonitoring in spinal cord stimulation. *Stereotact Funct Neurosurg*. 2015;**93**(5):348–354. https://pubmed .ncbi.nlm.nih.gov/26444517/.

27. Shils JL, Arle JE. Intraoperative neurophysiologic methods for spinal cord stimulator placement under general anesthesia. *Neuromodulation*. 2012;**15** (6):560–572. https://pubmed.ncbi.nlm.nih.gov/22672099/.

28. Falowski SM, Celii A, Sestokas AK et al. Awake vs. asleep placement of spinal cord stimulators: A cohort analysis of complications associated with

placement. *Neuromodulation*. 2011;**14**(2):130–135. https://pubmed
.ncbi.nlm.nih.gov/21992199/.

29. Tamkus AA, Scott AF, Khan FR. Neurophysiological monitoring during
spinal cord stimulator placement surgery. *Neuromodulation*. 2015;**18**
(6):460–464. https://pubmed.ncbi.nlm.nih.gov/25677059/.

30. Schoen N, Chieng LO, Madhavan K, Jermakowicz WJ, Vanni S. The use of
intraoperative electromyogram during spinal cord stimulator placement
surgery: A case series. *World Neurosurg*. 2017;**100**:74–84. https://pubmed
.ncbi.nlm.nih.gov/28034811/.

31. Medical Advisory Secretariat. Spinal cord stimulation for neuropathic pain:
An evidence-based analysis. *Ont Health Technol Assess Ser*. 2005;**5**(4):1–78.
https://pubmed.ncbi.nlm.nih.gov/23074473/.

32. Lind G, Meyerson BA, Winter J, Linderoth B. Intrathecal baclofen as adjuvant
therapy to enhance the effect of spinal cord stimulation in neuropathic pain:
A pilot study. *Eur J Pain*. 2004;**8**(4):377–383. https://pubmed
.ncbi.nlm.nih.gov/15207519/.

33. Schechtmann G, Lind G, Winter J, Meyerson BA, Linderoth B. Intrathecal
clonidine and baclofen enhance the pain-relieving effect of spinal cord
stimulation: A comparative placebo-controlled, randomized trial.
*Neurosurgery*. 2010;**67**(1):173–181. https://pubmed.ncbi.nlm.nih.gov/20559
103/.

34. Gee L, Smith HC, Ghulam-Jelani Z et al. Spinal cord stimulation for the
treatment of chronic pain reduces opioid use and results in superior clinical
outcomes when used without opioids. *Neurosurgery*. 2019;**84**(1):217–226.
https://pubmed.ncbi.nlm.nih.gov/29538696/.

# Chapter 40

# Regenerative Medicine

Nazir Noor and Clay Gibb

## Discogenic Low Back Pain

- A chronic pain condition that involves one or more intervertebral discs (1)
- Most common type of low back pain due to attributable causes (2)
- Exact causes of the disc degeneration are difficult to pinpoint even with modern-day diagnostic and imaging techniques (3)

## Epidemiology and Risk Factors

- Primarily adults between the ages of 20 and 50 years are affected by discogenic back pain (4)
- Common risk factors
  - Aging
  - Genetic predisposition
  - Nutritional factors such as obesity
  - Mechanical trauma
  - Smoking (3,5)

## Pathophysiology

- The pathophysiology is just beginning to be understood (1)
- The adult intervertebral disc is an avascular organ with poor inherent healing potential. The organ relies on passive diffusion from adjacent endplate vessels for nutrition (3)
- Decreases in supplied oxygen from the disc and decreased ability to respond to stressors such as load or injury weakens the tissue (6)
- Weakened tissue and extracellular matrix changes push the cell toward catabolic turnover (6)
- The main components that make up the strength of the IVD are the central type II collagen, proteoglycan-rich nucleus pulposus and the peripheral fibrous type I collagen-rich annulus fibrosis.

The degeneration of the disc causes a type II to type I shift, which decreases the swelling pressures needed for support (7)

- Upregulation of inflammatory cytokines and degradative enzymes cause changes in the microcomposition, growth factors, and cell composition, ultimately leading to lack of function of the IVD (1)

## Current Treatments

- There are a few different approaches to treating discogenic low back pain. There is the conservative route and the surgical approach. There is little consensus as to which approach is best
- The underlying issue is not treated by either the surgical approach or the pharmacological approach (1)
- Stem cell therapy and platelet-rich plasma both address the underlying issue of IVD degeneration (1,8)

## Stem Cell Therapy

- This type of treatment is still relatively young, but has promising data that encourages further research (3)
  - *Type of Cells*
    - There are two main possible types of stem cells: mesenchymal stem cells (MSC) or embryonic stem cells (ESC). Percutaneously delivered MSC has been the most proposed cell type to use (1,7)
    - ESC has disadvantages due to ethical concerns, disease, teratoma, or immune rejection after transplant
    - MSC can possibly reverse or halt the disc degeneration process by promoting synthesis of proteoglycans and type II collagen (1)
  - *Advantages of Stem Cell*
    - Due to the anatomy of the IVD (cartilaginous and avascular), natural regeneration is very difficult when the homeostatic environment is disrupted. Stem cell therapy gives a boost to the body's natural healing with minimal invasion (9)
    - Accomplishes the three objectives of treating disc pathology: pain relief, improved disc microenvironment, and tissue regeneration (9)

- ○ *Disadvantages of Stem Cell*
  - Harvesting process for bone marrow MSC involves aspirating from the posterior iliac crest which can be a cumbersome process (9)
  - Most studies have been on animal models which may not be an optimal surrogate for humans due to differences in size and height between the animal models and human discs (1,3)
- ○ *Route of Administration*
  - Current route of administration is image assisted percutaneous injection through the annulus fibrosus. To maximize both safety and efficacy the optimal needle size and dosage are needed (3)
  - Current route shows damage to AF, backflow of cells through injection site, and low survival rate of implanted cells, so an alternative delivery route through the pedicles has been proposed (3)
- ○ *Further research*
  - Stem cell therapy has very promising implications, but further work needs to be done. Improvements in efficacy, isolation, culture, delivery, and realistic use in human models are expected in the future (1,3)

# Platelet-Rich Plasma (PRP) Treatment

- Limited small studies have demonstrated that platelet-rich plasma may be another effective alternative treatment to low back pain
  - ○ *Overview*
    - Platelets are important for homeostasis and wound healing through their high concentration of growth factors. PRP is beneficial for soft tissue healing, bone regeneration, and vascularization of grafts (8)
    - Studies have discovered that the ideal therapeutic platelet concentration is four to six times greater than whole blood (8,10)
  - ○ *Advantages of PRP*
    - The growth factors (PDGF and TGF-β) released by RPR are strongly associated with cellular remodeling and tissue

repair. They were shown to increase cell proliferation, matrix synthesis/repair, and nucleus pulposus survival (11)

- Autologous PRP therapy is cheaper than growth factor injections, allowing the treatment to be more accessible to those in need (8)

○ *Disadvantages of PRP*

- A small number of studies have been conducted and in those studies the sample sizes are small (8)
- Lack of standardization of preparation and administration of PRP (12)

○ *Route of Administration*

- Preparation and administration of PRP is a stepwise process that lends to get variability within each step. This can range from choice of anticoagulants to how the platelets are activated (12)
- The concentrated platelet solution is then injected directly into the injured or degrading body tissue (8)

○ *Further Research*

- The first step in research for PRP is focusing on increasing sample size within studies. The lack of large studies is impeding the growth and popularity of this treatment (8)
- Research into the most effective and efficient way to prepare the PRP for injection will help to standardize the process which encourages repeatable and measurable studies. Tracking of efficacy within patient treatment would also be helped by standardization (12)

# References

1. Urits I, Capuco A, Sharma M et al. Stem cell therapies for treatment of discogenic low back pain: A comprehensive review. *Curr Pain Headache Rep.* 2019;**23**(9):1–12. https://doi.org/10.1007/S11916-019-0804-Y.

2. Zhang YG, Guo TM, Guo X, Wu SX. Clinical diagnosis for discogenic low back pain. *Int J Biol Sci.* 2009;**5**(7):647–658. https://doi.org/10.7150/IJBS .5.647.

3. Barakat AH, Elwell VA, Lam KS. Stem cell therapy in discogenic back pain. *J Spine Surg.* 2019;**5**(4):561–583. https://doi.org/10.21037/JSS.2019.09.22.

4. Fujii K, Yamazaki M, Kang JD et al. Discogenic back pain: Literature review of definition, diagnosis, and treatment. *JBMR Plus.* 2019;**3**(5):e10180. https:// doi.org/10.1002/JBM4.10180.

5. Hong C, Lee CG, Song H. Characteristics of lumbar disc degeneration and risk factors for collapsed lumbar disc in Korean farmers and fishers. *Ann Occup Environ Med*. 2021;**33**(1):e16. https://doi.org/10.35371/AOEM .2021.33.E16.

6. Dowdell J, Erwin M, Choma T et al. Intervertebral disk degeneration and repair. *Clin Neurosurg*. 2017;**80**(3):S46–S54. https://doi.org/10.1093/NEUR OS/NYW078.

7. Richardson SM, Kalamegam G, Pushparaj PN et al. Mesenchymal stem cells in regenerative medicine: Focus on articular cartilage and intervertebral disc regeneration. *Methods*. 2016;**99**:69–80. https://doi.org/10.1016/J .YMETH.2015.09.015.

8. Urits I, Viswanath O, Galasso AC et al. Platelet-rich plasma for the treatment of low back pain: A comprehensive review. *Curr Pain Headache Rep*. 2019;**23** (7):1–11. https://doi.org/10.1007/s11916-019-0797-6.

9. Zeckser J, Wolff M, Tucker J, Goodwin J. Multipotent mesenchymal stem cell treatment for discogenic low back pain and disc degeneration. *Stem Cells Int*. 2016;**2016**. https://doi.org/10.1155/2016/3908389.

10. Dhillon M, Behera P, Patel S, Shetty V. Orthobiologics and platelet rich plasma. *Indian J Orthop*. 2014;**48**(1):1–9. https://doi.org/10.4103/0019-5413 .125477.

11. Wang S-z, Chang Q, Lu J, Wang C. Growth factors and platelet-rich plasma: Promising biological strategies for early intervertebral disc degeneration. *Int Orthop*. 2015;**39**(5):927–934. https://doi.org/10.1007/S00264-014-2664-8.

12. Pachito DV, Bagattini AM, de Almeida AM, Mendrone-Júnior A, Riera R. Technical procedures for preparation and administration of platelet-rich plasma and related products: A scoping review. *Front Cell Dev Biol*. 2020;**8**:598816. https://doi.org/10.3389/FCELL.2020.598816/FULL.

**Chapter 41**

# Cognitive Therapy

Clay Gibb and Elyse M. Cornett

- Patients with chronic pain have psychosocial factors that play a significant role in their condition. Addressing these factors through psychological strategies such as cognitive behavioral therapy and cognitive functional therapy may provide benefit (1)

## Cognitive Behavioral Therapy (CBT)

- The belief is that behaviors, thought patterns, and situations contribute to psychiatric dysfunction and lead to progression of pain. CBT aims to identify and change maladaptive behaviors, thought patterns, and situations to stop that progression of pain
- Primarily been studied and used to treat psychiatric disorders such as depression, anxiety, and PTSD (1)
  - Goals of CBT
    - Increase the patient's ability to deal with the variety of challenges that chronic pain brings into their lives by
      - Reducing pain
      - Increasing function
      - Increased independence
      - Greater ability to complete activities of daily life
    - Patients are asked to set a goal at the onset of treatment, and majority of patients (75%) set physical activity and functional status goals (2)
  - Mechanism of effect – neurological
    - CBT treatments correlate with changes in a variety of areas of the brain including the prefrontal cortex. The prefrontal cortex is activated by acute pain and is involved in the process of responding to painful stimuli (3)

- The connection between the prefrontal cortex, limbic system, and basal ganglia is increased in patients with chronic pain. Downregulation of these abnormal connections occurred after CBT treatment was seen to correlate with better pain-coping mechanisms (4,5)
- Reduced dorsal posterior cingulate cortex activity after treatment with CBT correlated with improvements in anxiety related to pain and pain intensity (1,6)

○ Uses

- As discussed, CBT can be applied outside the conventional use in psychiatric disorders to help with chronic pain. Areas of management in which this technique has been proved useful are as follows:
  - Migraines – adult and pediatric (7,8)
  - Gynecological pain (9,10)
  - Fibromyalgia (11)
  - Arthritic pain (12)
  - Abdominal pain (1)

# Cognitive Functional Therapy (CFT)

- Based on a three-step process, beginning with cognitive training, progresses to function movement training with exposure control and then ending with physical activity and lifestyle changes (1)
- Incorporating foundational behavioral psychology and neuroscience within physical therapy (13,14)
- Biopsychosocial factors are considered barriers to recovery in patients with chronic pain, and this therapy aims at targeting these barriers to alleviate the pain (13)

○ Goals

- Modify different aspects of pain such as:
  - Causes that drive pain
  - Pain-related distress
  - Disability (13)

- Eliminate the perceived threat of pain by normalizing provocative movements (1,13)

○ Mechanism of effect

- Patient must be helped to understand their pain. Learning the circumstances in which they experience pain, and how they change their lifestyle (activities and movements) in response to this cycle of pain and distress (1)

- Techniques of body and mind relaxation are practiced to help the individual promote control of their sympathetic and fear response during behaviors that would normally elicit a painful response (13)
- The focus of body control and relaxation helps direct the patient's focus away from the pain and invalidates their fear-avoidance beliefs associated with that activity (13)
- Personalized exercise and strength plans are developed to help the patient deal with any deficits that have occurred because of avoidance and to normalize these movements (1)
  ◦ Uses
    - Chronic low back pain (13,14)
    - Neck pain
    - Disability due to fear of movement because of pain (1)

## Access to Treatment

- CBT and CFT have classically been performed face to face, but with technological advancements through internet communication the barriers of access have been decreasing. This is promising for many reasons such as location independence, cost-effectiveness, and decreased therapist time (13)

## References

1. Urits I, Hubble A, Peterson E et al. An update on cognitive therapy for the management of chronic pain: A comprehensive review. *Curr Pain Headache Rep.* 2019;**23**(8):1–7. https://doi.org/10.1007/s11916-019-0794-9.

2. Heapy AA, Wandner L, Driscoll MA et al. Developing a typology of patient-generated behavioral goals for cognitive behavioral therapy for chronic pain (CBT-CP): Classification and predicting outcomes. *J Behav Med.* 2017;**41**(2):174–185. https://doi.org/10.1007/S10865-017-9885-4.

3. Nascimento SS, Oliveira LR, DeSantana JM. Correlations between brain changes and pain management after cognitive and meditative therapies: A systematic review of neuroimaging studies. *Complement Ther Med.* 2018;**39**:137–145. https://doi.org/10.1016/J.CTIM.2018.06.006.

4. Shpaner M, Kelly C, Lieberman G et al. Unlearning chronic pain: A randomized controlled trial to investigate changes in intrinsic brain connectivity following cognitive behavioral therapy. *Neuroimage Clin.* 2014;5:365–376. https://doi.org/10.1016/J.NICL.2014.07.008.

5. Yuan M, Zhu H, Qiu C et al. Group cognitive behavioral therapy modulates the resting-state functional connectivity of amygdala-related network in patients with generalized social anxiety disorder. *BMC Psychiatry.* 2016;16 (1):1–9. https://doi.org/10.1186/S12888-016-0904-8/TABLES/2.

6. Yoshino A, Okamoto Y, Okada G et al. Changes in resting-state brain networks after cognitive-behavioral therapy for chronic pain. *Psychol Med.* 2018;48(7):1148–1156. https://doi.org/10.1017/S0033291717002598.

7. Ng QX, Venkatanarayanan N, Kumar L. A systematic review and meta-analysis of the efficacy of cognitive behavioral therapy for the management of pediatric migraine. *Headache.* 2017;57(3):349–362. https://doi.org/10.1111/HEAD.13016.

8. Cousins S, Ridsdale L, Goldstein LH et al. A pilot study of cognitive behavioural therapy and relaxation for migraine headache: A randomised controlled trial. *J Neurol.* 2015;262(12):2764–2772. https://doi.org/10.1007/S00415-015-7916-Z.

9. Haugstad GK, Kirste U, Leganger S, Haakonsen E, Haugstad TS. Somatocognitive therapy in the management of chronic gynaecological pain: A review of the historical background and results of a current approach. *Scand J Pain.* 2011;2(3):124–129. https://doi.org/10.1016/J.SJPAIN.2011.02.005/MACHINEREADABLECITATION/RIS.

10. Haugstad GK, Haugstad TS, Kirste UM et al. Continuing improvement of chronic pelvic pain in women after short-term Mensendieck somatocognitive therapy: Results of a 1-year follow-up study. *Am J Obstet Gynecol.* 2008;199 (6):615.e1–615.e8. https://doi.org/10.1016/j.ajog.2008.06.019.

11. Menga G, Ing S, Khan O et al. Fibromyalgia: Can online cognitive behavioral therapy help? *Ochsner J.* 2014;14(3):343. /pmc/articles/PMC4171792/.

12. Ismail A, Moore C, Alshishani N, Yaseen K, Alshehri MA. Cognitive behavioural therapy and pain coping skills training for osteoarthritis knee pain management: A systematic review. *J Phys Ther Sci.* 2017;29(12):2228. https://doi.org/10.1589/JPTS.29.2228.

13. O'Sullivan PB, Caneiro JP, O'Keeffe M et al. Cognitive functional therapy: An integrated behavioral approach for the targeted management of disabling low back pain. *Phys Ther.* 2018;98(5):408–410. https://doi.org/10.1093/PTJ/PZY022.

14. O'Sullivan K, Dankaerts W, O'Sullivan L, O'Sullivan PB. Cognitive functional therapy for disabling nonspecific chronic low back pain: Multiple case-cohort study. *Phys Ther.* 2015;95(11):1478–1488. https://doi.org/10.2522/PTJ.20140406.

# Alternative Therapy
Ajay Kurup and Ruben Schwartz

## Alternative Therapies

- Up to 12 million American adults suffer from chronic pain (1)
- Chronic pain of a variety of origins leads to significant emotional and physical disability costing up to $635 billion annually (2)
- NSAIDs, acetaminophen, and several anticonvulsants and antidepressants have shown minimal success in management of chronic pain (3)
- Approximately 6% of Americans aged 15–64 have abused opioids, and 115 deaths per year are related to opioid overdose (4)
- Acetaminophen/hydrocodone is one of the top ten most prescribed medicines in the United States (5)
- Risk factors for chronic pain requiring daily therapy include advanced age, diabetes, obesity, mental health concerns, among many other modifiable, and several non-modifiable factors (6)
- Between 60 and 90% of chronic musculoskeletal pain patients report using and benefiting from complementary, non-pharmaceutical therapies (7)
- Acupuncture is a common eastern alternative therapy for pain control with demonstrated effective pain relief over sham and control, although the consistency and magnitude of results is debated (8,9)
- Tai chi incorporates the combination of slow movements, meditation, and breathing exercises to achieve chronic pain relief (10)
- Osteopathic manipulative therapy (OMT) is a technique of musculoskeletal manipulation practiced by osteopathic physicians that has shown moderate pain control in certain populations and conditions (11)
- Chiropractic therapy is a popular form of chronic musculoskeletal pain control with a controversial methodology and pool of evidence (12)

# Epidemiology and Risk Factors for Chronic Pain

- 2016 Global Burden of Disease study reports that chronic pain and related syndromes are the leading causes of disability in the world (13)
  - 1.9 billion affected by recurrent tension-headaches
  - Neck, back, and other causes of musculoskeletal pain consistently in the top 10 causes of disability around the world
- 2022 study shows that 20.5% of American adults report pain on most or every day of the week (14)
  - Back, hip, knee, and foot pain were the most common locations of pain
  - Chronic pain respondents missed an average of 10.3 days of work per year vs. 2.8 days in respondents without chronic pain
- While the risk factors associated with various etiologies of chronic pain are as diverse as the etiologies themselves, several predispositions stand out as prominent risks (6)
  - Advanced age stands out, with one systematic review reporting an average of 62% of respondents 75 and older reporting chronic pain vs. 14.3% in respondents aged 18–25 (15)
  - Female gender is associated with increased reporting of chronic pain to healthcare providers as well as greater intensity of pain perception (16–18)
  - Income is inversely related to chronic pain prevalence, intensity, and attributable disability (19)
  - Increased physical activity is also inversely related to chronic pain severity and positively correlated with quality of life in chronic pain sufferers (20)
  - A preexisting site of pain is a strong indicator of developing greater severity of chronic pain in a new location (21)
  - Up to 50% of chronic pain patients report depression, and severity of chronic pain is positively correlated with reported depression (22–24)
  - Increasing BMI is also associated with higher prevalence of chronic pain with BMI of 25–29 at 20% relative increased prevalence, BMI of 30–35 at 68%, BMI of 36–40 at 136%, and BMI of >40 at 254% (25)

# Traditional Understanding of Alternative Therapies

- Acupuncture (26–29)
  - The practice of acupuncture in traditional Chinese medicine dates back over 3,000 years and has been studied extensively for its efficacy and mechanism
  - Traditional practitioners cite the existence of "Qi," a type of life-sustaining energy that exists in the body, that flows along channels called "meridians" and can be disrupted, leading to illness and pain
  - Meridians can be opened and closed through manipulation of over 400 described superficial "acupoints" located all over the body
  - Manipulation of the acupoints is achieved through a variety of techniques:
    - Inserting 32–36 gauge needles superficially over the understood location of acupoints
    - Running an electric current through one or more inserted needles simultaneously
    - Utilizing non-thermal laser irradiation on acupoints
    - Burning "moxa" superficially on the skin overlying acupoints
    - Creating a vacuum seal on the skin overlying acupuncture points
- Tai chi (30)
  - Also derived from traditional Chinese medicine, tai chi incorporates constant and deliberate movement combined with deep breathing patterns to allow for the proper flow of "Qi" through the body
  - Similar to the idea of manipulating specific points of Qi flow along the path of meridians in acupuncture, the purposeful and meditative movements of tai chi are designed to normalize the flow of Qi and aid in pain relief among many other health claims
- OMT (31–33)
  - Invented in the United States during the nineteenth century as a diagnostic and therapeutic option for physicians to provide a holistic treatment of body, mind, and spirit
  - Largely consists of manual manipulation techniques used primarily by osteopathic physicians to treat, among many

ailments, chronic pain through an interconnected understanding of anatomical elements of the body

- ○ The four primary principles of OMT are:
  - ▪ The human body is a dynamic unit of function
  - ▪ The body possesses self-regulatory mechanisms that are healing in nature
  - ▪ Structure and function are interrelated at all levels
  - ▪ Rational treatment is based on these principles

- Chiropractic (12,34)
  - ○ Developed out of the early teachings of OMT, chiropractic adjustments are predicated on the belief that vertebral subluxations are at the root of many types of chronic pain
  - ○ While many chiropractors incorporate other mainstream therapies into their overall practice, the original practice of spinal adjustment remains a cornerstone of the philosophy

    - ▪ Other therapies within nutrition, exercise, and applied kinesiology are among the most successful used by chiropractors

# Efficacy of Alternative Therapies

- Acupuncture
  - ○ In a 2020 Cochrane review of 33 trials evaluating the use of acupuncture vs. sham treatment, no treatment, and standard therapy in the treatment of nonspecific low-back pain, studies showed heterogeneous results, low quality of evidence, and high risk of bias in most studies (35)

    - ▪ Acupuncture yields better quality of life and pain relief than no treatment up to 1 week following treatment
    - ▪ No significant benefit was found in trials comparing acupuncture to sham or standard therapy

  - ○ A 2017 systematic review of 16 trials comparing acupuncture and electro-acupuncture to standard interventions such as physical therapy or pain medication in the treatment of neck pain revealed pain relief in trials with unclear allocation concealment where acupuncture was subsequently added on to the control (36)

    - ▪ Electroacupuncture added on to the control treatment option resulted in even higher pain relief than standard acupuncture

- Acupuncture treatments vs. control alone did not result in any significant benefit in pain relief, quality of life, or disability
  ○ In a 2016 systematic review of 7 trials comparing acupuncture to sham therapy or standard pharmaceutical therapy in the treatment of chronic prostatitis and chronic pelvic pain syndrome in men, acupuncture was found to decrease general pain, pain with voiding, and improve quality of life compared to sham therapy (37)
    - Acupuncture did not result in any significant benefits vs. levofloxacin, ibuprofen, and tamsulosin, and showed weak evidence to support potential similar effects
  ○ 2018 systematic review of 4 trials comparing acupuncture to conventional therapy in the treatment of chronic pelvic pain in women shows a small, but significant, decrease in pain when acupuncture was combined with conventional therapy (38)
    - Ultimately there were too few studies and too little methodologic homogeneity to support the review's results with any confident recommendations
  ○ 2015 Cochrane review evaluating efficacy of various alternative therapies on pregnancy-related pains shows that acupuncture significantly improves pregnancy-related pelvic pain (39)
    - A 2017 study also showed significant pain relief in patients receiving electroacupuncture during labor (40)
  ○ A 2017 systematic review of 17 trials assessing the efficacy of acupuncture as a sole or adjunct treatment for chronic knee pain shows significant reduction in visual analog scale (VAS) and Western Ontario and McMaster Universities Osteoarthritis Index (WOMAC) pain scores (41)
    - Significant heterogeneity between studies limited generalizability and clinical recommendations; however, acupuncture's safety profile was comparable to control
  ○ In a 2019 systematic review of 12 trials comparing acupuncture to sham therapy or standard pain-relief medicine in the treatment of fibromyalgia, acupuncture shows significantly superior pain relief and improvement in the quality of life in short- and long-term follow-up (42)

- A 2017 Cochrane review of 6 trials comparing various forms of acupuncture alone or as an adjuvant to sham therapy or standard medical treatment of neuropathic pain shows at best that acupuncture as an adjunct to standard medical therapy improves perceived pain relief and quality of life in participants with mild neuropathic pain scores at baseline (43)

  - The majority of studies showed significant methodological uncertainty and high risk for bias

- 2016 systematic review of 13 trials assessing the effectiveness of acupuncture in combination with other traditional Chinese medicine therapies on palliative cancer care shows small, but significant, improvements in pain and quality of life with various cancer etiologies vs. conventional medical therapies alone (44)

- A 2016 Cochrane review of 22 trials evaluated the benefits of acupuncture on episodic migraine pain and found several significant results (45)

  - Regular acupuncture therapy with symptomatic treatment vs. no acupuncture cut the frequency of migraines in half in 41% of participants

  - True acupuncture vs. sham acupuncture halved the frequency of migraines in 50% and 41% of participants respectively

  - Strong evidence shows migraine frequency was halved in 57% of those receiving acupuncture vs. 46% of those receiving standard prophylactic drugs at 3 months and 59% and 54% respectively at 6 months

- Tai chi

  - 2017 systematic review of 15 trials studying chronic osteoarthritis pain, back pain, and headache shows moderate-quality evidence to support tai chi as a mild, but significantly effective, treatment vs. no treatment or usual care in the short term for pain and functionality (30)

  - A 2022 systematic review of 17 trials assessed the efficacy of tai chi, yoga, and qigong in treating various chronic musculoskeletal pains in middle- and old-aged participants (46)

    - Significant pain relief and functional improvement was observed in the tai chi groups compared to physically active and nonactive controls

- ▪ Knee osteoarthritis had some of the strongest evidence to support tai chi as an intervention for improving functionality
- ○ A 2017 systematic review including 2 trials on tai chi for the treatment of chronic low back pain shows significant improvement in pain scores vs. controls (47)
- ○ In a 2019 systematic review of 7 trials on tai chi's effect on pain control and functionality in rheumatoid arthritis, there was insufficient evidence to support any conclusive benefit of the practice (48)

  - ▪ Two studies report a significant average of 22% improvement over 12 weeks
  - ▪ The majority of trials were not randomized and rated as very-low-quality evidence

- ○ A 2022 systematic review of 14 trials studying alternative exercise's impact on fibromyalgia shows that tai chi stood out as one of the most profound improvements in pain relief vs. control (49)
- ○ 2021 systematic review of 8 other systematic reviews and 21 trials studying various exercises' effects on neuropathic pain reports that tai chi is an effective intervention for pain reduction and mobility improvement in Parkinson's patients (50)

  - ▪ Two other trials evaluating tai chi's effect on multiple sclerosis-related pain, fatigue, and mobility resulted in significant benefits vs. control (51,52)

- ○ In a 2016 systematic review of 33 trials assessing the effectiveness of tai chi on 6-minute walking distance and knee-extension strength in patients with COPD, cancer, heart failure, and osteoarthritis, tai chi alone was found to significantly improve distance and strength in all groups (53)

- • OMT
  - ○ A 2021 systematic review of 10 trials evaluating OMT, myofascial release, craniosacral treatment, and osteopathic visceral manipulation for chronic nonspecific low back pain shows significantly reduced pain and improved functional mobility vs. control interventions (54)
  - ○ 2017 systematic review of OMT for pregnancy-related low back pain reports 5 trials showing significant pain relief and functional improvement during pregnancy and 3 trials showing the same for postpartum pain (55)

- A 2022 systematic review of 5 trials studying the effect of osteopathic interventions on chronic nonspecific neck pain shows significant moderate pain relief and functional improvement vs. sham therapy or no therapy (56)

    - These studies were rated as very-low-quality evidence

- 2015 randomized controlled trial studying the effect of OMT on migraines in 105 participants shows that OMT significantly reduced HIT-6 score, amount of medication use, number of days with migraines, severity of migraine pain, and disability contributed to migraines when compared to sham OMT (57)

- Chiropractic

    - In a 2019 systematic review of 47 trials, spinal manipulation was assessed for efficacy and potential harm in the treatment of chronic low back pain (58)

        - Spinal manipulation results in similar improvements to pain and functionality when compared to other recommended treatments; however, it is slightly superior to non-recommended or alternative therapies

        - Risk of adverse events was substantial across the studies; however, most events were transient, musculoskeletal, and self-limited

    - Another 2019 systematic review of 6 trials studying spinal manipulation's effects on chronic nonspecific neck pain shows a small, but significant, improvement in pain and disability in those receiving "thrust" technique with neck exercises vs. exercise alone at 1, 3, and 6 months post-intervention (59)

        - Twenty-five additional studies were evaluated for adverse events where only minor complications were reported

    - 2019 systematic review of 6 trials studying spinal manipulation for the treatment of migraine showed a mild decrease in the total number of migraine days as well as a decrease in migraine severity up to 6-month follow-up (60)

        - These studies showed significant heterogeneity with variable methods

## Conclusions

- Chronic pain of various etiologies presents a massive problem for healthcare with little-to-no obvious, efficacious, and innocuous solutions
- The exhaustion of conventional pharmaceutical therapies for conservative chronic pain management is a danger not only for their side effect profile when abused, but also for the risk of opioid dependence as a next step in pain control
- While many lifestyle interventions and alternative therapies have shown to be beneficial for prevention and treatment of mild pain, a critical evaluation of popular options must be kept up-to-date as new information is released
- Acupuncture has shown mixed results for a number of conditions, but with its substantial anecdotal presence in healthcare and albeit limited efficacy from hard evidence, it has proven to be a relatively safe and potentially effective sole or adjunct treatment for several etiologies of chronic pain
- Tai chi is another heavily anecdotal pain therapy that appears to have some benefit at least as an adjunct to conventional therapy and with a tremendous safety profile
- OMT has consistently shown to be at least minimally effective in a variety of pain etiologies with a solid safety profile when compared to some other manual therapy
- Chiropractic manipulation has mixed results with at least similar benefits to some other conservative therapies; however, the tenuous safety profile should be considered before recommendation

## References

1. Califf RM, Woodcock J, Ostroff S. A proactive response to prescription opioid abuse. *New Engl J Med*. 2016;**374**:1480–1485.

2. Stanos S, Brodsky M, Argoff C et al. Rethinking chronic pain in a primary care setting. *Postgrad Med*. 2016;**128**(5):502–515.

3. Kroenke K, Cheville A. Management of chronic pain in the aftermath of the opioid backlash. *JAMA*. 2017;**317**(23):2365.

4. Theisen K, Jacobs B, Macleod L et al. The United States opioid epidemic: A review of the surgeon's contribution to it and health policy initiatives. *BJU Int*. 2018;**122**:754–759.

5. Fuentes AV, Pineda MD, Venkata KCN. Comprehension of top 200 prescribed drugs in the US as a resource for pharmacy teaching, training and practice. *Pharmacy (Basel)*. 2018;**6**(2):43.

6.  Mills SEE, Nicolson KP, Smith BH. Chronic pain: A review of its epidemiology and associated factors in population-based studies. *Br J Anaesth.* 2019;123(2):e273–e283.

7.  Simpson CA. Complementary medicine in chronic pain treatment. *Phys Med Rehabil Clin North Am.* 2015;26(2):321–347.

8.  Vickers AJ, Cronin AM, Maschino AC et al. Acupuncture for chronic pain: Individual patient data meta-analysis. *Arch Intern Med.* 2012;172 (19):1444–1453.

9.  Patil S, Sen S, Bral M et al. The role of acupuncture in pain management. *Curr Pain Headache Rep.* 2016;20(4):22. doi: 10.1007/s11916-016-0552-1.

10. Hall A, Copsey B, Richmond H et al. Effectiveness of tai chi for chronic musculoskeletal pain conditions: Updated systematic review and meta-analysis. *Phys Ther.* 2017;97(2):227–238.

11. Bodine WA. Osteopathic manipulative treatment: A primary care approach. *Am Fam Physician.* 2019;99(4):214. PMID: 30763051.

12. Hawk C, Whalen W, Farabaugh RJ et al. Best practices for chiropractic management of patients with chronic musculoskeletal pain: A clinical practice guideline. *J Altern Complement Med.* 2020;26(10):884–901.

13. Vos T, Allen C, Arora M. Global, regional, and national incidence, prevalence, and years lived with disability for 328 diseases and injuries for 195 countries, 1990–2016: A systematic analysis for the Global Burden of Disease study 2016. *Lancet.* 2017;390:1211–1259.

14. Yong RJ, Mullins PM, Bhattacharyya N. Prevalence of chronic pain among adults in the United States. *Pain.* 2022;163(2):e328–e332.

15. Fayaz A, Croft P, Langford RM, Donaldson LJ, Jones GT. Prevalence of chronic pain in the UK: A systematic review and meta-analysis of population studies. *BMJ Open.* 2016;6(6):e010364. doi: 10.1136/bmjopen-2015-010364.

16. Greenspan J, Craft R, LeResche L. Studying sex and gender differences in pain and analgesia: A consensus report. *Pain.* 2007;132:S26–S45.

17. Ferreira Kdos S, Speciali J. Epidemiology of chronic pain in the office of a pain specialist neurologist. *Arq Neuropsiquiatr.* 2015;73:582–585.

18. Malon J, Shah P, Koh WY et al. Characterizing the demographics of chronic pain patients in the state of Maine using the Maine all payer claims database. *BMC Public Health.* 2018;18:810. doi: 10.1186/s12889-018-5673-5.

19. Janevic MR, McLaughlin SJ, Heapy AA, Thacker C, Piette JD. Racial and socioeconomic disparities in disabling chronic pain: Findings from the health and retirement study. *J Pain.* 2017;18:1459–1467.

20. Geneen LJ, Moore RA, Clarke C et al. Physical activity and exercise for chronic pain in adults: An overview of Cochrane Reviews. *Cochrane Database Syst Rev.* 2017;1(1):CD011279.

21. Elliott A, Smith B, Hannaford P. The course of chronic pain in the community: Results of a 4-year follow-up study. *Pain*. 2002;**99**:299–307.

22. McIntosh AM, Hall LS, Zeng Y et al. Genetic and environmental risk for chronic pain and the contribution of risk variants for major depressive disorder: A family-based mixed-model analysis. *PLoS Med*. 2016;**13**(8): e1002090.

23. Barnett K, Mercer SW, Norbury M et al. Epidemiology of multimorbidity and implications for health care, research, and medical education: A cross-sectional study. *Lancet*. 2012;**380**:37–43.

24. de Heer E, Ten Have M, van Marwijk HWJ. Pain as a risk factor for common mental disorders. Results from the Netherlands mental health survey and incidence study-2: A longitudinal population-based study. *Pain*. 2018;**159**:712–718.

25. Stone AA, Broderick JE. Obesity and pain are associated in the United States. *Obesity*. 2012;**20**:11491–11495.

26. Zhuang Y, Xing JJ, Li J, Zeng BY, Liang FR. History of acupuncture research. *Int Rev Neurobiol*. 2013;**111**:1–23.

27. Lim T-K, Ma Y, Berger F, Litscher G. Acupuncture and neural mechanism in the management of low back pain-an update. *Medicines*. 2018;**5**(3):63. doi: 10.3390/medicines5030063.

28. Wilkinson J, Faleiro R. Acupuncture in pain management. *Contin Educ Anaesth Crit Care Pain*. 2007;**7**(4):135–138.

29. Lao L. Acupuncture techniques and devices. *J Altern Complement Med*. 1996;**2**(1):23–25.

30. Hall A, Copsey B, Richmond H et al. Effectiveness of tai chi for chronic musculoskeletal pain conditions: Updated systematic review and meta-analysis. *Phys Ther*. 2017;**97**(2):227–238.

31. Slattengren AH, Nissly T, Blustin J, Bader A, Westfall E. Best uses of osteopathic manipulation. *J Fam Pract*. 2017;**66**(12):743–747.

32. Seffinger MA, Hruby RJ, Rogers FJ et al. Philosophy of osteopathic medicine. In Seffinger MA, Hruby R, Willard FH, Licciardone J, eds. *Foundations of osteopathic medicine: Philosophy, science, clinical applications, and research*. 4th ed. Wolters Kluwer; 2018. pp. 2–18.

33. Licciardone JC, Schultz MJ, Amen B. Osteopathic manipulation in the management of chronic pain: Current perspectives. *J Pain Res*. 2020;**13**:1839–1847.

34. Ernst E. Chiropractic: A critical evaluation. *J Pain Symptom Manage*. 2008;**35**(5):544–562.

35. Mu J, Furlan AD, Lam WY et al. Acupuncture for chronic nonspecific low back pain. *Cochrane Database Syst Rev*. 2020;**12**(12):CD013814.

36. Seo SY, Lee KB, Shin JS et al. Effectiveness of acupuncture and electroacupuncture for chronic neck pain: A systematic review and meta-analysis. *Am J Chin Med.* 2017;45(8):1573–1595.

37. Qin Z, Wu J, Zhou J, Liu Z. Systematic review of acupuncture for chronic prostatitis/chronic pelvic pain syndrome. *Medicine (Baltimore).* 2016;95(11): e3095.

38. Sung SH, Sung AD, Sung HK et al. Acupuncture treatment for chronic pelvic pain in women: A systematic review and meta-analysis of randomized controlled trials. *Evid Based Complement Alternat Med.* 2018:9415897. doi: 10.1155/2018/9415897.

39. Liddle SD, Pennick V. Interventions for preventing and treating low-back and pelvic pain during pregnancy. *Cochrane Database Syst Rev.* 2015;9: CD001139.

40. Schlaeger JM, Gabzdyl EM, Bussell JL et al. Acupuncture and acupressure in labor. *J Midwifery Womens Health.* 2017;62(1):12–28.

41. Zhang Q, Yue J, Golianu B, Sun Z, Lu Y. Updated systematic review and meta-analysis of acupuncture for chronic knee pain. *Acupunct Med.* 2017;35 (6):392–403.

42. Zhang XC, Chen H, Xu WT et al. Acupuncture therapy for fibromyalgia: A systematic review and meta-analysis of randomized controlled trials. *J Pain Res.* 2019;12:527–542.

43. Ju ZY, Wang K, Cui HS et al. Acupuncture for neuropathic pain in adults. *Cochrane Database Syst Rev.* 2017;12(12):CD012057.

44. Lau CHY, Wu X, Chung VCH et al. Acupuncture and related therapies for symptom management in palliative cancer care: Systematic review and meta-analysis. *Medicine (Baltimore).* 2016;95(9):e2901.

45. Linde K, Allais G, Brinkhaus B et al. Acupuncture for the prevention of episodic migraine. *Cochrane Database Syst Rev.* 2016;6:CD001218.

46. Wen YR, Shi J, Wang YF et al. Are mind-body exercise beneficial for treating pain, function, and quality of life in middle-aged and old people with chronic pain? A systematic review and meta-analysis. *Front Aging Neurosci.* 2022;14:921069. doi: 10.3389/fnagi.2022.921069.

47. Chou R, Deyo R, Friedly J et al. Nonpharmacologic therapies for low back pain: A systematic review for an American college of physicians clinical practice guideline. *Ann Intern Med.* 2017;166(7):493–505.

48. Mudano AS, Tugwell P, Wells GA, Singh JA. Tai chi for rheumatoid arthritis. *Cochrane Database Syst Rev.* 2019;9(9):CD004849.

49. Vasileios P, Styliani P, Nifon G et al. Managing fibromyalgia with complementary and alternative medical exercise: A systematic review and meta-analysis of clinical trials. *Rheumatol Int.* 2022;42(11):1909–1923.

50. Zhang YH, Hu HY, Xiong YC et al. Exercise for neuropathic pain: A systematic review and expert consensus. *Front Med (Lausanne)*. 2021;8:756940. doi: 10.3389/fmed.2021.756940.

51. Burschka JM, Keune PM, Oy UH, Oschmann P, Kuhn P. Mindfulness-based interventions in multiple sclerosis: Beneficial effects of tai chi on balance, coordination, fatigue and depression. *BMC Neurol*. 2014;14:165. doi: 10.1186/s12883-014-0165-4.

52. Tavee J, Rensel M, Planchon SM, Butler RS, Stone L. Effects of meditation on pain and quality of life in multiple sclerosis and peripheral neuropathy: A pilot study. *Int J MS Care*. 2011;13(4):163–168.

53. Chen YW, Hunt MA, Campbell KL, Peill K, Reid WD. The effect of tai chi on four chronic conditions-cancer, osteoarthritis, heart failure and chronic obstructive pulmonary disease: A systematic review and meta-analyses. *Br J Sports Med*. 2016;50(7):397–407.

54. Dal Farra F, Risio RG, Vismara L, Bergna A. Effectiveness of osteopathic interventions in chronic non-specific low back pain: A systematic review and meta-analysis. *Complement Ther Med*. 2021;56:102616.

55. Franke H, Franke JD, Belz S, Fryer G. Osteopathic manipulative treatment for low back and pelvic girdle pain during and after pregnancy: A systematic review and meta-analysis. *J Bodyw Mov Ther*. 2017;21(4):752–762.

56. Dal Farra F, Buffone F, Risio RG et al. Effectiveness of osteopathic interventions in patients with non-specific neck pain: A systematic review and meta-analysis. *Complement Ther Clin Pract*. 2022;49:101655.

57. Cerritelli F, Ginevri L, Messi G et al. Clinical effectiveness of osteopathic treatment in chronic migraine: 3-armed randomized controlled trial. *Complement Ther Med*. 2015;23(2):149–156.

58. Rubinstein SM, de Zoete A, van Middelkoop M et al. Benefits and harms of spinal manipulative therapy for the treatment of chronic low back pain: Systematic review and meta-analysis of randomised controlled trials. *BMJ*. 2019;364:l689. doi: 10.1136/bmj.l689.

59. Coulter ID, Crawford C, Vernon H et al. Manipulation and mobilization for treating chronic nonspecific neck pain: A systematic review and meta-analysis for an appropriateness panel. *Pain Physician*. 2019;22(2):E55–E70.

60. Rist PM, Hernandez A, Bernstein C et al. The impact of spinal manipulation on migraine pain and disability: A systematic review and meta-analysis. *Headache*. 2019;59(4):532–542.

# Chapter 43

# Role of CBD in Chronic Pain

Zohal Sarwary and Nazir Noor

## Introduction to Cannabidiol (CBD)

- CBD is one of the most studied compounds in the cannabis family (1)
- No psychoactive properties
- Commonly utilized in the treatment of certain childhood epilepsies
  - Epidiolex = pure cannabidiol FDA approved for childhood seizures
- Mechanism of CBD in pain management is not fully understood (2)
- Indications:
  - Nociceptive pain
  - Neuropathic pain
  - Inflammatory pain
- There are variable preparations ranging from different THC:CBD ratios to highly purified cannabidiol (CBD)
  - Standard = nabiximols (1:1 ratio of THC:CBD) (3)

## Routes of Administration

- Types (4):
  - Smoking/vaporization
    - Onset: 5–10 min
    - Duration: 2–4 hours
    - Rapid action
  - Oral:
    - Onset: 60–180 min
    - Duration: 6–8 hours

- Less odor, convenient
- Delayed onset – titration challenges
  - Oromucosal:
    - Onset 15–45 min
    - Duration: 6–8 hours
    - Pharmaceutical form available (nabixomol)
  - Topical:
    - Onset: variable
    - Duration: variable
    - Local effects
  - Suppositories
- Non-inhalation + inhalation administration routes have shown to be more efficacious in pain management and is associated with more medication substitutions (5)

## Adverse Effects of CBD
- Generally well tolerated with a good safety profile and does not have abuse potential (6)
- Most reported side effects (84%) are considered mild (6)
- Side effects include:
  - Hyperemesis syndrome
  - Dry mouth
  - Drowsiness/somnolence
  - Increased or decreased appetite
  - Dry eyes
  - Impaired concentration
  - Dizziness
  - Headache
  - Digestive complaints

## Role of CBD and Chronic Pain Management
- Few clinical trials exist exploring the analgesic effects of CBD in humans (7)
- Both animal and human studies have shown early positive results with limited minor side effects with respect to the safety and efficacy of oral and topical CBD for treating pain (8,9)

- Various studies have shown that CBD is a potential alternative to opioids for the treatment of arthritic pain and chronic migraines (6,10)
- Combination therapy:
  - CBD (30 mg/kg) and morphine (1 mg/kg) have an enhanced antinociceptive effect compared to morphine alone (1 mg/kg)
  - Treatment with CBD partially attenuates morphine-induced tolerance
  - CBD is useful an adjuvant to opioid therapy for the attenuation of neuropathic pain and opioid-induced analgesic tolerance (11)
- In a novel animal model of tonic pain, CBD microinjection into the NAc attenuated persistent inflammatory pain (12)
- Factors leading to higher rates of pain reduction and cessation of other medications:
  - Increased dose of CBD
  - Using CBD more frequently (≥once a day)
  - Using CBD over a prolonged period of time
    - Patients taking CBD for a period of more than 3 years were 3.6 times more likely to reduce or cease other medications, when compared to those taking CBD for less than 30 days (6)

## Summary

- CBD is the only cannabinergic medication available at present that does not cause the typical "cannabis high" and is not a "controlled substance" (13)
- More clinical trials should be done to prove CBD's significance clinically and statistically (14)
- There is either no study or no well-conducted, head-to-head, comparison available between different cannabis cultivars, between pure cannabinoids, and between pure cannabinoids and extracts
- Although there is some evidence showing that CBD has analgesic effects, further studies are required to further explore its role in chronic pain management (3)

## References

1. Häuser W, Welsch P, Klose P, Radbruch L, Fitzcharles MA. Efficacy, tolerability and safety of cannabis-based medicines for cancer pain: A systematic review with meta-analysis of randomised controlled trials. *Schmerz.* 2019;33(5):424–436 Published online 2019. https://doi.org/10.1007/s00482-019-0373-3.

2.  Louis-Gray K, Tupal S, Premkumar LS. TRPV1: A common denominator mediating antinociceptive and antiemetic effects of cannabinoids. *Int J Mol Sci.* 2022;23(17):10016. Published online 2022. https://doi.org/10.3390/ijms231710016.

3.  Köstenberger M, Nahler G, Jones TM, Neuwersch S, Likar R. The role of cannabis, cannabidiol and other cannabinoids in chronic pain: The perspective of physicians. *J Neuroimmune Pharmacol.* 2022;17(1–2):38–333. https://doi.org/10.1007/s11481-021-10010-x.

4.  MacCallum CA, Russo EB. Practical considerations in medical cannabis administration and dosing. *Eur J Intern Med.* 2018;49:12–19. https://doi.org/10.1016/j.ejim.2018.01.004.

5.  Boehnke KF, Yakas L, Scott JR et al. A mixed methods analysis of cannabis use routines for chronic pain management. *J Cannabis Res.* 2022;4(1):1–11. https://doi.org/10.1186/S42238-021-00116-7.

6.  Frane N, Stapleton E, Iturriaga C et al. Cannabidiol as a treatment for arthritis and joint pain: An exploratory cross-sectional study. *J Cannabis Res.* 2022;4(1):47. https://doi.org/10.1186/s42238-022-00154-9.

7.  Henderson LA, Kotsirilos V, Cairns EA et al. Medicinal cannabis in the treatment of chronic pain. *Aust J Gen Pract.* 2021;50. www.abs.gov.au/statistics/people/population/national-state-and-territory-population/dec-2020.

8.  Stephens KL, Heineman JT, Forster GL, Timko MP, Degeorge BR. Cannabinoids and pain for the plastic surgeon: What is the evidence? *Ann Plast Surg.* 2022;88(5 Suppl 5):S508–S511. https://doi.org/10.1097/SAP.0000000000003128.

9.  Yu CHJ, Rupasinghe HPV. Cannabidiol-based natural health products for companion animals: Recent advances in the management of anxiety, pain, and inflammation. *Res Vet Sci.* 2021;140:38–46. https://doi.org/10.1016/J.RVSC.2021.08.001.

10. Baraldi C, lo Castro F, Negro A et al. Oral cannabinoid preparations for the treatment of chronic migraine: A retrospective study. *Pain Med.* 2022;23(2):396–402. https://doi.org/10.1093/PM/PNAB245.

11. Jesus CHA, Ferreira MV, Gasparin AT et al. Cannabidiol enhances the antinociceptive effects of morphine and attenuates opioid-induced tolerance in the chronic constriction injury model. *Behav Brain Res.* 2022;435:114076. https://doi.org/10.1016/J.BBR.2022.114076.

12. Razavi Y, Rashvand M, Sharifi A et al. Cannabidiol microinjection into the nucleus accumbens attenuated nociceptive behaviors in an animal model of tonic pain. *Neurosci Lett.* 2021;762:136141. https://doi.org/10.1016/J.NEULET.2021.136141.

13. Chou R, Wagner J, Ahmed AY et al. Living systematic review on cannabis and other plant-based treatments for chronic pain. Rockville (MD): Agency for

Healthcare Research and Quality (US). Published online October 27, 2021. www.ncbi.nlm.nih.gov/books/NBK586045/. https://doi.org/10.23970 /AHRQEPCCER250.

14. Campos RMP, Aguiar AFL, Paes-Colli Y et al. Cannabinoid therapeutics in chronic neuropathic pain: From animal research to human treatment. 2021;12:785176. Published online 2021. https://doi.org/10.3389/fphys .2021.785176.

# Index

Index

diagnosis, 160
epidemiology, 157
management, 161
symptoms, 157
tic douloureux, *see* trigeminal
        neuralgia (TN).
tizanidine
    as treatment for CP pain and
            spasticity, 55, 257
    as treatment for MPS, 269
toll-like receptors (TLRs), and opioid-
        related dysbiosis, 28
topical administration of medication,
        49–51
    indications, 49
    *see also* capsaicin; diclofenac;
        lidocaine.
topiramate, as treatment for LBP, 101
tramadol
    as treatment for OA-related pain,
            167, 177
    as treatment for PHN, 215
transcranial direct current
        stimulation (tDCS)
    for neuropathic pain control, 9
    as treatment for CPSP, 283
transcranial magnetic
        stimulation (TMS)
    in diagnosis of MPS, 263
    for neuropathic pain control, 9
    potential for mitigation of MS
            symptoms, 250
    as treatment for CPSP, 282–283
transcranial stimulation, as treatment
        for CPSP, 282
transcutaneous electrical nerve
        stimulation (TENS)
    as treatment for LBP, 100,
            266–267
    as treatment for MPS, 266
    as treatment for PHN, 215
tricyclic antidepressants (TCAs)
    contraindications, 64
    dosage/routes of administration, 63
    mechanism of action, 62
    side effects/adverse reactions, 63–64

as treatment for LBP, 100
as treatment for MPS, 268
as treatment for ON, 89
as treatment for PHN, 215
as treatment for TN, 84
trigeminal neuralgia (TN), 81–84
    characteristics, 81, 83
    diagnosis, 83–84
    epidemiology, 81–82
    imaging tests and alternatives,
            82–83, 84
    as indicator for antineuropathic
            medication, 62
    MS-related, 248–249
    pathophysiology, 82–83
    prevalence, 81
    risk factors, 81–82
    treatment, 84

ulcers, gastric and duodenal, as cause
        of CAP, 289
urticaria, diclofenac contraindicated
        for, 51

vaccines, for prevention of Shingles
        rash, 214
venlafaxine
    dosage/routes of administration, 62
    mechanism of action, 62
    side effects/adverse reactions,
            63–64
    as treatment for LBP, 100
vertebral compression fractures
        (VCFs), 107–113
    atypical light chain
            amyloidosis, 109
    diagnosis, 109–111
    epidemiology, 107
    gestation, 109
    low estrogen effects, 108
    osteoporosis, 108
    pathophysiology, 108
    risk factors, 107
    treatment
        conservative, 111
        research and guidelines, 112–113